Sport-Related Concussion

Editor

PETER K. KRIZ

CLINICS IN SPORTS MEDICINE

www.sportsmed.theclinics.com

Consulting Editor
MARK D. MILLER

January 2021 • Volume 40 • Number 1

ELSEVIER

1600 John F. Kennedy Boulevard • Suite 1800 • Philadelphia, Pennsylvania, 19103-2899

http://www.theclinics.com

CLINICS IN SPORTS MEDICINE Volume 40, Number 1
January 2021 ISSN 0278-5919, ISBN-13: 978-0-323-75545-0

Editor: Lauren Boyle
Developmental Editor: Donald Mumford

Clinics in Sports Medicine (ISSN 0278-5919) is published quarterly by Elsevier Inc., 360 Park Avenue South, New York, NY 10010-1710. Months of issue are January, April, July, and October. Business and Editorial Offices: 1600 John F. Kennedy Blvd., Ste. 1800, Philadelphia, PA 19103-2899. Customer Service Office: 3251 Riverport Lane, Maryland Heights, MO 63043. Periodicals postage paid at New York, NY and additional mailing offices. Subscription prices are $364.00 per year (US individuals), $931.00 per year (US institutions), $100.00 per year (US students), $405.00 per year (Canadian individuals), $964.00 per year (Canadian institutions), $100.00 (Canadian students), $475.00 per year (foreign individuals), $964.00 per year (foreign institutions), and $235.00 per year (foreign students). Foreign air speed delivery is included in all *Clinics* subscription prices. All prices are subject to change without notice. **POSTMASTER:** Send address changes to *Clinics in Sports Medicine*, Elsevier Health Sciences Division, Subscription Customer Service, 3251 Riverport Lane, Maryland Heights, MO 63043. Customer Service (orders, claims, online, change of address): Elsevier Health Sciences Division, Subscription Customer Service, 3251 Riverport Lane, Maryland Heights, MO 63043. **Tel: 1-800-654-2452 (U.S. and Canada); 314-447-8871 (outside U.S. and Canada). Fax: 314-447-8029. E-mail: journalscustomerservice-usa@elsevier.com (for print support); journalsonlinesupport-usa@ elsevier.com (for online support).**

Reprints. For copies of 100 or more of articles in this publication, please contact the Commercial Reprints Department, Elsevier Inc., 360 Park Avenue South, New York, NY 10010-1710. Tel.: 212-633-3874; Fax: 212-633-3820; E-mail: reprints@elsevier.com.

Clinics in Sports Medicine is covered in *MEDLINE/PubMed (Index Medicus) Current Contents/Clinical Medicine, Excerpta Medica,* and *ISI/Biomed.*

Contributors

CONSULTING EDITOR

MARK D. MILLER, MD
S. Ward Casscells Professor, Head, Department of Orthopaedic Surgery, Division of
Sports Medicine, University of Virginia, Charlottesville, Virginia, USA; Team Physician,
Miller Review Course, Harrisonburg, Virginia, USA

EDITOR

PETER K. KRIZ, MD
Associate Professor (Clinical), Division of Sports Medicine, Departments of Orthopaedics
and Pediatrics, Warren Alpert Medical School, Brown University, Rhode Island Hospital/
Hasbro Children's Hospital, East Providence, Rhode Island, USA

AUTHORS

KATHRYN E. ACKERMAN, MD, MPH, FACSM
Assistant Professor, Medicine, Harvard Medical School, Boston Children's Hospital,
Massachusetts General Hospital, Sports Medicine, Boston, Massachusetts, USA

BJØRN BAKKEN, MD
Sports Medicine Fellow, Department of Medicine, Albany Medical Center, Cohoes, New
York, USA

KATHLEEN COHEN, DO
Sports Medicine Fellow, Rutgers-Robert Wood Johnson Medical School, New Brunswick,
New Jersey, USA; University Health Services, Princeton University, Princeton, New
Jersey, USA

CHRISTY COLLINS, PhD
President, Datalys Center for Sports Injury Research and Prevention, Indianapolis,
Indiana, USA

MICHAEL W. COLLINS, PhD
Clinical and Executive Director, Department of Orthopedics, UPMC Sport Medicine
Concussion Program, Pittsburgh, Pennsylvania, USA

PRACHI DUBEY, MD, MPH
Neuroradiology, Houston Methodist Hospital, Houston, Texas, USA

CARRIE ESOPENKO, PhD
Department of Rehabilitation and Movement Sciences, School of Health Professions,
Rutgers Biomedical and Health Sciences, Rutgers University, Newark, New Jersey, USA

PETER D. FABRICANT, MD, MPH
Department of Orthopaedic Surgery, Hospital for Special Surgery, New York, New York,
USA

RAJAN R. GADHIA, MD
Assistant Professor of Neurology, Medical Director of Houston Methodist Concussion Center, Stanley H. Appel Department of Neurology, Houston Methodist Hospital, Houston, Texas, USA

ANDREW GREGORY, MD
Associate Professor of Orthopedics, Neurosurgery and Pediatrics, Vanderbilt University Medical Center, Vanderbilt Sports Medicine, Nashville, Tennessee, USA

MOHAMMAD NADIR HAIDER, MD
UBMD Department of Orthopaedics and Sports Medicine, Concussion Management Clinic and Research Center, University at Buffalo, The State University of New York, Buffalo, New York, USA

LENORE HERGET, PT, DPT, SCS, MEd, CSCS
Massachusetts General Hospital, MGH Sports Medicine, Neurotrauma Consultant, New England Patriots, Boston Bruins, Boston Celtics, New England Revolution and Boston Red Sox, Boston, Massachusetts, USA

THOMAS BLAINE HOSHIZAKI, PhD
Professor Neurotrauma Impact Science Laboratory, University of Ottawa, Ottawa, Ontario, Canada

GREGORY HOUSE, MD
Family Medicine Resident, Department of Family and Community Medicine, Albany Medical Center, Cohoes, New York, USA

DAVID R. HOWELL, PhD, ATC
Sports Medicine Center, Children's Hospital Colorado, Department of Orthopedics, University of Colorado School of Medicine, Aurora, Colorado, USA

SABRINA JENNINGS, PhD
Neuropsychology Fellow, Department of Orthopedics, UPMC Sport Medicine Concussion Program, Pittsburgh, Pennsylvania, USA

GAURAV JINDAL, MD
Assistant Professor of Diagnostic Imaging, Warren Alpert School of Medicine, Brown University, Rhode Island Hospital, Providence, Rhode Island, USA

JACOB C. JONES, MD
Department of Sports Medicine, Texas Scottish Rite Hospital for Children, Department of Orthopaedic Surgery and Pediatrics, University of Texas Southwestern, Dallas, Texas, USA

CLARA KARTON, PhD
Neurotrauma Impact Science Laboratory, University of Ottawa, Ottawa, Ontario, Canada

HAMISH KERR, MD, MSc, FAAP, FACSM, CAQSM
Fellowship Director, Sports Medicine, Professor, Department of Medicine, Albany Medical College, Cohoes, New York, USA

PETER K. KRIZ, MD
Associate Professor (Clinical), Division of Sports Medicine, Departments of Orthopaedics and Pediatrics, Warren Alpert Medical School, Brown University, Rhode Island Hospital/Hasbro Children's Hospital, East Providence, Rhode Island, USA

KYLE N. KUNZE, MD
Department of Orthopaedic Surgery, Hospital for Special Surgery, New York, New York, USA

ADAM G. LAMM, MD
Department of Physical Medicine and Rehabilitation, Spaulding Rehabilitation Hospital, Massachusetts General Hospital, Brigham and Women's Hospital, Harvard Medical School, Boston, Massachusetts, USA

JOHN J. LEDDY, MD
UBMD Department of Orthopaedics and Sports Medicine, Concussion Management Clinic and Research Center, University at Buffalo, The State University of New York, Buffalo, New York, USA

ROBERT G. MARX, MD, MSc
Department of Orthopaedic Surgery, Hospital for Special Surgery, New York, New York, USA

JAMES P. MacDONALD, MD, MPH
Associate Professor (Clinical), Division of Sports Medicine, Department of Pediatrics, Ohio State University, College of Medicine, Nationwide Children's Hospital, Columbus, Ohio, USA

CHRISTINA L. MASTER, MD, FAAP, CAQSM, FACSM
Co-Director, Minds Matter Concussion Program, Pediatric and Adolescent Sports Medicine, Division of Pediatric Orthopedics, Professor of Clinical Pediatrics, Perelman School of Medicine, University of Pennsylvania, The Children's Hospital of Philadelphia, Philadelphia, Pennsylvania, USA

WILLIAM P. MEEHAN III, MD
Director, The Micheli Center for Sports Injury Prevention, Division of Sports Medicine, Boston Children's Hospital, Associate Professor of Pediatrics and Orthopedics, Harvard Medical School, Waltham, Massachusetts, USA

BENEDICT U. NWACHUKWU, MD, MBA
Department of Orthopaedic Surgery, Hospital for Special Surgery, New York, New York, USA

MICHAEL J. O'BRIEN, MD
The Micheli Center for Sports Injury Prevention, Division of Sports Medicine, Department of Orthopedics, Boston Children's Hospital, Assistant Professor, Department of Orthopaedic Surgery, Harvard Medical School, Boston Children's Sports Medicine, Boston, Massachusetts, USA

TATIANA PATSIMAS, MD
Pediatric Resident, Department of Pediatrics, University of Colorado School of Medicine, Aurora, Colorado, USA

LAUREN A. PIERPOINT, PhD
Hip Research Manager, Steadman Philippon Research Institute, Vail, Colorado, USA

SOURAV PODDAR, MD
Associate Professor, Family Medicine and Orthopedics, University of Colorado School of Medicine, CU Sports Medicine Center, Denver, Colorado, USA

MARGOT PUTUKIAN, MD, FACSM, FAMSSM
Director of Athletic Medicine, Assistant Director of Medical Services, Princeton University, University Health Services, Associate Clinical Professor, Rutgers-Robert Wood Johnson Medical School, Princeton, New Jersey, USA

KATHERINE H. RIZZONE, MD, MPH
Assistant Professor, Orthopaedics and Pediatrics, University of Rochester Medical Center, Rochester, New York, USA

WILLIAM O. ROBERTS, MD, MS
Professor, Department of Family Medicine and Community Health, University of Minnesota, Minneapolis, Minnesota, USA

JULIA SOUTHARD, BS
Sports Medicine Center, Children's Hospital Colorado, Department of Psychology and Neuroscience, Regis University, Denver, Colorado, USA

ALEX M. TAYLOR, PsyD
Brain Injury Center, Boston's Children Center, Boston, Massachusetts, USA

MICHAEL TURNER, MBBS
International Concussion and Head Injury Foundation, ISEL-UCL, London, United Kingdom

BRIAN T. VERNAU, MD, FAAP, CAQSM
Pediatric and Adolescent Sports Medicine, Division of Pediatric Orthopedics, The Children's Hospital of Philadelphia, Philadelphia, Pennsylvania, USA

CHARLES WILBER, MD
UBMD Department of Orthopaedics and Sports Medicine, Concussion Management Clinic and Research Center, University at Buffalo, The State University of New York, Buffalo, New York, USA

BARRY S. WILLER, PhD
Department of Psychiatry, Jacobs School of Medicine and Biomedical Sciences, Director of Research, Concussion Management Clinic and Research Center, University at Buffalo, The State University of New York, Buffalo, New York, USA

JULIE C. WILSON, MD, FAAP
Co-Director, Concussion Program, Children's Hospital Colorado, Assistant Professor, Departments of Orthopedics and Pediatrics, University of Colorado School of Medicine, Aurora, Colorado, USA

BONNIE M. WONG, MD
Department of Physical Medicine and Rehabilitation, Spaulding Rehabilitation Hospital, Massachusetts General Hospital, Brigham and Women's Hospital, Harvard Medical School, Boston, Massachusetts, USA

ROSS D. ZAFONTE, DO
Department of Physical Medicine and Rehabilitation, Spaulding Rehabilitation Hospital, Massachusetts General Hospital, Brigham and Women's Hospital, Harvard Medical School, Boston, Massachusetts, USA

STESSIE DORT ZIMMERMAN, MD, FAAP
Physician, Urgent Care, Seattle Children's Hospital, Seattle, Washington, USA

Contents

Sport-related concussions are common in the United States. Concussion rates have increased over time, likely due to improved recognition and awareness. Concussion rates vary across level (high school vs college), sex, and sport. Concussion rates are the highest among men, particularly in football, wrestling, ice hockey, and lacrosse where collisions and contact are inherent to the sports, although girls'/women's soccer rates are high. In gender-comparable sports, women have higher concussion rates. Continued data collection will increase understanding of sport-related concussion and provide areas for targeted prevention in the future.

As awareness on the short-term and long-term consequences of sports-related concussions and repetitive head impacts continues to grow, so too does the necessity to establish biomechanical measures of risk that inform public policy and risk mitigation strategies. A more precise exposure metric is central to establishing relationships among the traumatic experience, risk, and ultimately clinical outcomes. Accurate exposure metrics provide a means to support evidence-informed decisions accelerating public policy mandating brain trauma management through sport modification and safer play.

After a concussion, a series of complex, overlapping, and disruptive events occur within the brain, leading to symptoms and behavioral dysfunction. These events include ionic shifts, damaged neuronal architecture, higher concentrations of inflammatory chemicals, increased excitatory neurotransmitter release, and cerebral blood flow disruptions, leading to a neuronal crisis. This review summarizes the translational aspects of the pathophysiologic cascade of postconcussion events, focusing on the role of excitatory neurotransmitters and ionic fluxes, and their role in neuronal disruption. We review the relationship between physiologic disruption and behavioral alterations, and proposed treatments aimed to restore the balance of disrupted processes.

prescribe targeted rehabilitation therapies to treat postconcussion symptoms. Evidence-based rehabilitation approaches include cervical rehabilitation, vestibulo-ocular rehabilitation, and sub–symptom threshold aerobic exercise.

Mild traumatic brain injuries, or concussions, often result in transient brain abnormalities not readily detected by conventional imaging methods. Several advanced imaging studies have been evaluated in the past couple decades to improve understanding of microstructural and functional abnormalities in the brain in patients suffering concussions. The thought remains a functional or pathophysiologic change rather than a structural one. The mechanism of injury, whether direct, indirect, or rotational, may drive specific clinical and radiological presentations. This remains a dynamic and constantly evolving area of research. This article focuses on the current status of imaging and future directions in concussion-related research.

The medications used in postconcussion syndrome are typically used to help manage or minimize disruptive symptoms while recovery proceeds. These medications are not routinely used in most concussions that recover within days to weeks. However, it is beneficial to be aware of medication options that may be used in athletes with prolonged concussion symptoms or for those that have symptom burdens that preclude entry into basic concussion protocols. Medications and supplements remain a small part of the concussion treatment plan, which may include temporary academic adjustments, physical therapy, vestibular and ocular therapy, psychological support, and graded noncontact exercise.

Female athletes are participating in collision sports in greater numbers than previously. The overall incidence of concussion is known to be higher in female athletes than in male athletes participating in similar sports. Evidence suggests anatomic, biomechanical, and biochemical etiologies behind this sex disparity. Future research on female athletes is needed for further guidance on prevention and management of concussion in girls and women.

Pediatric patients with concussions have different needs than adults throughout the recovery process. Adolescents, in particular, may take longer to recover from concussion than adults. Initially, relative rest from academic and physical activities is recommended for 24 to 48 hours to allow symptoms to abate. After this time period, physicians should guide the return to activity and return to school process in a staged fashion using published guidelines. Further concussion research in pediatric patients, particularly those younger than high-school age, is needed to advance the management of this special population.

Concussion remains a common injury among sports participants. Implementing risk-reduction strategies for sport-related concussion (SRC) should be a priority of medical professionals involved in the care of athletes. Over the past few decades, a multifaceted approach to reducing SRC risk has been developed. Protective equipment, rule and policy change/enforcement, educational programs, behavioral modifications, legislation, physiologic modifications, and sport culture change are a few of the programs implemented to mitigate SRC risk. In this article, the authors critically review current SRC risk-reduction strategies and offer insight into future directions of injury prevention for SRC.

This article presents a brief history and literature review of chronic traumatic encephalopathy (CTE) in professional athletes that played contact sports. The hypothesis that CTE results from concussion or sub-concussive blows is based largely on several case series investigations with considerable bias. Evidence of CTE in its clinical presentation has not been generally noted in studies of living retired athletes. However, these studies also demonstrated limitation in research methodology. This paper aims to present a balanced perspective amidst a politically charged subject matter.

The recommendation to retire from sport after concussion has evolved with the understanding of concussion. Age, sport, position, level of play, relevant medical and concussion history, severity and duration of symptoms, neuroimaging and neuropsychological testing should all be considered. Susceptibility to injury, persistence of symptoms, psychological distress, and personal values and support may also play a role. Pediatric athletes may require a more conservative approach, given ongoing growth and development. For professional and/or elite athletes, financial or career implications may be considerations. When possible, retirement should be a shared decision among the athlete, the family, and the health care team.

Hamish Kerr, Bjørn Bakken, and Gregory House

This article focuses on 3 concepts that continue to be investigated in the search for the holy grail of concussion—a valid diagnostic test. Imaging advances are discussed with optimism that functional MRI and diffusion tensor imaging may be available clinically. Biomarkers and the use of genetic tests are covered. Sideline accelerometer use may help steer discussions of head trauma risk once technology exists to accurately estimate acceleration of the brain. In the meantime, strategies including allowing athletes to be substituted out of games for an evaluation and video review in elite sports can improve recognition of sports-related concussion.

Special Article

Kyle N. Kunze, Peter D. Fabricant, Robert G. Marx, and Benedict U. Nwachukwu

As the COVID-19 (Coronavirus disease 2019) pandemic continues, the paradigm of treatment continues to rapidly evolve, especially for sports medicine surgeons, because treatment before the pandemic was considered predominantly elective. This article provides subjective and objective data on the changes implicated by the COVID-19 pandemic with regard to the interactions and practices of sports medicine surgeons. This perspective also considers the potential impact on the patients and athletes treated by sports medicine surgeons. This article discusses the impact of the COVID-19 pandemic on sports medicine and provides thoughts on how the landscape of the field may continue to change.

CLINICS IN SPORTS MEDICINE

SERIES OF RELATED INTERESTED

Orthopedic Clinics
Foot and Ankle Clinics
Hand Clinics
Physical Medicine and Rehabilitation Clinics

THE CLINICS ARE AVAILABLE ONLINE!
Access your subscription at:
www.theclinics.com

Foreword
Sport-Related Concussion: Heads Up!

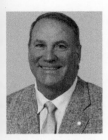

Mark D. Miller, MD
Consulting Editor

There has been a lot of progress since the last time we covered this topic in *Clinics in Sports Medicine* a decade ago, including new research, an emphasis on no return to play the same day, and a better understanding of chronic traumatic encephalopathy. Nevertheless, there is still a great deal that we don't know. Thank you to Dr Kriz for putting together this treatise outlining the current state-of-the-art on sport-related concussion (SRC). This issue covers the entirety of this topic, beginning with the basics and bringing in both research and clinical management. The editor addresses all populations, including females, kids, and athletes, at all levels. But he didn't stop there, prevention, long-term effects, and future directions are all covered as well. In sum, this is an excellent update on SRC that I encourage all to read and incorporate into their sideline game bag!

Mark D. Miller, MD
Division of Sports Medicine
Department of Orthopaedic Surgery
University of Virginia
James Madison University
400 Ray C. Hunt Drive, Suite 330
Charlottesville, VA 22908-0159, USA

E-mail address:
MDM3P@hscmail.mcc.virginia.edu

Clin Sports Med 40 (2021) xiii
https://doi.org/10.1016/j.csm.2020.10.001
0278-5919/21/© 2020 Published by Elsevier Inc.

sportsmed.theclinics.com

Preface

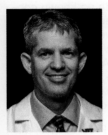

Peter K. Kriz, MD
Editor

It has been nearly a decade since Drs Meehan and Micheli were guest editors of an issue of *Clinics in Sports Medicine* dedicated entirely to sport-related concussion (SRC). It is an honor to follow these giants in their respective fields and provide an update on a condition that continues to impact millions of athletes annually in the United States. Recent data utilizing emergency department visits estimate that 1.0 to 1.8 million SRCs occur each year in individuals 18 years old and younger, with approximately 400,000 of these injuries occurring in high-school athletes. Over this time frame, there has been an increase in recognition of the injury and improved symptom reporting, due at least in part to national education efforts. There has also been a parallel and exponential increase in the number of clinical studies dedicated to SRC. A quick PubMed query using the search terms "sport + concussion" demonstrates an annual publication count of 211 in 2011 increasing to 713 in 2019. Well-designed clinical studies have enhanced our understanding of SRC, spawned emerging and promising diagnostic tools and rehabilitative programs, and furthered the evolution of concussion care.

While the decade has seen significant strides in SRC management, there are still no readily available objective tests to confirm diagnosis. A quest for the "ideal" biomarker for SRC, a point-of-care serologic or salivary test that can be performed easily with high sensitivity and reasonable specificity within hours of a head injury, remains elusive. Similarly, while advanced neuroimaging studies, including functional MRI and diffusion tensor imaging, show promise in detecting subtle, clinically relevant brain activation patterns and white matter changes, respectively, following a traumatic brain injury, these studies remain research tools and likely cost-prohibitive options for routine neuroimaging in the setting of SRC.

There have admittedly been setbacks over this decade. The public perception of SRC and its potential complications has been influenced less by the research than the media's interpretation of the scientific findings. Hollywood has even weighed in on the subject with the movie, *Concussion*. Despite no evidence supporting the association between suicide and brain pathologies in former athletes, societal fears remain pervasive that collision sport participation, even in small participation doses, markedly

Clin Sports Med 40 (2021) xv–xvi
https://doi.org/10.1016/j.csm.2020.09.002
0278-5919/21/© 2020 Published by Elsevier Inc.

increases an athlete's risk of chronic traumatic encephalopathy (CTE). As of 2020, standardized criteria for CTE have yet to be adopted by neuropathologists, and emerging evidence demonstrates that unique CTE neuropathology may continue to be elusive, as CTE pathology has been identified in individuals with no known contact/collision sport participation or known exposure to repetitive neurotrauma.

It is our hope that the ensuing decade provides additional answers regarding the risks and benefits of contact and collision sport participation, which continue to contribute to SRC incidence in our youth and adult populations. We are grateful to the contributing authors of this issue of *Clinics in Sports Medicine*, a diverse group of expert clinicians and researchers from across North America, who have volunteered their time and effort to contribute to this comprehensive resource and update on SRC.

Peter K. Kriz, MD
Division of Sports Medicine
Departments of Orthopaedics and Pediatrics
Warren Alpert Medical School
Brown University
1 Kettle Point Avenue
East Providence, RI 02915, USA

E-mail address:
Peter_Kriz@brown.edu

Twitter: @DrPKrizBrownU (P.K. Kriz)

Epidemiology of Sport-Related Concussion

Lauren A. Pierpoint, PhD[a],*, Christy Collins, PhD[b]

KEYWORDS

- Concussion • High school • College • Sport • Epidemiology • Traumatic brain injury

KEY POINTS

- Concussion rates vary across sport and age, with college athletes generally having higher concussion rates than high school athletes.
- Across gender-comparable sports, females have higher concussion rates than males in both college and high school.
- Concussion rates have increased over time, likely due to an increase in awareness and recognition.
- Although data collection efforts have improved over time, continued and increased data collection is necessary to fully understand the burden of sport-related concussion.

INTRODUCTION

Participation in sports occurs across the life span. In 2018, 56% of children aged 6 to 12 years in the United States played a team sport, with 38% of these children participating on a regular basis.[1] In addition to club sports and travel leagues, during the 2018/19 academic year, 7.9 million athletes participated in school-sanctioned high school sports, and more than 500,000 collegiate athletes participated in National Collegiate Athletic Association (NCAA) championship and emerging sports.[2,3] Approximately 1 in 4 adults in the United States (US) play sports, with 18% of adults participating in sports and exercise on an average day.[4,5] **Table 1** presents changes in participation numbers between the 2009/10 and 2018/19 seasons for select high school and college sports.

Being active in sports is one way to maintain a physically fit, healthy lifestyle. In addition to helping maintain a healthy weight, sports participation can increase strength, endurance, and flexibility.[6,7] Regular physical activity has also been shown to improve psychological well-being, increase self-esteem, reduce depression and anxiety, and improve academic performance.[6,8]

[a] Steadman Philippon Research Institute, 181 West Meadow Drive, Suite 100, Vail, CO 81657, USA; [b] Datalys Center for Sports Injury Research and Prevention, 401 West Michigan Street, Suite 500, Indianapolis, IN 46202, USA
* Corresponding author.
E-mail address: lpierpoint@sprivail.org

Clin Sports Med 40 (2021) 1–18
https://doi.org/10.1016/j.csm.2020.08.013
0278-5919/21/© 2020 Elsevier Inc. All rights reserved.

Table 1
Participation changes 2009/10 and 2018/19 by sport and sex for select high school and college sports

		High School[a]			College[a]		
		2009/10	2018/19	% Change	2009/ 10	2018/ 19	% Change
Men's sports	American football	1,109,278	1,006,013	−9%	66,313	73,712	11%
	Baseball	472,644	482,740	2%	30,365	36,011	19%
	Basketball	540,207	540,769	0%	17,008	18,816	11%
	Ice hockey	36,475	35,283	−3%	3945	4323	10%
	Lacrosse	90,670	113,702	25%	9844	14,603	48%
	Soccer	391,839	459,077	17%	21,770	25,499	17%
	Wrestling	272,890	247,441	−9%	6397	7300	14%
Women's sports	Basketball	439,550	399,067	−9%	15,423	16,509	7%
	Field hockey	63,719	60,824	−5%	5634	6119	9%
	Lacrosse	68,768	99,750	45%	7683	12,452	62%
	Soccer	356,116	394,105	11%	23,650	28,310	20%
	Softball	391,776	368,640	−6%	17,726	20,419	15%
	Volleyball	403,985	452,808	12%	15,133	17,780	17%
Co-ed[b]	Cheerleading	126,390	165,296	31%			

[a] High school data from the annual NFHS participation report; college data from the annual NCAA participation report.
[b] Cheerleading is not an NCAA-sanctioned sport.
Data from National Federation of State High School Associations. 2018-19 High School Athletics Participation Survey. 2019; https://www.nfhs.org/media/1020412/2018-19_participation_survey. pdf. Accessed 11/27/2019 and National Collegiate Athletic Association. NCAA Sports Sponsorship and Participation Rates Report Student-Athlete Participation 1981-82 - 2018-19 2019; https:// ncaaorg.s3.amazonaws.com/research/sportpart/2018-19RES_ SportsSponsorshipParticipationRatesReport.pdf. Accessed 11/27/2019.

Despite the numerous health benefits, athletes are at risk of sports-related injury, as a certain endemic level of injury can be expected among participants of any physical activity. A wide variety of injuries occur during sports participation including concussion, the definition of which may vary across studies. The Berlin Consensus Statement on Concussion in Sport defines a sports-related concussion as a "traumatic brain injury (TBI) induced by biomechanical forces."[9] The Centers for Disease Control and Prevention defines a concussion as a "type of TBI caused by a bump, blow, or jolt to the head or by a hit to the body that causes the head and brain to move rapidly back and forth."[10] A concussion results in a range of clinical symptoms that vary individual to individual that may or may not include a loss of consciousness. Most symptoms of concussion resolve in 1 to 3 weeks; however, some symptoms may persist for a month or longer.[11]

The burden of sports-related concussion has been measured in various settings, such as emergency departments (EDs), hospitals/inpatient, clinics, schools, and sports organizations. One study found that an estimated 283,000 children aged 18 years and younger are treated in US EDs for a sports- or recreation-related TBI each year.[12] In 2017, 2.5 million high school students reported sustaining at least one sport or activity-related concussion in the past year, and one million high school students reported sustaining more than one sport- or activity-related concussion in the past year.[13] Of the 3.42 million sports- and recreation-related TBIs seen in US ED from 2001 to 2012, 30% occurred among adults aged 20 years and older.[14] The incidence of concussion is certainly underestimated, as these numbers do not include concussions in which the injured athlete did not seek medical treatment or the concussion was not properly diagnosed. Current data sources may capture only 1 out of every 9 concussions sustained in the United States.[15]

Just as the definition of concussion and source of data varies from study to study, so does how the burden of concussion was measured. The most commonly used metric of injury occurrence in sports injury research is a rate or the total number of injuries divided by some measure of exposure such as team-season, team-games, player-season, player-games, player-minutes, player-plays, or athlete-exposure.[16] Other common metrics used in sports injury research include injury risk and injury odds.[16] Injury risk is calculated as the number of injured athletes in a given time period divided by the number of athletes at risk of being injured in the same time period. Odds of injury, which is a function of risk, is calculated by dividing the risk of injury by one minus the risk. When making direct comparisons of results across studies, it is important to consider how the burden of concussion was measured.

Recently, direct comparisons between sports and age groups were made possible through data collected via 2 national sports injury surveillance systems, High School Reporting Information Online (RIO) and the NCAA Injury Surveillance Program (NCAA-ISP). Both systems are web-based and rely on athletic trainers to enter in injury and athlete exposure (AE) information on a weekly basis. **Tables 2** and **3** display comparative data collected during the 2004/05 to 2013/14 seasons. National estimates of concussions presenting to US EDs are also available from the National Electronic Injury Surveillance System (NEISS) using a nationally representative sample of 100 US hospitals with EDs.

In general, previous studies using the abovementioned surveillance systems have found that the incidence of sports-related concussions has increased significantly in the last 15 years.[14,17] This may be due, in part, to increased recognition of concussion symptoms, better reporting practices, and state legislation regarding concussion and return to play.[18] The risk of concussion varies by sport, which is presented later in the sport-specific findings.

SPORT-SPECIFIC FINDINGS
American Football

In the United States, football is the most popular sport with 73,712 participants across all divisions at the collegiate level and 1,006,013 participants at the high school level in 2018/19.[2,3] Because of the high number of participants and the level of contact inherent to the game, concussions remain a significant concern in football. Football continues to have the highest number of catastrophic TBIs and one of the highest concussion rates across many years and multiple studies comparing football with other sports.

Between 2013 and 2018, the National Center for Catastrophic Sport Injury Research (NCCSIR) reported a total of 45 catastrophic brain injuries, 41 of which occurred at the middle or high school level, 2 at the youth level, 1 at the collegiate level, and 1 at the professional or semiprofessional level. Further, the 5-year average number of brain injuries with incomplete neurologic recovery has more than doubled since 1982 (4.2 in 1982 vs 8.8 in 2018).[19]

A study of the 2013/14 to 2017/18 seasons comparing concussion rates across 20 high school sports found that football had the highest concussion rates overall (10.4 per 10,000 AE), during competitions (35.8) and practices (5.0).[20] Across the study period, competition concussions increased from 33.2 to 39.1 per 10,000 AE.

In contrast to high school, collegiate football has the fourth highest concussion rate out of 25 sports under surveillance by the NCAA-ISP (behind men's wrestling, men's

Table 2
Concussion rates per 10,000 AE and rate ratios comparing competitions versus practices in high school and college sports

		High School[a]				College[a]			
		Overall Rate	Competition Rate	Practice Rate	Rate Ratio Competition vs Practice (95% CI)	Overall Rate	Competition Rate	Practice Rate	Rate Ratio Competition vs Practice (95% CI)
Men's sports	American football[30]	7.28	25.73	3.54	7.27 (6.78, 7.79)	6.31	30.09	3.99	7.53 (6.89, 8.24)
	Baseball[32]	0.69	1.33	0.34	3.87 (2.59, 5.79)	1.13	2.25	0.53	4.22 (2.70, 6.58)
	Basketball[35]	1.53	3.27	0.79	4.14 (3.27, 5.23)	6.18	12.62	4.52	2.79 (2.35, 3.32)
	Ice hockey[44]	6.83	17.66	1.50	11.74 (8.24, 16.72)	6.95	22.88	2.06	11.12 (8.76, 14.12)
	Lacrosse[47]	4.87	12.18	1.63	7.46 (5.76, 9.66)	4.51	16.98	2.19	7.75 (5.74, 10.47)
	Soccer[72]	2.78	7.68	0.68	11.28 (8.81, 14.45)	4.02	12.36	1.73	7.16 (5.58, 9.19)
	Wrestling[77]	3.13	5.85	2.17	2.70 (2.24, 3.25)	6.72	27.95	4.10	6.81 (5.05, 9.18)
Women's sports	Basketball[36]	2.98	7.39	1.08	6.82 (5.55, 8.38)	4.99	9.99	3.54	2.82 (2.31, 3.44)
	Field hockey[40]	2.67	5.94	1.16	5.14 (3.63, 7.29)	4.19	11.29	1.86	6.08 (3.80, 9.73)
	Lacrosse[55]	3.67	8.34	1.57	5.33 (3.85, 7.36)	5.07	14.23	2.88	4.94 (3.56, 6.83)
	Soccer[73]	4.50	12.84	0.92	13.92 (11.13, 17.40)	6.44	19.11	2.33	8.19 (6.73, 9.98)
	Softball[34]	1.40	2.20	0.97	2.26 (1.66, 3.07)	2.61	4.19	1.50	2.80 (2, 3.92)
	Volleyball[75]	1.18	1.90	0.80	2.39 (1.77, 3.23)	2.29	3.26	1.88	1.73 (1.22, 2.46)

High School Reporting Information Online (2005/06–2013/14) and the National Collegiate Athletic Association Injury Surveillance Program (2004/05–2013/14).
Abbreviations: AE, athlete exposure, one athlete participating in one practice or competition; CI, confidence interval.
[a] HS RIO and the NCAA-ISP collect injury and exposure data from national samples of high school and collegiate sports programs, respectively. Data presented in this table were collected from each surveillance system during the same time periods. HS RIO began data collection of lacrosse, ice hockey, and field hockey in 2008/09.

Table 3
Concussion numbers and percentage of all practice and competition injuries in high school and college sports

		High School[a]				College[a]			
		Practice		Competition		Practice		Competition	
		n	%	n	%	n	%	n	%
Men's sports	American football[30]	1337	15.8	1966	20.4	1136	8.4	834	9.4
	Baseball[32]	35	5.1	74	8.8	28	2.5	63	4.4
	Basketball[35]	110	7.2	192	12.6	312	10.3	225	14.3
	Ice hockey[44]	36	21.8	208	31.4	87	10.1	297	17.0
	Lacrosse[47]	75	13.8	248	28.8	72	6.3	104	14.3
	Soccer[72]	76	6.6	366	20.9	93	3.8	183	7.9
	Wrestling[77]	226	11.3	218	15.9	94	5.9	79	10.1
Women's sports	Basketball[36]	122	9.6	357	21.7	215	8.7	176	12.4
	Field hockey[40]	45	8.8	107	22.7	26	4.3	52	13.3
	Lacrosse[55]	52	15.2	125	35.0	67	10.2	79	21.2
	Soccer[73]	90	8.6	537	24.5	136	5.2	361	14.6
	Softball[34]	75	11.5	89	12.8	51	5.4	100	11.0
	Volleyball[75]	77	7.8	96	15.1	75	5.0	54	8.5

High School Reporting Information Online (2005/06–2013/14) and the National Collegiate Athletic Association Injury Surveillance Program (2004/05–2013/14).

[a] HS RIO and the NCAA-ISP collect injury and exposure data from national samples of high school and collegiate sports programs, respectively. Data presented in this table were collected from each surveillance system during the same time periods. HS RIO began data collection of lacrosse, ice hockey, and field hockey in 2008/09.

ice hockey, and women's ice hockey), although football accounted for most of the concussions sustained across all sports.[21] During 2009/10 to 2013/14, a total of 603 concussions were reported to NCAA-ISP, corresponding to a rate of 6.7 per 10,000 AE. Football also had the second highest competition concussion rate (30.1).

A 2013 study using ED data collected from the NEISS showed that the estimated number of youth football players aged 13 years or younger who were treated for a concussion in US EDs increased from 1784 in 2002 to 10,797 in 2012.[22] A study collecting data from 9 middle schools in Virginia during the 2015/16 to 2017/18 seasons found a concussion rate of 3.7 per 1000 AE in competitions and 1.0 in practices.[23] A meta-analysis including 5 studies of youth football concussions found a pooled estimate of 0.5 per 1000 AE.[24] Other studies found rates ranging from 1.8 per 1000 AE[25] to 2.0 per 1000 AE.[26] In a 2016-2017 study in which 863 youth were followed, 51 sustained a football-related concussion corresponding to an athlete level incidence of 5.1% per season.[27] Another study of youth football players in Hawaii found the risk of concussion was 7.8%.[28]

One 2015 study comparing concussion rates across the US youth, high school, and collegiate levels using data collected from athletic trainers (AT) found that game rates were highest at the collegiate level (3.7 per 10,000 AE) followed by youth (2.4) then high school (2.0), though youth and high school rates were not statistically different.[29] Another study comparing data collected from 2004/05 through 2013/14 at the high school and collegiate levels also found that concussion rates were significantly higher at the collegiate level compared with the high school level for both practices (4.0 vs 3.5 per 10,000 AE) and competitions (30.1 vs 25.7).[30]

Baseball and Softball

Baseball continues to increase in popularity, with 482,740 high school participants and 36,011 college participants in the 2018/19 seasons.[2,3] In general, baseball exhibits low concussion rates compared with other popular sports. At the high school level, baseball concussion rates are among the lowest with a 2013/14 to 2017/18 estimate of 1.0 per 10,000 AE. Only swimming, track and field, and cross-country had lower concussion rates.[20,31] Overall rates were similar at the collegiate level (0.9–1.1 per 10,000 AE).[21,32] Rates of competition concussion were higher than in practice for high school (2.1 vs 0.5; incidence rate ratio [IRR] = 4.4; 95% confidence interval [CI], 3.1–6.4) and for college (2.2 vs 0.5, IRR = 4.2; 95% CI, 2.7–6.6).[20,32] College players had higher concussion rates than high school athletes (IRR=1.6; 95% CI, 1.2–2.2).[32] Concussions accounted for 5.1% of practice injuries and 8.8% of competition injuries in high school and 2.5% of practice injuries and 4.4% of competition injuries in college.[32] During 1994 to 2006, 91,877 baseball-related concussions/closed head injuries in children younger than 18 years presented to US EDs, representing 5.8% of all baseball-related injuries.[33]

In 2018/19 there were 368,640 participants in high school girls' softball (a 6% decline from 2009/10) and 20,419 in college softball (a 15% increase).[2,3] During the 2013/14 to 2017/18 seasons, the overall concussion rate in high school was 2.3 per 10,000 AE, with higher rates during competition (3.9) than practice (1.4; IRR = 2.7; 95% CI, 2.1–3.6).[20] During 2008/09 to 2013/14, the overall concussion rate in college softball was 3.3 per 10,000 AE, with higher rates in competition (5.6) compared with practice (1.8, IRR = 3.2; 95% CI, 2.1-6.4).[21] Concussion rates were higher in college softball players compared with high school players (IRR=1.9; 95% CI, 1.5-2.3).[34]

Although there are distinct differences between baseball and softball, they are considered sex-comparable sports. Several studies have shown that softball players experience at least twice the concussion rates of baseball players across age groups.[20,21,31,34] In high school during the 2008/09 to 2009/10 academic years, concussions also represented a greater proportion of injuries among softball players (13.4%) than baseball players (5.4%) (IPR= 2.5; 95% CI, 1.6–3.9). In college, most concussions in softball and baseball were due to ball contact (baseball: 54.4%; softball: 66.7%) followed by player contact (baseball: 37.5%; softball: 25.8%).[21] In baseball, 7.2% of concussions occurred during precompetition warmups compared with 26.3% of softball concussion, highlighting an area for concussion prevention in softball.

Basketball

In the 2018/19 season, 540,769 men participated in high school basketball and 18,816 in collegiate basketball.[2,3] During the 2013/14 to 2017/18 academic years, the concussion rate in high school boys' basketball was 2.1 per 10,000 AE with a higher rate in competitions (4.1) compared with practices (1.2; IRR = 3.3; 95% CI, 2.7–4.1).[20] In collegiate basketball, rates were higher in competition versus practice (overall = 3.9 per 10,000 AE, competition = 5.6, practice = 3.4; IRR = 1.6; 95% CI, 1.0–2.6).[21] Across studies, concussion rates have been higher among collegiate basketball players compared with high school, with one study including 10 years of surveillance data showing an IRR = 4.1; 95% CI, 3.5 to 4.7.[35]

Women's basketball at the collegiate level experienced a 7% increase in participants since 2009/10 with 16,509 participants in 2018/19. Conversely, high school girls' basketball declined by 9%, but its 399,067 participants in 2018/19 still made it one of the most popular high school sports. A 5-year study of concussions among high school athletes found a concussion rate of 4.9 per 10,000 AE, with higher rates in competition (12.1) compared with practice (1.6; IRR = 7.8 ; 95% CI, 6.5–9.4).[20] Similar findings were observed at the college level where the overall concussion rate was 6.0 per 10,000 AE and rates were higher in competitions (10.9) compared with practices (4.4) (IRR = 2.5; 95%, CI 1.7-3.6).[21] When comparing college with high school, collegiate basketball had higher concussion rates than high school (IRR = 1.7; 95% CI, 1.5–1.9).[36] A study of US ED visits for sports- and recreation-related TBIs found that among women younger than 18 years, basketball was the third most common cause, contributing 10,617 TBIs (11.9% of all TBIs) reported during 2010 to 2016.[12]

In both high school and college, women had higher concussion rates than men (high school IRR = 2.3; 95% CI, 2.1–2.6; college IRR = 1.5; 95% CI, 1.2–2.0).[20,21] Mechanism of injury was similar between men and women at the high school and collegiate level with most concussions due to player contact (college: men = 77.4%, women = 68.1%; high school: boys = 65.7%, girls = 55.4%).

Cheerleading

Cheerleading is becoming an increasingly popular sport. In 2018/19, there were 161,358 female and 3938 male athletes participating in cheerleading at the high school level, corresponding to an overall 31% increase in participation since 2009/10.[2] In conjunction with its increase in popularity, more catastrophic injuries have been associated with cheerleading.

Cheerleading is a technical sport involving stunts and aerial maneuvers such as basket tosses, which place athletes at risk. The 36th Annual NCCSIR Report found that between the 182/83 and the 2017/18 seasons, cheerleading had the second highest number of catastrophic injuries behind football, and the highest rate accounting for overall participation.[19] Between 1990 and 2012, there were 35,079 concussion/closed head injuries treated in US EDs among 5- to 18-year-olds. During 2001-2012, the rate of concussions increased by 290%.[37] The same study found that stunts were more likely to result in concussions than other maneuvers (RR = 2.4; 95% CI, 2.1–2.8). A study of high school and collegiate cheerleading injuries recorded 54 catastrophic injuries between 2002 and 2017, 28 (52%) of which involved the brain/head.[38] During the 2009/10 to 2013/14 seasons, a study on high school cheerleading injuries found that concussions were the most common cheerleading injury (31.1% of injuries) but that cheerleading concussion rates (2.2 per 10,000 AE) were lower than all other sports combined during that time frame (IRR = 0.6; 95% CI, 0.5–0.7).[39] However, practice rates (2.5 per 10,000 AE) ranked third behind boys' football and wrestling. Most concussions occurred during stunts (69.0%) and resulted from contact with another person (58.9%). In contrast to most other sports, cheerleading concussion rates are lower in competition than they are in practices (IRR = 0.6; 95% CI, 0.5–0.8).[20]

Field Hockey

Compared with other sports, participation in field hockey is generally lower. In 2018/19, there were 60,824 girls' field hockey participants in high schools and 6119 college participants.[2,3] Despite lower participation, concussions in field hockey are still a concern, particularly during competitions.

During the 2013/14 to 2018/19 seasons, the overall high school field hockey concussion rate was 2.7 per 10,000 AE, with competitions (6.5 per 10,000 AE) having 7.5 (95% CI, 4.7–12.0) times the rate of practices (0.9 per 10,000 AE).[20] Collegiate field hockey showed a similar pattern during the 2008/09 and 2013/14 seasons, with an overall concussion rate of 4.0 per 10,000 AE, a competition rate 6.3 times higher than in practice (competition = 11.1, practice rate = 1.8; IRR = 6.3; 95% CI, 2.2–18.4). Concussion rates were higher in college field hockey compared with high school (IRR = 1.6; 95% CI, 1.2–2.1).[40] At the national level between 1990 through 2003, less than 5% of the estimated 64,070 pediatric (2-18 years) field hockey-related injuries treated in US EDs were concussions.[41] In a comparative study of field hockey injuries in high school and college, during competitions, concussions represented 22.7% of high school injuries and 13.3% of collegiate injuries.[40] During practices, concussions represented 8.8% and 4.3% of high school and college injuries, respectively. The most common injury mechanisms at the high school level were contact with equipment (eg, stick, ball) (46.5%) and player contact (41.4%). In college, player contact accounted for 53.3% of concussions.

Ice Hockey

As with field hockey, ice hockey has fewer participants compared with other sports. In 2018/19, there were 35,283 participants at the high school level for boys, 4,323 at the college level for men, and 2,531 at the college level for women.[2,3] Across multiple studies of varying age groups, ice hockey consistently has had high concussion rates.

Twenty-two percent of high school boys ice hockey injuries are concussions, the highest of any sport under High School RIO surveillance during the 2008/09 through 2009/10 academic years.[31] Ice hockey also represents 13% of all concussions in NCAA collegiate athletics, with a 6.9% risk of sustaining a concussion.[42] A study of 20 high school sports across the 2013/14 to 2017/18 seasons found ice hockey to have the third highest concussion rate overall (7.7 per 10,000 AE) and in competitions (19.5).[20] However, the high school ice hockey practice rate of 1.2 per 10,000 AE was relatively low (IRR = 16.2; 95% CI 10.3–25.5). In college, men's ice hockey had the second highest overall rate (7.9 per 10,000 AE) and women the third highest rate (7.5) behind men's wrestling.[21] There was also a large difference between competition and practice rates for men (IRR=9.9; 95% CI, 7.3-13.5) and women (IRR=6.7; 95% CI,

4.2-10.7). Youth data from the 2011 to 2012 season in Alberta, Canada showed similar concussion incidence between males and females (IRR= 1.0; 95% CI, 0.7-1.3), as did NCAA-ISP data from 2004/05 to 2013/14 (IRR=1.0; 95% CI, 0.8-1.2).[43,44] The high concussion rates seen in high school and college may be a product of the collision nature of the sport. Most high school ice hockey concussions were due to player contact (47.7%) and glass/boards contact (31.9%).[45] Most (73.2% for men, 49.4% for women) concussions in college ice hockey were due to player contact.[21]

Lacrosse

Lacrosse is one of the fastest growing team sports at the high school and college level for both men and women. Among men in 2018/19, there were 113,702 high school participants and 14,603 college participants. Among women there were 99,750 high school and 12,452 college participants.[2,3]

Boys' and men's lacrosse are collision sports (although youth lacrosse only permits limited checking) that mandate extensive wear of protective equipment including gloves, arm pads, shoulder pads, mouth guards, and a hard shell helmet.[46] Despite such protective equipment, concussions remain a concern. During the 2013/14 to 2017/18 academic years, high school boys' lacrosse had the fourth highest concussion rate (4.9 per 10,000 AE) behind boys' football, boys' ice hockey, and girls' soccer.[20] At the collegiate level, men's lacrosse ranks somewhat lower, at 13 among 25 collegiate sports.[21] When compared during the same time frame, overall concussion rates were similar between high school and college lacrosse (IRR 1.1; 95% CI, 0.8-1.2).[47] Although youth data are limited, a study comparing youth versus high school versus collegiate lacrosse found the concussion rate in youth was higher than both high school (0.7 vs 0.3 per 1000 AEs) and the NCAA (0.7 vs 0.3 per 1000 AEs).[48]

Across all levels in boys' and men's lacrosse, concussion rates are generally consistently higher in competition than in practice.[21,31,49] Concussions accounted for a greater proportion of injuries at the high school level (13.8% in practices, 28.8% in games) than collegiate level (6.3% in practices, 14.3% in games).[47] Across many studies, the primary mechanism of injury for concussions was contact with another player, with estimates of up to 80% of concussions sustained in college athletes and 50% sustained in high school athletes.[48,50-52] Two studies of youth lacrosse players found that at least 50% were due to player contact.[48,53]

In contrast to males, female lacrosse players are only required to wear a mouth guard and protective eyewear and hard shell helmets are prohibited. Full body contact and direct stick checking are also not allowed.[54] In high school, girls' lacrosse had the seventh highest rate of concussion out of 20 different sports (4.2 per 10,000 AEs). In college, women's lacrosse also had the seventh highest rate of 25 different sports (5.2 per 10,000 AEs).[21,31] As with boys, surveillance data on youth girls' lacrosse is limited. One study of boys' and girls' youth lacrosse players only recorded 2 concussions among females during the 2015 and 2016 seasons.[53] When comparing across age groups, concussion rates were higher in college athletes (5.1 per 10,000 AE) than high school athletes (3.7; IRR = 1.4; 95% CI, 1.1-1.7).[54] At the high school level, concussions represented 15.2% of injuries in practice and 35.0% in competitions. In college, concussions accounted for 10.2% of practice injuries and 21.2% in competitions. Competitions were associated with greater risk of injury in both high school (IRR = 5.2) and college (IRR = 4.9). The most common mechanisms of concussion were contact with the stick/ball at both the high school (72.2%) and college (65.5%) levels.[20,49]

Although the vast differences in protective equipment and game rules preclude making direct sex comparisons between male and female lacrosse, recent studies found no differences in concussion rates between women and men at the high school level (IRR = 1.2; 95% CI, 1.0-1.4) but higher rates among women at the collegiate level (IRR = 1.6; 95% CI, 1.1-2.4).[20,21]

Rugby

In the 2018/19 academic year, 2389 boys and 678 girls competed in high school rugby and 164 men and 530 women competed in college rugby.[2,3] However, many athletes play rugby outside of the school setting. USA Rugby reported 30,255 registered college players and 28,711 registered high school players in 2019.[56]

A meta-analysis of 12 youth sports in the United States found that rugby had the highest incidence of concussion (4.18 injuries per 1000 athlete-exposures), followed by hockey (1.20) and football (0.53).[57] A systematic review of adolescent rugby injuries in multiple countries found the incidence of concussion ranged from 0.19 to 1.45 injuries per 1000 playing hours and from 3.8 to 5.7 injuries per 1000 AE.[24] At the high school level, a study of 121 boys' and girls' US high school rugby clubs found that 15.8% of all injuries were concussions, and boys and girls sustained a similar proportion of concussions (16.1% and 14.3%, respectively).[58] Three activities, including being tackled (33.0%), tackling (31.9%), and rucks (22.3%) were associated with 87.2% of concussions. In another study at the high school level in the United States, concussions accounted for 25% of all injuries with an incidence rate of 3.8 injuries per 1000 AE or 11.3 injuries per 100 player seasons.[59]

Of all rugby injuries treated in US emergency rooms from 1978 through 2004, 3.4% were concussions.[60] Rugby players aged 18 years and younger were significantly more likely to be diagnosed with a concussion than rugby players older than 18 years (IPR: 1.62, 95% CI: 1.06–2.50; P<.001). When this study was replicated by a different group of researchers using the same source of data but from 2004 to 2013, the number of rugby concussions had doubled.[61] This study also found that college-aged people of 19 to 24 years of age had the highest number of rugby-related injuries.

In a prospective cohort study of more than 13,500 players aged 13 to 49 years who participated in 28 US Rugby 7s tournaments, the overall incidence of concussion was 7.7 injuries per 1000 player-hours, and there was no difference in incidence of concussion between men and women (7.6 and 8.1, respectively).[62]

Skiing and Snowboarding

Skiing and snowboarding are popular recreational sports, with over 10 million participants annually in the US. At the organized high school level 10,999 athletes participated in skiing at the high school level (boys = 5,484; girls = 4,615) and 972 in snowboarding (boys=638; girls=334). At the collegiate level, 388 men and 431 women participated in skiing.[2,3] Overall, concussions represent approximately 5-10% of injuries among both recreational skiers and snowboarders, though estimates range up to 20%.[63,64] Between 2010 and 2014, 5,388 skiing-related concussions and 5,558 snowboarding-related concussions presented to US EDs. There was a higher incidence of concussion among skiers and snowboarders aged 0-19 years compared to 20 years and older.[65] A study of skiing and snowboarding-related head injuries to children and adolescents from 1996-2010 estimated that 78,538 head injuries were treated in US EDs, 77.2% of which were TBIs (including concussion). The annual incidence of head injury also increased during the time period.[66] Further, TBIs also account for 50-88% of the skiing and snowboarding deaths in the US each year.[67] Although some reports find that among recreational skiers men sustain more concussions than women, a world cup analysis found that women had a higher head injury incidence (5.8 per 100 athletes) than men (3.9) during the 2006-2013 seasons

(IRR = 1.5%, 95% CI, 1.2-1.9).[68,69] However, no sex differences were observed among world cup snowboarders during the 2007-2012 seasons.[70] A 2013-2015 study of skiers and snowboarders diagnosed and admitted for TBI found that the most common mechanism of injury was falls (54%) followed by collision (18%).[71] The most severe TBIs were associated with collisions with objects.

Soccer

In 2018/19, there were 459,077 athletes participating in high school boys' soccer and 25,499 participating in men's collegiate soccer, representing a 17% increase at both levels since 2009/10.[2,3] A study including data from the 2013/14 to 2017/18 seasons showed an overall concussion rate of 3.4 per 10,000 AE, an increase from 1.9 calculated in a similar study of the 2008/09 to 2009/10 school years.[20,31] Men's soccer concussion rates have also increased. College men have higher concussion rates than their high school counterparts (IRR = 1.5; 95% CI 1.3–1.7).[72] Concussions accounted for a larger proportion of injuries sustained during competitions at the high school level (high school=20.9%, college=7.9%).

The number of female soccer players also increased, with 394,105 high school participants and 28,310 college participants, a 11% and 20% increase from the 2009/10 season, respectively.[2,3] Data from 2013/14 to 2017/18 showed that high school girl soccer players have the second highest concussion rate (8.2 per 10,000 AE) among 20 high school sports, behind boys' football.[20] Competition rates (21.8 per 10,000 AE) were 10.2 times higher than practice rates (2.1). Collegiate women's soccer showed similar trends (overall rate = 6.3 per 10,000 AE, competition = 19.4, practice = 2.1) with significantly higher rates in competition (IRR = 9.1, 95% CI 6.1–13.3). Concussion rates were higher at the collegiate level (IRR = 1.5; 95% CI, 1.3–1.7).[73] Concussions accounted for a greater proportion of injuries in competitions in high school athletes (24.5%) than college athletes (14.6%).

Female soccer players sustain concussions at a higher rate than male players. Studies from 2004/05 to 2013/14 found both high school and college female athletes had a 1.6 times higher rate of concussion compared with male athletes.[74] More recent data show greater differences in high school girls versus boys (IRR = 2.3; 95% CI, 2.1–2.6).[20,21] A study of the 2005/06 to 2013/14 seasons found that in high school athletes, contact with another player was the most common concussion mechanism overall for both boys (68.8%) and girls (51.3%).[74] Heading was the most common activity during which concussions were sustained in boys (30.6%) and girls (25.3%), and player contact was the most common mechanism among heading-related concussions (boys=78.1%, girls=61.9%). Similar findings were observed in college soccer—most concussions were due to player contact (men = 70.9%, women = 52.9%), with the most common activity-mechanism combination being player contact while heading the ball (men = 23.6%, women = 19.9%).[21]

Volleyball

Participation in girls'/women's volleyball has grown over the past decade. The 2018/19 season saw 452,808 high school participants and 17,780 college participants, an 12% and 17% increase since 2009/10, respectively.[2,3] As seen with some other sports, the concussion rate in volleyball has increased over time. In 2005/06, the concussion rate in high school volleyball was 0.5 per 10,000 AE, whereas the 2013/14 to 2017/18 seasons saw rates of 3.1 per 10,000 AE.[20,75] Similarly, collegiate volleyball had a concussion rate of 1.8 per 10,000 AE in 2005/06 compared with 3.6 during 2009/10 to 2013/14.[21] Competition rates were higher than practice in both high school (IRR = 2.6, 95% CI, 2.1–3.1) and in college (IRR = 2.1; 95% CI, 1.3–3.6). Concussion rates were higher in college volleyball compared with high school (IRR = 2.0, 95% CI, 1.6–2.4).[75] Ball contact (high school = 53.9%, college = 39.3%) and surface contact (high school = 24.8%, college = 23.2%) were the most common concussion mechanisms.[20,21] In high school, 27.5% of competition concussions occurred during pre-competition warmups, highlighting a area for future concussion prevention efforts.[20]

Wrestling

Wrestling is a popular sport, with 247,441 high school and 7300 college participants during 2018/19.[2,3] Wrestling also carries a large concussion burden, yet it receives comparatively little attention to other contact sports such as American football. During 2000-2006, 10,113 wrestling related TBIs presented to US EDs in youth ages 5-17 years.[76] In a study of 12 sports in grades 8-12 in Hawaii, wrestling carried the highest concussion risk (20.8%).[28] During 2013/14-2017/18, the overall concussion rate in high school wrestling was 4.8 per 10,000 AE, with higher rates in competitions (9.9) compared to practices (3.1, IRR=3.2; 95% CI, 2.7-3.8).[20] In college, wrestling has the highest concussion rate out of 25 sports (10.9 per 10,000 AE), with a competition rate nearly 10 times that in practice (IRR=9.8; 95% CI, 6.4-14.9).[21] Further, an estimated 7.9% of male NCAA wrestlers sustain a concussion per season, the highest risk of all collegiate sports.[42] Data from 2004/05 to 2013/14 showed that concussion rates were significantly higher at the college level (IRR=2.1; 95% CI, 1.8-2.6), with an even larger difference observed during competitions (27.9 vs 5.8 per 10,000 AE), possibly reflecting increases in athlete body mass and therefore impact forces with age.[77] Concussions accounted for 11.3% of injuries in practices and 15.9% in competitions in high schoolers, and 5.9% during practices and 10.1% during competitions in college athletes. Takedowns were the most common activity during which concussions were sustained, although mechanism of injury differed between high school and college. High school athletes most frequently sustained concussions due to contact with the playing surface during takedown (32.6%), whereas collegiate athletes sustained theirs via contact with an opponent during takedown (31.4%).[20,21]

SUMMARY

Across sports and age groups, concussion rates have increased over the past decade. Much of the increase is attributed to increased concussion knowledge, leading to better recognition and treatment. There is recent evidence that state-mandated TBI laws, now implemented in all 50 states and Washington D.C., may be influencing concussion rates.[18] Only continued data collection will enable researchers to evaluate the long-term effects of legislation and whether concussion rates will decrease in the future.

There are several trends that were observed across many sports and age groups. In general, concussion rates are higher in competitions compared with practices. Some sports, such as ice hockey, have low rates of concussion in practices compared with competitions. Determining why ice hockey has relatively low practice concussion rates may help other collision/contact sports reduce rates during practices. In gender-comparable sports, women reported higher rates of concussion compared with men. This finding has been well established in the literature and may be due to physiologic and biomechanical differences or sociocultural differences in reporting.

Despite improvements in data collection and the ability to directly compare high school and college data during the same time frames using similar collection methods, gaps in data collection, particularly at the youth level, still exist. In addition, athletes who do not seek medical care are not accounted for and there are few systematic studies of injuries that occur in nonsanctioned or recreational sports. Therefore, current reported numbers and rates of concussions are likely underestimates of the true burden. Improvement and expansion of data collection efforts are necessary to further understand the burden of concussion. Continued monitoring of rates, patterns, and trends of concussion will be essential for driving injury prevention efforts and reducing concussion burden.

DISCLOSURE

The authors have nothing to disclose.

REFERENCES

1. The Aspen Institute Project Play. State of play 2019: trends and developments in youth sports. 2019. Available at: https://assets.aspeninstitute.org/content/uploads/2019/10/2019_SOP_National_Final.pdf?_ga=2.78766999.2089146329.1600396237-1441157283.1600396237. Accessed November 27, 2019.
2. National Federation Of State High School Associations. 2018-19 high school athletics participation Survey. 2019. Available at: https://www.nfhs.org/media/1020412/2018-19_participation_survey.pdf. Accessed November 27, 2019.
3. National Collegiate Athletic Association. NCAA sports sponsorship and participation rates report student-athlete participation 1981-82 - 2018-19 2019. Available at: https://ncaaorg.s3.amazonaws.com/research/sportpart/2018-19RES_SportsSponsorshipParticipationRatesReport.pdf. Accessed November 27, 2019.
4. National Public Radio, Robert Wood Johnson Foundation, Harvard T.H. Chan School of Public Health. Sports and Health in America. 2015. Available at: https://www.rwjf.org/content/dam/farm/reports/reports/2015/rwjf420908. Accessed November 27, 2019.
5. Woods RA. Division of labor force statistics, U.S. Bureau of labor statistics. Spotlight on statistics, sports and exercise 2017. Available at. https://www.bls.gov/spotlight/2017/sports-and-exercise/home.htm. Accessed January 15, 2020.
6. Physical Activity Guidelines Advisory Committee. Physical activity guidelines advisory committee report, 2008. 2008. Available at: https://health.gov/sites/default/files/2019-10/CommitteeReport_7.pdf. Accessed November 27, 2019.
7. Janssen I, Leblanc AG. Systematic review of the health benefits of physical activity and fitness in school-aged children and youth. Int J Behav Nutr Phys Act 2010;7:40.
8. Rasberry CN, Lee SM, Robin L, et al. The association between school-based physical activity, including physical education, and academic performance: a systematic review of the literature. Prev Med 2011;52(Suppl 1):S10–20.
9. McCrory P, Meeuwisse W, Dvorak J, et al. Consensus statement on concussion in sport-the 5(th) international conference on concussion in sport held in Berlin, October 2016. Br J Sports Med 2017;51(11):838–47.
10. Centers for Disease Control and Prevention. Brain injury basics, what is a concussion? Available at: https://www.cdc.gov/headsup/basics/concussion_whatis.html. Accessed January 16, 2020.
11. Centers for Disease Control and Prevention. Brain injury basics, recovery from concussion. Available at: https://www.cdc.gov/headsup/basics/concussion_recovery.html. Accessed January 16, 2020.
12. Sarmiento K, Thomas KE, Daugherty J, et al. Emergency department visits for sports- and recreation-related traumatic brain injuries among children - United States, 2010-2016. MMWR Morb Mortal Wkly Rep 2019;68(10):237–42.

13. DePadilla L, Miller GF, Jones SE, et al. Self-reported concussions from playing a sport or being physically active among high school students - United States, 2017. MMWR Morb Mortal Wkly Rep 2018;67(24):682–5.

14. Coronado VG, Haileyesus T, Cheng TA, et al. Trends in sports- and recreation-related traumatic brain injuries treated in us emergency departments: the national electronic injury surveillance system-all injury program (NEISS-AIP) 2001-2012. J Head Trauma Rehabil 2015;30(3):185–97.

15. Centers for Disease Control and Prevention. National concussion surveillance system. Available at: https://www.cdc.gov/traumaticbraininjury/ncss/index.html. Accessed January 16, 2020.

16. Wasserman EB, Herzog MM, Collins CL, et al. Fundamentals of sports analytics. Clin Sports Med 2018;37(3):387–400.

17. Centers for Disease Control and prevention. Concussion at play: opportunities to reshape the culture around concussion. Available at: https://www.cdc.gov/headsup/pdfs/resources/concussion_at_play_playbook-a.pdf.   Accessed January 16, 2020.

18. Yang J, Comstock RD, Yi H, et al. New and recurrent concussions in high-school athletes before and after traumatic brain injury laws, 2005-2016. Am J Public Health 2017;107(12):1916–22.

19. Kucera KL, Cantu RC. Catastrophic sport injury research 36th annual report: fall 1982-spring 2008. National Center for Catastrophic Injury Research at the University of North Carolina at Chapel Hill. Available at: https://nccsir.unc.edu/reports/. Accessed November 30, 2019.

20. Kerr ZY, Chandran A, Nedimyer AK, et al. Concussion Incidence and Trends in 20 High School Sports. Pediatrics 2019;144(5):e20192180.

21. Zuckerman SL, Kerr ZY, Yengo-Kahn A, et al. Epidemiology of sports-related concussion in NCAA athletes from 2009-2010 to 2013-2014: incidence, recurrence, and mechanisms. Am J Sports Med 2015;43(11):2654–62.

22. Jacobson NA, Buzas D, Morawa LG. Concussions from youth football: results from NEISS hospitals over an 11-year time frame, 2002-2012. Orthop J Sports Med 2013;1(7). 2325967113517860.

23. Kerr ZY, Cortes N, Ambegaonkar JP, et al. The epidemiology of injuries in middle school football, 2015-2017: the advancing healthcare initiatives for underserved students project. Am J Sports Med 2019;47(4):933–41.

24. Pfister T, Pfister K, Hagel B, et al. The incidence of concussion in youth sports: a systematic review and meta-analysis. Br J Sports Med 2016;50(5):292–7.

25. Kontos AP, Elbin RJ, Fazio-Sumrock VC, et al. Incidence of sports-related concussion among youth football players aged 8-12 years. J Pediatr 2013; 163(3):717–20.

26. Kerr ZY, Yeargin SW, Djoko A, et al. Examining play counts and measurements of injury incidence in youth football. J Athl Train 2017;52(10):955–65.

27. Chrisman SPD, Lowry S, Herring SA, et al. Concussion incidence, duration, and return to school and sport in 5- to 14-year-old american football athletes. J Pediatr 2019;207:176–84.e1.

28. Tsushima WT, Siu AM, Ahn HJ, et al. Incidence and risk of concussions in youth athletes: comparisons of age, sex, concussion history, sport, and football position. Arch Clin Neuropsychol 2019;34(1):60–9.

29. Dompier TP, Kerr ZY, Marshall SW, et al. Incidence of concussion during practice and games in youth, high school, and collegiate american football players. JAMA Pediatr 2015;169(7):659–65.

30. Kerr ZY, Wilkerson GB, Caswell SV, et al. The first decade of web-based sports injury surveillance: descriptive epidemiology of injuries in United States high school football (2005-2006 through 2013-2014) and national collegiate athletic association football (2004-2005 through 2013-2014). J Athl Train 2018;53(8): 738–51.

31. Marar M, McIlvain NM, Fields SK, et al. Epidemiology of concussions among United States high school athletes in 20 sports. Am J Sports Med 2012;40(4): 747–55.

32. Wasserman EB, Sauers EL, Register-Mihalik JK, et al. The first decade of web-based sports injury surveillance: descriptive epidemiology of injuries in United States high school boys' baseball (2005-2006 Through 2013-2014) and National Collegiate Athletic Association men's baseball (2004-2005 through 2013-2014). J Athl Train 2019;54(2):198–211.

33. Lawson BR, Comstock RD, Smith GA. Baseball-related injuries to children treated in hospital emergency departments in the United States, 1994-2006. Pediatrics 2009;123(6):e1028–34.

34. Wasserman EB, Register-Mihalik JK, Sauers EL, et al. The first decade of web-based sports injury surveillance: descriptive epidemiology of injuries in United States high school girls' softball (2005-2006 through 2013-2014) and National Collegiate Athletic Association women's softball (2004-2005 through 2013-2014). J Athl Train 2019;54(2):212–25.

35. Clifton DR, Onate JA, Hertel J, et al. The first decade of web-based sports injury surveillance: descriptive epidemiology of injuries in United States high school boys' basketball (2005-2006 through 2013-2014) and National Collegiate Athletic Association men's basketball (2004-2005 through 2013-2014). J Athl Train 2018; 53(11):1025–36.

36. Clifton DR, Hertel J, Onate JA, et al. The first decade of web-based sports injury surveillance: descriptive epidemiology of injuries in United States high school girls' basketball (2005-2006 through 2013-2014) and National Collegiate Athletic Association women's basketball (2004-2005 through 2013-2014). J Athl Train 2018;53(11):1037–48.

37. Naiyer N, Chounthirath T, Smith GA. Pediatric cheerleading injuries treated in emergency departments in the United States. Clin Pediatr (Phila) 2017;56(11): 985–92.

38. Yau RK, Dennis SG, Boden BP, et al. Catastrophic high school and collegiate cheerleading injuries in the United States: an examination of the 2006-2007 basket toss rule change. Sports Health 2019;11(1):32–9.

39. Currie DW, Fields SK, Patterson MJ, et al. Cheerleading injuries in United States high schools. Pediatrics 2016;137(1):2015–447.

40. Lynall RC, Gardner EC, Paolucci J, et al. The First Decade of Web-Based Sports Injury Surveillance: Descriptive Epidemiology of Injuries in US High School Girls' Field Hockey (2008-2009 Through 2013-2014) and National Collegiate Athletic Association Women's Field Hockey (2004-2005 Through 2013-2014). J Athl Train 2018;53(10):938–49.

41. Yard EE, Comstock RD. Injuries sustained by pediatric ice hockey, lacrosse, and field hockey athletes presenting to United States emergency departments, 1990-2003. J Athl Train 2006;41(4):441–9.

42. Kerr ZY, Roos KG, Djoko A, et al. Epidemiologic measures for quantifying the incidence of concussion in National Collegiate Athletic Association sports. J Athl Train 2017;52(3):167–74.

43. Schneider KJ, Nettel-Aguirre A, Palacios-Derflingher L, et al. Concussion burden, recovery, and risk factors in elite youth ice hockey players. Clin J Sport Med 2018. https://doi.org/10.1097/JSM.0000000000000673.

44. Lynall RC, Mihalik JP, Pierpoint LA, et al. The First Decade of Web-Based Sports Injury Surveillance: Descriptive Epidemiology of Injuries in US High School Boys' Ice Hockey (2008-2009 Through 2013-2014) and National Collegiate Athletic Association Men's and Women's Ice Hockey (2004-2005 Through 2013-2014). J Athl Train 2018;53(12):1129–42.

45. Kerr ZY, Pierpoint LA, Rosene JM. Epidemiology of Concussions in High School Boys' Ice Hockey, 2008/09 to 2016/17 School Years. Clin J Sport Med 2018. https://doi.org/10.1097/JSM.0000000000000697.

46. McCulloch PC, Bach BR Jr. Injuries in men's lacrosse. Orthopedics 2007;30(1): 29–34.

47. Pierpoint LA, Lincoln AE, Walker N, et al. The First Decade of Web-Based Sports Injury Surveillance: Descriptive Epidemiology of Injuries in US High School Boys' Lacrosse (2008-2009 Through 2013-2014) and National Collegiate Athletic Association Men's Lacrosse (2004-2005 Through 2013-2014). J Athl Train 2019;54(1): 30–41.

48. Kerr ZY, Roos KG, Lincoln AE, et al. Injury incidence in youth, high school, and NCAA Men's Lacrosse. Pediatrics 2019;143(6):e20183482.

49. Marshall SW, Guskiewicz KM, Shankar V, et al. Epidemiology of sports-related concussion in seven US high school and collegiate sports. Inj Epidemiol 2015; 2(1):13.

50. Dick R, Romani WA, Agel J, et al. Descriptive epidemiology of collegiate men's lacrosse injuries: National Collegiate Athletic Association Injury Surveillance System, 1988-1989 through 2003-2004. J Athl Train 2007;42(2):255–61.

51. Lincoln AE, Hinton RY, Almquist JL, et al. Head, face, and eye injuries in scholastic and collegiate lacrosse: a 4-year prospective study. Am J Sports Med 2007;35(2):207–15.

52. Kerr ZY, Quigley A, Yeargin SW, et al. The epidemiology of NCAA men's lacrosse injuries, 2009/10-2014/15 academic years. Inj Epidemiol 2017;4(1):6.

53. Kerr ZY, Lincoln AE, Dodge T, et al. Epidemiology of Youth Boys' and Girls' Lacrosse Injuries in the 2015 to 2016 Seasons. Med Sci Sports Exerc 2018; 50(2):284–91.

54. Hinton RY, Lincoln AE, Almquist JL, et al. Epidemiology of lacrosse injuries in high school-aged girls and boys: a 3-year prospective study. Am J Sports Med 2005; 33(9):1305–14.

55. Pierpoint LA, Caswell SV, Walker N, et al. The First Decade of Web-Based Sports Injury Surveillance: Descriptive Epidemiology of Injuries in US High School Girls' Lacrosse (2008-2009 Through 2013-2014) and National Collegiate Athletic Association Women's Lacrosse (2004-2005 Through 2013-2014). J Athl Train 2019; 54(1):42–54.

56. USA Rugby. Year in Reveiw 2019. 2019. Available at: https://www.usa.rugby/about-usa-rugby/. Accessed February 3, 2020.

57. Bleakley C, Tully M, O'Connor S. Epidemiology of adolescent rugby injuries: a systematic review. J Athl Train 2011;46(5):555–65.

58. Collins CL, Micheli LJ, Yard EE, et al. Injuries sustained by high school rugby players in the United States, 2005-2006. Arch Pediatr Adolesc Med 2008; 162(1):49–54.

59. Marshall SW, Spencer RJ. Concussion in Rugby: The Hidden Epidemic. J Athl Train 2001;36(3):334–8.

60. Yard EE, Comstock RD. Injuries sustained by rugby players presenting to United States emergency departments, 1978 through 2004. J Athl Train 2006;41(3): 325–31.
61. Sabesan V, Steffes Z, Lombardo DJ, et al. Epidemiology and location of rugby injuries treated in US emergency departments from 2004 to 2013. Open Access J Sports Med 2016;7:135–42.
62. Lopez V Jr, Ma R, Weinstein MG, et al. Concussive Injuries in Rugby 7s: An American Experience and Current Review. Med Sci Sports Exerc 2016;48(7):1320–30.
63. Summers Z, Teague WJ, Hutson JM, et al. The spectrum of pediatric injuries sustained in snow sports. J Pediatr Surg 2017;52(12):2038–41.
64. Russell K, Selci E. Pediatric and adolescent injury in snowboarding. Res Sports Med 2018;26(sup1):166–85.
65. Gil JA, DeFroda SF, Kriz P, et al. Epidemiology of Snow Skiing- Versus Snowboarding-Related Concussions Presenting to the Emergency Department in the United States from 2010 to 2014. Clin J Sport Med 2017;27(5):499–502.
66. Graves JM, Whitehill JM, Stream JO, et al. Emergency department reported head injuries from skiing and snowboarding among children and adolescents, 1996-2010. Inj Prev 2013;19(6):399–404.
67. Xiang H, Stallones L, Smith GA. Downhill skiing injury fatalities among children. Inj Prev 2004;10(2):99–102.
68. Steenstrup SE, Bere T, Bahr R. Head injuries among FIS World Cup alpine and freestyle skiers and snowboarders: a 7-year cohort study. Br J Sports Med 2014;48(1):41.
69. Fukuda O, Takaba M, Saito T, et al. Head Injuries in Snowboarders Compared with Head Injuries in Skiers: A Prospective Analysis of 1076 patients from 1994 to 1999 in Niigata, Japan. Am J Sports Med 2001;29(4):437–40.
70. Major DH, Steenstrup SE, Bere T, et al. Injury rate and injury pattern among elite World Cup snowboarders: a 6-year cohort study. Br J Sports Med 2014;48(1): 18–22.
71. Bailly N, Afquir S, Laporte J-D, et al. Analysis of Injury Mechanisms in Head Injuries in Skiers and Snowboarders. Med Sci Sports Exerc 2017;49(1):1–10.
72. Kerr ZY, Putukian M, Chang CJ, et al. The First Decade of Web-Based Sports Injury Surveillance: Descriptive Epidemiology of Injuries in US High School Boys' Soccer (2005-2006 Through 2013-2014) and National Collegiate Athletic Association Men's Soccer (2004-2005 Through 2013-2014). J Athl Train 2018; 53(9):893–905.
73. DiStefano LJ, Dann CL, Chang CJ, et al. The First Decade of Web-Based Sports Injury Surveillance: Descriptive Epidemiology of Injuries in US High School Girls' Soccer (2005-2006 Through 2013-2014) and National Collegiate Athletic Association Women's Soccer (2004-2005 Through 2013-2014). J Athl Train 2018;53(9): 880–92.
74. Comstock RD, Currie DW, Pierpoint LA, et al. An evidence-based discussion of heading the ball and concussions in high school soccer. JAMA Pediatr 2015; 169(9):830–7.
75. Kerr ZY, Gregory AJ, Wosmek J, et al. The First Decade of Web-Based Sports Injury Surveillance: Descriptive Epidemiology of Injuries in US High School Girls' Volleyball (2005-2006 Through 2013-2014) and National Collegiate Athletic Association Women's Volleyball (2004-2005 Through 2013-2014). J Athl Train 2018; 53(10):926–37.

76. Myers RJ, Linakis SW, Mello MJ, et al. Competitive wrestling-related injuries in school aged athletes in U.S. Emergency Departments. West J Emerg Med 2010;11(5):442–9.

77. Kroshus E, Utter AC, Pierpoint LA, et al. The First Decade of Web-Based Sports Injury Surveillance: Descriptive Epidemiology of Injuries in US High School Boys' Wrestling (2005-2006 Through 2013-2014) and National Collegiate Athletic Association Men's Wrestling (2004-2005 Through 2013-2014). J Athl Train 2018;53(12): 1143–55.

Biomechanics of Sport-Related Neurological Injury

Clara Karton, PhD*, Thomas Blaine Hoshizaki, PhD

KEYWORDS

- Injury mechanism • Sport-related concussion • Repetitive head impact
- Tissue response • Clinical outcome • Cumulative exposure • Measurement metrics
- Brain trauma profiling • Risk mitigation

KEY POINTS

- Improved metrics of cumulative exposure to repetitive head impacts are needed to draw relationships between trauma and risk of neurologic injury.
- Routine symptom-based assessments are not designed to capture the range of trauma experienced within sport defined by structural and functional changes within the brain.
- Brain trauma profiling is an objective measurement method of quantifying cumulative exposure by incorporating the characteristics that associate with risk to brain injury.

INTRODUCTION

As knowledge of short-term and long-term consequences of sports-related concussions (SRC) continues to grow, so too does the necessity of establishing measures of brain trauma that inform public policy and risk mitigation strategies. Cumulative exposure from repetitive head impacts (RHI) pose a variety of risks, including increased concussion susceptibility, mental health disorders, cognitive impairments, and brain disease pathologies, including chronic traumatic encephalopathy (CTE).[1] Physical trauma to neurons disrupts a number of processes, many with acute and chronic consequences that may not express as immediately recognizable injury,[2,3] but rather develop over time.[4,5] Clinical definitions of concussion depend on immediate and transient expression, and recognition and documentation of signs and symptoms. Incidence estimates of SRC therefore account for recognized and reported symptoms; however, fail to account for underreporting and cumulative RHI and provide limited understanding of the injury itself defined by functional and structural cellular changes. As a result, relying on reported and incidence rates of SRC as an indicator of risk and injury is inconsistent, subjective, and only captures one level of trauma. As the appreciation of the complexity of the mechanisms and neurologic

Neurotrauma Impact Science Laboratory, University of Ottawa, A106-200 Lees Avenue, Ottawa, ON K1N 6N5, Canada
* Corresponding author.
E-mail address: ckarton@uottawa.ca

outcomes of traumatic brain injury (TBI) in sport is realized, there has come a broader recognition of the public health problem being faced.[6] Large-scale questions remain regarding population-based and individual risks, dose-response relationships, and evidence-informed strategies for risk reduction.

This article describes the need to develop improved biomechanical metrics of brain trauma including cumulative exposure. Advances in understanding brain injury in sport continue as evidence reveals the inadequacy of using single-event metrics, acute clinical expression, or concussion incidence as measures of trauma. A review of the neurobiological underpinnings of neurotrauma is presented, described, and incorporated into redefining the biomechanics of neurologic injury beyond the current, rather ambiguous, definitions. An objective method of capturing and quantifying RHI exposure by identifying and integrating the biomechanical characteristics that associate with risk of neurologic injury is needed. A more precise measure of exposure is central to establishing relationships between the traumatic event(s), risk and clinical outcomes. Accurate exposure metrics provide a means to support evidence-informed decisions accelerating public policy mandating RHI management through sport modification and safer play.

SPORTS-RELATED CONCUSSION

The challenge in establishing a universal consensus on SRC is complicated by the subjective nature of its definition.[7] The result is that SRC largely remain underreported and undiagnosed,[8,9] estimated at as little as 1 in 6.[10] In many cases, recognizing symptoms and reporting a concussion is primarily the responsibility of the athlete, including young athletes with limited knowledge and resources.[8] Educational programs may have limited reach, as self-reporting requires the athlete not only to recognize the injury but disclose symptoms. Kroshus and colleagues[11] demonstrated that educating National Collegiate Athletic Association (NCAA) hockey players was an ineffective intervention to increasing player safety, as minimal behavior change in voluntary reporting was observed. Young athletes face social and performance pressures that discourage reporting, such as fear of being removed from the game, letting down teammates and coaches, missing practice, and looking weak.[8,12] Challenges in recognizing, reporting, and diagnosing concussion, limits the use of concussion data as an accurate measure for trauma in sport. Acute symptoms following an impact often represent an individual response to trauma and do not account for asymptomatic expression or cumulative RHI. Cumulative RHI associates with microstructural changes within the brain and presents as changes in function, connectivity, activation, and cognition in athletes playing various sports in the absence of diagnosed injury.[2–5] The consequence is that many athletes experience unrecognized RHI throughout the season, where they continue to participate seemingly unharmed. The most severe consequence of RHI is its association with CTE, progressive brain disease affecting the integrity of cell proteins. Incomplete reporting, ambiguous presentation, and poor definition of what is regarded as a tissue "injury" presents a challenge when defining relationships between trauma and risk. Establishing these relationships largely relies on how exposure is measured.

BIOMECHANICS OF TRAUMATIC BRAIN INJURY
Mechanisms and Metrics of Head Injury

Biomechanics of head injury aim to understand the mechanical circumstances leading to the initial trauma and are the starting point to addressing global TBI pathophysiology. Injury mechanism describes the mechanical and physical changes that result in structural and/or functional damage.[13] Biomechanical research on TBI is rooted in historic investigations using cadaver and animal models examining the head's mechanical response to impact and ascertained the mechanisms associated with brain injury.[14–17] As momentum and energy are transferred to the head during a direct impact, causing change in head motion, this leads to deformation of soft tissues involving the scalp, skull, and brain. Translational or linear head motion predominantly associates with focal injuries that are localized, and more severe in nature, such as intracranial bleeds and skill fracture. Focal injuries typically result from high-magnitude, short-duration loading, caused from pressure gradients throughout the brain and/or skull deformation.[15,18] As linear head acceleration/deceleration was originally found to highly relate to internal pressure changes, it became a primary metric in TBI research.[19] This led to the development of integrations using peak linear acceleration and its time curve, specifically the Gadd Severity Index and Head Impact Criterion to evaluate safety performance of head protection.[20,21] These metrics are simple measures representing a single-axis resultant acceleration curve from impacts of one direction and location. The success of linear acceleration-based metrics is demonstrated in the ability of helmets to mitigate risk and reduce life-threatening injuries in contact/collision sport.[22] Many challenges faced today in sport pertain to injuries caused by brain motion within the skull and the integrity of axons including SRC and cumulative RHI, which more closely associate with rotational head motion.[16,23] Holbourn[16] initially suggested that shear strains within the brain are the main cause of injury. As linear acceleration forces produced compressional strains, they do not have an injurious effect because of the near incompressibility of neural tissue. They concluded that rotation had a far greater influence on brain damage than translation, and only shear stresses/strains were responsible for injury. Research later demonstrated this theory, showing that controlled rotational, or angular acceleration, was the primary source of shear strain and brain displacement capable of producing a range of injury severities including cerebral hematoma and diffuse axonal injury.[15,18] To address risks associated with SRC, a number of rotation-based injury risk metrics exist, which include peak rotational acceleration, peak rotational velocity, the Generalized Head Acceleration Model for Brain Injury Threshold (GAMBIT) and Head Impact Power (HIP).[24,25] GAMBIT was developed to consider both linear and rotational acceleration, and direct and indirect impacts in head injury criterion. HIP integrates directional components, which may be an advantageous target for safety standards helmet design[26]; however, because the final criterion established is a single value, it provides little explanation for the cause of any change (ie, impact location) and lacks predictive capacity, as there is no direct link to injury mechanism. Metrics that incorporate rotational head motion account for more variables; however, no one metric exists that sufficiently captures all relevant characteristics, including component head motion and time curve duration and shape. Due to the viscoelastic mechanical properties of neural tissue, damage may incur at low peak acceleration magnitudes with extended durations of dynamic loading. The brain is less resistant to rotationally induced shearing as the duration of the event increases.[27] For example, a helmet may reduce the peak acceleration to a level deemed "low" risk; however, as energy attenuation is prolonged, the increased duration of loading leads to injurious tissue stress and strains.[27–30] Although there have been many iterations of kinematics-driven brain injury predictor metrics, as a whole, they are not widely used in injury research. Their predictive capacity is limited and do not reflect the tissue level mechanisms of injury. With the development of improved computational power, finite element modeling of the human brain affords a detailed analysis of how kinematics affects brain tissue. The newest approaches incorporate tissue strain in their predictive metrics, such as DAMAGE (Diffuse Axonal Multi-Axis General Evaluation).[31] Although these approaches are certainly improvements on past metrics, establishing a link between different levels of brain tissue and injury outcomes (ie, metabolic, structural) is complex.

Brain Tissue Deformation

Tissue deformation caused by head motion from direct impact is considered a primary measure in biomechanical head injury research. Sophisticated computational modeling provides an important and useful tool for measuring brain tissue response to ascertain relationships between local mechanical deformation and brain injury. Maximum principal strain (MPS) is a frequent brain deformation metric used in the biomechanical evaluation of injury prediction and risk, as it is in close agreement with anatomic failure testing and measurement of brain function.[32,33] MPS describes tissue elongation relative to its original length along one of the principal axes.[34] A summary of strain values associated with a spectrum of head impact severities, injury risk, and outcomes are presented in **Fig. 1**. A general severity scale can be observed from this research reflective of the range of trauma experienced in sport environments. Risk probability estimates to injury outcomes are calculated using logistic regression curves from combined injury and "no" injury data sets. A 50% risk probability of sustaining a concussion is estimated below 0.27 MPS within cerebrum gray and white matter,[29,30,35] and trend toward lower estimates than reported average strain values.[27,36] High reported strains associate with risk of loss of consciousness and persistent post-concussion symptoms.[37,38] Lower strain values are documented

Author(s)	Sport/Activity	Injury	Brain Region	Strain Value	Severity Scale
Karton et al 2016	kendo	asymptomatic	cerebrum	0.05–0.07	
Clark et al 2018	lacrosse	asymptomatic	cerebrum	0.05–0.15	
Kuo et al 2017	soccer	asymptomatic	-	0.085	
Giordano & Kleiven 2014	American football	mTBI (50% risk)	midbrain	0.11	
Zanetti et al 2013	American football (lineman)	asymptomatic	cerebrum	0.12	
Karton et al 2019	American football (lineman)	asymptomatic	cerebrum	0.08-0.17	
Patton et al 2013	rugby	mTBI (50% risk)	corpus callosum	0.15	
Zhang et al 2004	American football	mTBI (50% risk)	midbrain	0.19	
Giordano & Kleiven 2014	American football	mTBI (50% risk)	white matter	0.19	
Kleiven 2007	American football	mTBI (50% risk)	corpus callosum	0.21	
			gray matter	0.26	
Patton et al 2013	rugby	mTBI (50% risk)	white matter	0.26	
			gray matter	0.27	
McAllister et al 2012	American football/ ice hockey	mTBI (ave.)	corpus callosum	0.28	
Rousseau 2014	ice hockey	mTBI (ave.)	gray matter	0.3	
Deck & Willinger 2008	variable	mDAI (50% risk)	-	0.31	
Viano et al 2005	American football	mTBI (ave.)	cerebrum	0.32	
			midbrain	0.34	
Post et al 2014	variable	PCS (ave.)	white matter	0.38	
Cournoyer & Hoshizaki 2019a	American football	LOC (50% risk)	white matter	0.39	
			cerebral cortex	0.45	
Oeur et al 2015	variable	PCS (ave.)	cerebrum	0.45	
Post et al 2014	variable	PCS (ave.)	gray matter	0.48	
Cournoyer & Hoshizaki 2019b	boxing	LOC (ave.)	white matter	0.69	
			cerebral cortex	0.73	

Fig. 1. Severity scale from physical reconstructions of head impacts using MPS as an indicator of magnitude.

from event reconstructions of asymptomatic impacts with no acutely identifiable/reported injury.[39,40] Kendo sword strikes to multiple head locations using a Hybrid III headform elicited a 0.05 to 0.07 MPS response,[39] where no known reports of cumulative brain injury or abnormal rates of neurologic disorders are documented among practitioners. Clark and colleagues[41] reported similar, yet a wider range, of strain than Kendo strikes from various forms of a lacrosse stick slash to both a protected (0.05–0.11 MPS), and unprotected head (0.06–0.15 MPS), a common cause of head injury in lacrosse, especially in woman's leagues that do not require head protection.[42] Research on lower-magnitude impacts is immature and therefore distinguishing and interpreting implications for risks on the playing field is preliminary. Low magnitude may be influential in cumulative event scenarios potentially leading to changes in neuronal physiology and/or structure. Karton and colleagues[43] reported from a 32-game analysis that more than 90% of the head impacts experienced by lineman in professional American football (AF) caused strains ranging from 0.08 to 0.17. This level may correspond to changes in white matter microstructure and cumulative axonal injury measured in athletes following a season of play with no reported concussion.[3,44] Increasing evidence suggests that all magnitude levels within contact/collision sport should be considered, and therefore the full severity scale should be represented in overall exposure measurements.

DEFINING TISSUE RESPONSE AND NEUROLOGIC INJURY
Axonal Strain

The increasing rates of mild head injury in collision/contact sport has initiated ongoing research that uses tissue cultures to link various levels of head motion to localized axonal stretch that disrupt the structure and function of cell membranes. An understanding of pathophysiological mechanisms associated with head injury outcomes is important in biomechanics research, as it provides a platform for establishing the human tissue's biological response and tolerance criteria. Various axonal responses are observed from an applied strain, including swelling, electrophysiological impairment, morphologic responses, cytoskeleton disassociation, and axotomy.[45–47] Studies demonstrate the brain's biological response to mechanical loading, using strain as a measure of injury. A summary of strain values associated with functional and structural changes to the axon are presented in **Fig. 2**. Responses may be acute and transient; however, may also initiate chronic cellular dysfunction and death. Axonal failure occurs in 2 ways: the primary mode is mechanical rupture and the secondary mode is gradual failure via progressive degradation, in which mechanical tissue strain has been linked to both in the in vitro TBI models.[45,47–49] Smith and colleagues[45] demonstrated primary axotomy at 0.65 dynamic stretch, but when an axon is stretched below magnitude causing primary axotomy, morphologic changes develop, wavelike appearances caused by immediate breakage and buckling of microtubules, at periodic points along their length. Although axons will gradually recover their original prestretch straight orientation, these swellings are similar to those found in brain-injured humans.[45] Physical damage from direct mechanical failure triggers progressive disassembly of microtubules around breakage sites.[47] Low strains of 0.05 to 0.15 have been associated with functional impairment of signal transmission in the absence of structural damage.[46,50,51] Yuen and colleagues[52] used cell cultures to demonstrate 0.05 strain was the minimum injury threshold required to observe minor undulations and induce calcium influx. Further, significant increases in calcium were observed when 2 sub-threshold injuries were repeated within 24 hours. Weber[53] demonstrated that the extent of cumulative cell damage in vitro was also dependent

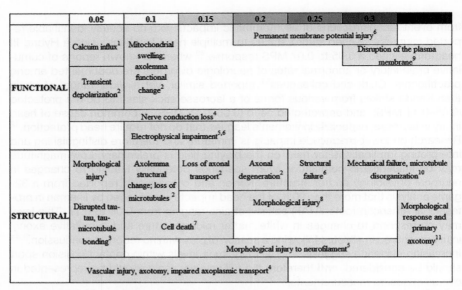

Fig. 2. Strain levels associated with functional and structural changes to an axon under dynamic stretch. (*Data from* Refs.[1–10])

on the time between repeated injuries. Injured cultures experienced more neuronal loss and released more neuron-specific enolase and S100-B from repeated stretch induced within shorter time intervals. Ahmadzadeh and colleagues[54] modeled macroscopic strains as low 0.05 causing microscopic changes in the form of protein unfolding, disrupting tau-tau bonding and tau-microtubule connections. Under dynamic loading conditions of rapid axon stretch, tau proteins behave more stiffly, resulting in primary breaking of microtubules,[54] which has been shown to lead to subsequent disassembly of microtubules and axon degeneration.[47]

Neuro-metabolism and Inflammation

Temporary neuronal dysfunction may express as ionic shifts with altered metabolism and inflammation.[55] Both responses demonstrate a window in which the brain is vulnerable to second impact. A state of decreased cerebral metabolic rate of glucose (CMRglc) that occurs following an injurious impact worsens if a second insult is experienced before recovery. After metabolic recovery, however, CMRglc depression resembles that of a single injury.[56] The precise duration of heightened vulnerability conceivably is not universally defined; however, 2 stretch injuries within 24 hours may exacerbate tissue injury. Subsequent insults during this time are often more severe, take longer to recover from, and the brain is less tolerable to impacts of lower severity.[56] An interinjury interval of 120 hours and 144 hours has demonstrated sufficient time to avoid repeat injury.[56,57] Posttraumatic metabolic changes in the immature brain appear to be shorter lasting than in adults,[58] but axonal vulnerability to injury may be more prominent in the young brain.[59] Chronic consequences of RHI could lead to excitotoxic processes from repeated indiscriminate presynaptic release of glutamate. Neurons can be particularly vulnerable to glutamate receptor activation,[55,60] and higher levels of glutamate have been measured in athletes with a history of RHI.[61] Further, a state of oxidative stress may lead to irreversible damage to neuronal membranes, causing secondary pathophysiological mechanisms leading to chronic neurologic deficits and cell death.[62]

Similarly, when a second injury is experienced during the acute inflammatory phase, the repair process is halted and neuroinflammation is enhanced.[63] However, if the secondary injury is experienced during the wound-healing phase, then normal processes continue.[63] Persistent proinflammation, manifested by extensive activation of microglia and astroglia, associates with the onset of depression,[64] and may contribute to posttraumatic neurodegeneration.[65] Prolonged microglial activation is measured in active and retired athletes with a history of RHI[66] and worsens brain disease pathology.[67] Neuroinflammatory response to physical trauma may contribute to phosphorylated tau (p-tau) pathology, specifically in the dorsolateral prefrontal cortex in those diagnosed with CTE, where the degree of neuroinflammation associates with longer duration of RHI exposure.[68]

Disruption of the Blood Brain Barrier

Blood brain barrier (BBB) dysfunction is observed in patients who have sustained severe TBI and milder forms of brain injury and RHI.[69,70] A breakdown of BBB components influences time course and extent of neuronal recovery, which may persist in individuals with RHI exposure.[70,71] BBB disruption allows peripheral immune cells to infiltrate into the brain, which leads to further complications of long-lasting inflammation and allows for the extravasation of plasma proteins into the brain.[72] Research on RHI shows that extravasation of systemic components is specifically found in regions associated with distinct areas of perivascular p-tau deposition in patients with CTE,[70,73] a similar disease course in other tauopathies.[74] Blair and colleagues[75] demonstrated using an animal model that perivascular p-tau deposition caused BBB dysfunction, but with a suppressed tau buildup, BBB integrity was recovered. In clinical studies, elevated serum S100 B concentrations, a biomarker of BBB dysfunction,[76] are detected in athletes exposed to RHI, including boxers, and soccer and football players.[77,78] Marchi and colleagues[79] studied a cohort of 67 college football athletes reporting serum S100-B levels were highest in athletes receiving the highest number of head impacts, and S100-B antibodies predicted lasting changes in mean white matter diffusivity. BBB disruption has been reported as early as 2 hours after RHI in adolescent rugby players and associates with their level of exposure.[80]

Neuroimaging

Subtle structural and/or functional abnormalities following head trauma can be identified using neuroimaging measurements. Changes within the microenvironment and axonal structure may contribute to long-term progressive changes and functional disturbances. Methodologies involving diffusion tensor imaging (DTI) show sensitivity in detecting microstructural damage via axonal mean diffusivity (MD) and fractional anisotropy (FA) in white matter integrity and gray-white matter junction after diagnosed mild brain injury, and asymptomatic RHI,[44,81] often involving the corpus callosum.[2,82] In several studies, changes in white matter structure and neuronal activity have been reported following a single season of play among athletes involved in contact/collision sport without diagnosed injury; in these studies, the frequency of head impacts is positively correlated with the extent of the measured changes.[2,44,83,84] Research regarding long-term RHI on white matter damage is immature; however, repeated mild head injury causes white matter thinning and reductions in myelin in animal model corpus callosum.[85] Further, experiencing trauma during periods of neurodevelopment may affect multiple processes including myelination, demonstrated in altered corpus callosum microstructure later in life.[86] Although less common to DTI, changes in brain activation following head trauma is measured using functional MRI (fMRI) in the form of cognitive task execution often involving working memory using auditory, visual, verbal, and motor performance.[87–89] Neurophysiological fluctuations from baseline and post season whole brain and region of interest activation have been observed in athletes sustaining RHI.[90] Higher-impact frequencies correspond with neurophysiological changes within various regions of the brain and associate with neurocognitive and neuropsychological outcomes in nonconcussed athletes.[90,91] For instance, the frequency of soccer headers associates with poorer test performance on psychomotor speed, attention and concentration, working memory, and memory.[91] Hypoconnectivity during resting state and hyperactivation of brain regions during cognitive tasks has also been measured in retired athletes with pronounced deficits.[92]

Cytoskeletal Disconnection and Biochemical Markers of Brain Injury

Axonal stretch may compromise the structural integrity of the cell through microtubule and neurofilament disruption. Various biomarkers have been associated with injury in patients with severe and mild TBI, and in symptomatic and asymptomatic athletes.[3,93,94] Kondo and colleagues[95] showed similar durations of elevated levels of pathogenic *cis* p-tau protein from repetitive trauma compared with single severe TBI, suggesting similar neurologic risks associated with repeated trauma to neural tissues. Serum biomarkers of axonal injury following single insult in ice hockey tend to return to baseline sooner (7–8 days) compared with repeated impact with knockout in boxing, which may take up to 36 weeks to return to baseline.[94–96] Biochemical biomarker concentrations are higher in those experiencing higher RHI frequencies in multiple sports, predominantly, neurofilament light polypeptide and total-tau.[3,94–99] Di Battista and colleagues[98] reported higher plasma-tau levels in male collision sport athletes (AF, ice hockey, lacrosse, rugby) to noncollision sport comparisons. Increased levels were also found in noncollision sport athletes, specifically following heading in soccer, which persisted for 1 month,[97] and significantly correlate with number of headers.[99] Higher plasma total-tau and exosomal tau levels are reported in retired AF athletes compared with controls.[100,101] In cases of CTE, neurofibrillary tangles are found throughout the brain tissue, indicative of continued disruption of microtubules and neurofilaments.[1]

Fluid Exchange and Prion Propagation in Tauopathy

There is exchange between cerebrospinal fluid (CSF) and interstitial fluid (ISF) facilitating metabolite and waste clearance through fluid drainage pathways. Physical trauma affects this system,[102] potentially leading to secondary pathophysiological mechanisms.[103] Iliff and colleagues[102] demonstrated that lymphatic pathway function is reduced following head trauma, persisting for at least 1 month after injury, and renders the brain vulnerable to tau aggregation. In CTE, p-tau deposition is initially found around perivascular spaces and along low-resistance interstitial pathways associated with CSF/ISF exchange.[1] Even with cessation from participation, studies indicate that biomarkers within CSF may take months to return to normal.[95] Elevated levels for weeks after trauma may lead to chronic levels of circulating waste, caused by continued RHI exposure without compensatory time for recovery. This potentially overwhelms flow and clearance leading to chronic impairment of glymphatic system, resulting in increased levels of interstitial tau.[102–104] Further, impediment of the CSF and ISF flow and drainage might play a role in the prionlike spread of abnormal p-tau. Prusiner's[105] work with biogenic mice identified a disease progression from a self-propagating process of tau prions, suggesting that brain trauma may cause prionlike spread of pathogenic protein. Misfolded tau proteins cause structural disruption of nearby native tau proteins eventually inhibiting cell-to-cell communication. The movement of self-propagating proteins is a slow process, explaining why even the most aggressive cases of disease often express decades after trauma.[1,101]

QUANTIFYING REPETITIVE HEAD IMPACTS USING BIOMECHANICAL METRICS
Duration of Exposure and Cognitive Impairment

Duration of athletic career and years of RHI exposure significantly contribute to behavioral and cognitive abnormalities.[1,5,106] Initially described in boxers, persistent poor mental health outcomes associate with the number of bouts and knockouts experienced.[107] Self-reported fight exposure scores of years of fighting and fights per year associates with lower brain volumes and greater cognitive impairments in professional boxers and fighters.[106] Similarly, cortical thinning in retired soccer players associates with decreased memory performance and RHI exposure.[108] Jordan[109] described risk for brain disease development and progression as high exposure, defined by career duration and age of retirement. In a convenience sample of deceased football players' brains, McKee and colleagues[1] found a positive correlation between years of contact sport participation and progressive stage of CTE. Interestingly, the same relationship was not found between the number of diagnosed concussions and pathologic progression.[1] Vulnerability of young developing brains to cumulative RHI is demonstrated through positive associations in predicting neuropsychological and cognitive impairments later in life. Participation in collision sport increases one's risk of depression, apathy, executive dysfunction, cognitive deficits, and lower mental functioning in adulthood, and participation at younger ages associates with greater deviations from normal functioning.[4,5] Similarly shown in noncollision sports, adult soccer players with the highest lifetime estimates of heading showed lower scores in attention and concentration, cognitive flexibility, and general intellectual functioning.[91] Many current studies reporting the relationship between RHI exposure and cognitive impairment are limited by subjective measures of exposure from participant recall in relation to objective outcomes.

Cumulative Exposure Measurement Metrics

Few studies have developed a metric for cumulative RHI drawing from impact sensors data. A cumulative head impact index (CHII) is derived from impact frequency in conjunction with self-reported history measures of number of seasons played, position played, and level of play to estimate exposure in former professional AF players. CHII positively correlates with plasma-tau levels and the degree of neurocognitive deficits in former athletes.[5,100] Risk weighted cumulative exposure (RWE), a metric developed using concussion injury risk curves of peak head acceleration was used to measure impact exposure in high school football.[110] Statistically significant linear relationships were found with RWE score and decreased FA after one season of play.[110] Munce and colleagues[111] measured the cumulative head impact exposure (HIE) defined as impact frequency (#) × impact magnitude of linear acceleration in youth football. Individual clinical measures of balance, oculomotor performance, reaction time, and self-reported symptoms of neurologic function were not correlated with HIE. Current indices estimating RHI provide limited information regarding event details (ie, mass, velocity, location, compliance), accurate head rotation, event duration, and strain, which are important for defining tissue response to trauma.[27–29,112]

Impact Sensor Technology

Wearable technologies have become popular for measuring head dynamic response by placing sensors in helmets, mouth/chin guards, on skin, or worn as headband/cap.

Sensors objectively measure exposure as impact frequency and acceleration magnitude during a game, practice, and/or season ranging from youth to collegiate levels within a number of sports, collecting large amounts of data in real-time.[113–116] Methods using these devices have supported biomechanical characteristics such as impact frequency and density as influential variables to neurobiological and neurocognitive outcomes.[117] Many studies have drawn from various modalities in conjunction with sensors to identify associations between a measured change within the brain and impact frequencies outside the boundaries of acute clinical expression.[44,83,84,91] Bazarian and colleagues[44] demonstrated that changes in white matter microstructure, specifically greater voxel percentage with decreased FA, was significantly correlated with head hit frequency throughout a season exceeding 2 magnitude values of peak rotational accelerations; impacts greater than 4500 rad/s2 exceeded 30 to 40, and impacts greater than 6000 rad/s2 exceeded 10 to 15. Information collected using these technologies is used by sports organization, coaches, and parents to support decisions about managing accumulated brain trauma. As an evaluation tool, sensors are limited in providing quantifiable evidence for the effectiveness of an intervention designed to decrease exposure. Head accelerations measured from helmet sensors during illegal collisions (23 g; 1530 rad/s2) were reported as significantly higher when compared with those considered legal (21 g; 1417 rad/s2); however, these differences provide limited information concerning safety, risk, and clinical relevance.[118] Evaluation of a helmetless-tackling football practice training intervention demonstrated an average of 30% fewer impact frequencies per athletic exposure compared with controls.[119] Their analysis showed this reduction happened at 2 time points, week 4 and week 7, and disappeared by the end of the season.[119] This analysis provides quantifiable information on decreased frequency; however, the decrease may have

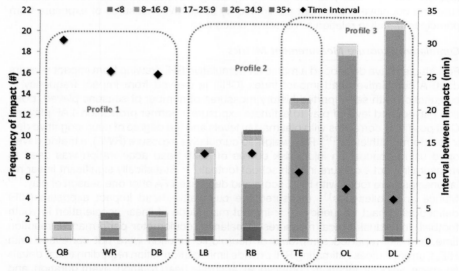

Fig. 3. Position-specific brain trauma profiles presented per game. Average head impact frequency count distributed by MPS magnitude. Interval is presented as an average time (measured in minutes) between impact frequency total (magnitude collapsed). (*From* Karton 2020 C, Hoshizaki TB, Gilchrist MD. A novel repetitive head impact exposure measurement tool differentiates player position in National Football League. Sci Rep 2020;10:1200; with permission.)

Table 1

Head impact frequency, per magnitude level, for head-to-ice and head-to-shoulder impact events per 1000 player hours, captured through game video of 6 youth ice hockey divisions

Magnitude Category	Weighting (*)	IP		Novice		Atom		Peewee Boys		Peewee Girls		Bantam		Midget	
		Freq.	Exp.	Freq.	Exp.	Freq.	Exp.	Freq.	Exp.	Freq.	Exp.	Freq.	Exp.	Freq.	Exp.
Very low	1	0	0	0.15	0.15	0.2	0.2	0.25	0.25	0	0	0.05	0.1	0.05	0.05
Low	2	2.3	4.6	0.9	1.8	0.4	0.8	0.5	1.0	0.2	0.4	0.25	0.5	0.35	0.7
Med	3	1.2	3.6	0.7	2.1	0.65	1.95	0.6	1.8	0.25	0.75	0.3	0.9	0	0
High	4	2.1	8.4	0	0	0.1	0.4	0.1	0.4	0	0	0.05	0.2	0.05	0.2
Very high	5	0	0	0	0	0	0	0	0	0	0	0	0	0	0
Event: head to ice		16.6		4.05		3.35		3.45		1.15		1.7		0.95	
Very low	1	1.8	1.8	2.6	2.6	1.35	1.35	1.2	1.2	0.8	0.8	1	1	1.85	1.85
Low	2	1.25	2.7	2.7	4	0.5	1	0.5	1	0.5	1	1.2	2.4	1.5	3
Med	3	0	0	0	0	0	0	0	0	0	0	0.2	0.6	0.25	0.75
High	4	0	0	0	0	0.06	0.24	0	0	0	0	0.25	1	0	0
Very high	5	0	0	0	0	0	0	0	0	0	0	0	0	0	0
Event: head to shoulder		4.5		6.6		2.59		2.2		1.8		5.0		5.6	
Exposure: TOTAL		21.1		10.65		5.94		5.65		2.95		6.7		6.55	

Abbreviations: Freq., frequency; IP, impact power; Exp, exposure. * indicates a multiplication symbol.

been influenced by multiple factors not limited to helmetless-tackling practice. Valid concerns have been raised regarding the accuracy of sensor technology for measuring dynamic magnitudes and duration, particularly evident for rotational head motion. Accurate measurements of rotational motion, a variable closely associated with brain tissue strain, is important when measuring brain trauma. Issues with helmet fit, sensor/skull coupling, and oblique impact events add further complication.[120,121] There is value in their relative readings, where higher magnitudes are interpreted as sustaining higher trauma, but connecting biomechanical measurements to the injury is difficult, as current technologies lack accuracy in predicting brain tissue response,[122] consequently making exposure results difficult to interpret and challenges their usefulness as a stand-alone measurement tool for exposure.

Primary Characteristics that Associate with Neurologic Injury

Various forms of neurobiological and neurocognitive changes consistently demonstrate recurrent associations with tissue strain magnitude, the frequency of damage, the time interval between events, and duration of exposure. Trauma-induced cellular changes are observed in athletes following symptomatic and asymptomatic head trauma,[2,3,81,83] and the degree of alteration associates with the impact intensity and frequency.[44,90,95] Moreover, time for neurobiological recovery from either frequent or intense impacts has been implicated in recurrent injury and brain health.[3,55,56,117] Exposure to RHI is not uniform and is created using various combinations of these characteristics.[123] Brain trauma profiling (BTP) is an objective approach to quantifying exposure by measuring and incorporating these primary characteristics that associate with neurologic risks. Strain magnitude, impact frequency, time interval between impacts, over a specified duration defines cumulative RHI exposure,[123] and has effectively described subtleties between exposure profiles within multiple sports and ability levels.[124–126] A metric, brain strain exposure over time (BSE/T), calculated using these characteristics distinguished player field position in professional AF, which identified 3 statistically unique profiles, a reflection of their different environmental conditions (**Fig. 3**).[43] Tight end was identified as a hybrid position of both lineman and short distance receiver, illustrating the sensitivity of BSE/T. AF players are at high risk for the spectrum of acute and chronic neurologic injury,[1,100,127] making them an important subset of individuals for establishing dose-response relationships between exposure in an uncontrolled environment (game play) and risk to various outcomes. BTP can be a useful tool in facilitating this knowledge. This approach describes differences in exposure profiles for individuals, teams, sports, age levels, gender, and competitive level, providing a platform for making informed decisions on effective risk-reduction practices.[124–126] **Table 1** presents the frequency and magnitude of head-to-ice and head-to-shoulder impacts documented in youth ice hockey. This analysis provides detailed objective evaluations of head contact characteristics that is valuable in establishing the most impactful intervention efforts for risk-reduction outcomes specific to level of play. Safer play can be achieved by effectively managing 1 or more trauma characteristic. How these characteristics are managed need to be based on the exposure profile, contextual definitions leading to contact,[128] and appropriate modification strategies for the sport application.

SUMMARY

Changes in brain cell structure and function associated with RHI sustained in contact/collision sport describe brain injury as an acute disorder and one that may develop into chronic impairment. The effects of dynamic tissue loading are observed through various cellular processes including microglia activation, ionic disturbances, BBB disruption, and structural disconnection within the cytoskeleton. In many cases, RHI exposure to low magnitude impacts without symptom expression elicits similar cellular responses. Routine symptom-based assessment diagnostic tools are not designed to capture the full range in cellular responses associated with all levels of trauma. Research describing biomechanical forces leading to cellular changes signifies an interaction of strain magnitude, impact frequency, time interval between impacts, and duration of exposure. Although recent research has begun to address the cumulative effect of RHI in contact/collision sports, little has been done to develop a metric to quantify exposure. To advance the understanding of how trauma leads to various brain injury outcomes, an objective and multidimensional approach is necessary to capture a more complete exposure profile during sport participation. Precise biomechanical measures can contribute to understanding TBI pathophysiology following trauma through an improved description of exposure.

CLINICS CARE POINTS

- Sport-related neurological injuries exist along a spectrum of severity.
- Acutely asymptomatic head impacts may lead to mental health disorders and brain damage.
- Damage to neural tissue occurs from both acute and chronic mechanisms and presents in patients as changes in cognition, behaviour and psychology.
- Head impact magnitude and the presence of acute symptoms do not reflect the entire spectrum of neurological injuries. Brain trauma characteristics of frequency, time interval, and duration of exposure also associate with clinical outcomes.
- Symptom resolution may not represent neurobiological recovery.

DISCLOSURE

The authors declare no competing commercial or financial interests.

REFERENCES

1. McKee AC, Stern RA, Nowinski CJ, et al. The spectrum of disease in chronic traumatic encephalopathy. Brain 2013;136:43–64.
2. McAllister TW, Ford JC, Flashman LA, et al. Effect of head impacts on diffusivity measures in a cohort of collegiate contact sport athletes. Neurology 2014; 82:63–9.
3. Oliver JM, Jones MT, Kirk KM, et al. Serum neurofilament light in American football athletes over the course of a season. J Neurotrauma 2016;33:1–19.
4. Alosco ML, Kasimis AB, Stamm JM, et al. Age of first exposure to American football and long-term neuropsychiatric and cognitive outcomes. Transl Psychiatry 2017;7:e1236.
5. Montenigro PH, Alosco ML, Martin BM, et al. Cumulative head impact exposure predicts later-life depression, apathy, executive dysfunction, and cognitive impairment in former high school and college football players. J Neurotrauma 2017;34:328–40.
6. Finkel AM, Bieniek KF. A quantitative risk assessment for chronic traumatic encephalopathy (CTE) in football: How public health science evaluates evidence. Hum Ecol Risk Assess 2018;25:564–89.

7. McCrory P, Meeuwisse W, Dvorak J, et al. Consensus statement on concussion in sport—the 5th international conference on concussion in sport held in Berlin, October 2016. Br J Sports Med 2017;51:838–47.

8. McCrea M, Hammeke T, Olsen G, et al. Unreported concussion in high school football players: implications for prevention. Clin J Sport Med 2004;14:13–7.

9. Meehan WP, Mannix RC, O'Brien MJ. The prevalence of undiagnosed concussions in athletes. Clin J Sport Med 2013;23:339–42.

10. Concussion Legacy Foundation. 2020. Available at: https://concussionfoundation.org/. Accessed January 2020.

11. Kroshus E, Daneshvar D, Baugh CM, et al. NCAA concussion education in ice hockey: An ineffective mandate. Br J Sports Med 2013;48:135–40.

12. Public Health Agency of Canada (PHAC). Understanding and awareness of sports-related concussion, with a focus on youth. Final Report. January 2019.

13. Viano DC, King AI, Melvin JW, et al. Injury biomechanics research: an essential element in the prevention of trauma. J Biomech 1989;22:403–17.

14. Gurdjian ES, Lissner HR, Latimer FR, et al. Quantitative determination of acceleration and intracranial pressure in experimental head injury. Neurology 1953;3: 417–23.

15. Gennarelli TA, Thibault LE, Ommaya AK. Pathophysiological responses to rotational and translational accelerations of the head. In Proceedings of the 16th Stapp Car Crash Conference, SAE Paper No. 720970, pp. 296-308. Detroit, MI, November 8-10, 1972.

16. Holbourn AH. Mechanics of head injuries. Lancet 1943;2:438–41.

17. Ommaya AK, Hirsch AE. Tolerances for cerebral concussion from head impact and whiplash in primates. J Biomech 1971;4:13–21.

18. King AI, Yang KH, Zhang L, et al. Is head injury caused by linear or angular acceleration? IRCOBI Conference, Lisbon, Portugal, pp.1–12. September 25-26, 2003.

19. Thomas LM, Roberts VL, Gurdjian ES. Impact-induced pressure gradients along three orthogonal axes in the human skull. J Neurosurg 1967;26:316–21.

20. Gadd CW. Use of a weighted-impulse criterion for estimating injury hazard. In Proceeding in the 10th Stapp Car Crash Conference, SAE Paper No. 660793. Hollomon Air Force Base, NM, November 8-9, 1996.

21. Versace J. A review of the severity index. In Proceedings of the 15th STAPP Car Crash Conference (Vol. 15, pp. 43-69). Coronado, CA, November 17-19, 1971.

22. Hoshizaki TB, Brien SF. The science and design of head protection in sport. Neurosurg 2004;55:956–67.

23. Gennarelli TA, Thibault LE, Adams H, et al. Diffuse axonal injury and traumatic coma in the primate. Ann Neurol 1982;12:564–74.

24. Newman J. A generalized acceleration model for brain injury threshold (GAMBIT). In Proceedings of the International Research Council on the Biomechanics of Injury Conference (Vol. 14, pp. 121-131). Zurich, CH, September 2-4, 1986.

25. Newman J, Barr C, Beusenberg M, et al. A new biomechanical assessment of mild traumatic brain injury. Part 2: results and conclusions. In Proceedings of the International Research Council on the Biomechanics of Injury Conference (Vol. 28, pp. 223-233). Montpellier, FR, September 20-22, 2000.

26. Taylor K, Hoshizaki TB, Gilchrist MD. The influence of impact force redistribution and redirection on maximum principal strain for helmeted head impacts. Comput Methods Biomech Biomed Engin 2019;22:1047–60.

27. Rousseau P. An analysis of concussion metrics associated with elite ice hockey elbow-to-head and shoulder-to-head collisions. Canada: Doctorate thesis, University of Ottawa; 2014.

28. Willinger R, Baumgartner D. Human head tolerance limits to specific injury mechanisms. Int J Crashworthiness 2003;8:605–17.

29. Zhang L, Yang KH, King AI. A proposed injury threshold for mild traumatic brain injury. J Biomech Eng 2004;126:226–36.

30. Kleiven S. Predictors for traumatic brain injuries evaluated through accident reconstruction. Stapp Car Crash J 2007;51:81–114.

31. Gabler LF, Crandall JR, Panzer MB. Development of a second-order system for rapid estimation of maximum brain strain. Ann Biomed Eng 2019;47:1971–81.

32. Zou H, Schmiedeler JP, Hardy WN. Separating brain motion into rigid body displacements and deformation under low-severity impacts. J Biomech 2007;40:1183–91.

33. McAllister TW, Ford JC, Ji S, et al. Maximum principal strain and strain rate associated with concussion diagnosis correlates with changes in corpus callosum white matter indices. Ann Biomed Eng 2012;40:127–40.

34. Silva VD. Mechanics and strength of materials. New York: Pringer; 2006.

35. Patton DA, McIntosh AS, Kleiven S. The biomechanical determinants of concussion: finite element simulations to investigate brain tissue deformations during sporting impacts to the unprotected head. J Appl Biomech 2013;29:721–30.

36. Viano DC, Pellman EJ. Concussion in professional football: biomechanics of the striking player – Part 8. Neurosurg 2005;56:266–80.

37. Post A, Kendall M, Koncan D, et al. Characterization of persistent concussive syndrome using reconstruction and finite element modelling. J Mech Behav Biomed Mater 2015;41:325–35.

38. Cournoyer J, Hoshizaki TB. Biomechanical comparison of concussions with and without a loss of consciousness in elite American football: implications for prevention. Sports Biomech 2019;17:1–17.

39. Karton C, Hoshizaki TB, Gilchrist MD. Frequency, magnitude, and rate of head impacts and risks to neurological disorders in sport. In Proceedings of Traumatic Brain Injury: Clinical, Pathological and Translational Mechanisms Conference, Santa Fe NM, January 24–27, 2016.

40. Zanetti K, Post A, Karton C, et al. Identifying risk profiles for three player positions in American football using physical and finite element modeling reconstructions. In Proceedings of IRCOBI, Gothenburg, Sweden. September 11–13, 2013.

41. Clark LM, Hoshizaki TB, Gilchrist MD. Assessing women's lacrosse head impacts using finite element modelling. J Mech Behav Biomed Mater 2018;80:20–6.

42. Marar M, McIlvain NM, Field SK, et al. Epidemiology of concussions among United States high school athletes in 20 sports. Am J Sports Med 2012;40:747–55.

43. Karton C, Hoshizaki TB, Gilchrist MD. A novel repetitive head impact exposure measurement tool differentiates player position in National Football League. Sci Rep 2020;10:1200.

44. Bazarian JJ, Zhu T, Zhong J, et al. Persistent, long-term cerebral white matter changes after sports-related repetitive head impacts. PLoS One 2014;9:e94734.

45. Smith DH, Wolf JA, Lusardi TA, et al. High tolerance and delayed elastic response of cultured axons to dynamic stretch injury. J Neurosci 1999;19:4263–9.

46. Bain A, Meaney D. Tissue-level thresholds for axonal damage in an experimental model of central nervous system white matter injury. J Biomech 2000; 122:615–22.
47. Tang-Schomer MD, Patel AR, Baas PW, et al. Mechanical breaking of microtubules in axons during dynamic stretch injury underlies delayed elasticity, microtubule disassembly, and axon degeneration. FASEB J 2010;24:1401–10.
48. Morrison B 3rd, Cater HL, Wang CC-B, et al. A tissue level tolerance criterion for living brain developed with an in vitro model of traumatic mechanical loading. Stapp Car Crash J 2003;47:93–105.
49. Elkin BS, Morrison B 3rd. Region-specific tolerance criteria for the living brain. Stapp Car Crash J 2007;51:127–38.
50. Galbraith JA, Thibault LE, Matteson DR. Mechanical and electrical responses of the squid giant axon to simple elongation. J Biomech Eng 1993;115:13–22.
51. Singh A, Lu Y, Chen C, et al. A new model of traumatic axonal injury to determine the effects of strain and displacement rates. Stapp Car Crash J 2006;50:601–23.
52. Yuen TJ, Browne KD, Iwata A, et al. Sodium channelopathy induced by mild axonal trauma worsens outcome after a repeat injury. J Neurosci Res 2009; 87:3620–5.
53. Weber JT. Experimental models of repetitive brain injuries. In: Weber JT, Mass AIR, editors. Progress in brain research, vol. 161. Amsterdam: Elsevier B.V; 2007. p. 253–61.
54. Ahmadzadeh H, Smith DH, Shenoy VB. Mechanical effects of dynamic binding between tau proteins on microtubules during axonal injury. Biophys J 2015;109: 2328–37.
55. Giza CC, Hovda DA. The new neurometabolic cascade of concussion. Neurosurgery 2014;75:S24–33.
56. Prins ML, Alexander D, Giza CC, et al. Repeated mild traumatic brain injury: mechanisms of cerebral vulnerability. J Neurotrauma 2013;30:30–8.
57. Effgen GB, Morrison B 3rd. Electrophysiological and pathological characterization of the period of heightened vulnerability to repetitive injury in an in vitro stretch model. J Neurotrauma 2017;34:914–24.
58. Thomas S, Prins ML, Samii M, et al. Cerebral metabolic response to traumatic brain injury sustained early in development: a 2-deoxy-D-glucose autoradiographic study. J Neurotrauma 2000;17:649–65.
59. Prins ML, Hales A, Reger M, et al. Repeat traumatic brain injury in the juvenile rat is associated with increased axonal injury and cognitive impairments. Dev Neurosci 2010;32:510–8.
60. Algattas H, Huang JH. Traumatic brain injury pathophysiology and treatments: early, intermediate, and late phases post-injury. Int J Mol Sci 2013;15:309–41.
61. Lin AP, Ramadan S, Stern RA, et al. Changes in the neurochemistry of athletes with repetitive brain trauma: preliminary results using localized correlated spectroscopy. Alzheimers Res Ther 2015;7:1–9.
62. Cornelius C, Crupi R, Calabrese V, et al. Traumatic brain injury: oxidative stress and neuroprotection. Antioxid Redox Signal 2013;19:836–53.
63. Russo MV, Latour LL, McGavern DB. Distinct myeloid cell subsets promote meningeal remodeling and vascular repair after mild traumatic brain injury. Nat Immunol 2018;19:442–52.
64. Fenn AM, Gensel JC, Huang Y, et al. Immune activation promotes depression one month after diffuse brain injury: a role for primed microglia. Biol Psychiatry 2014;76:575–84.

65. Xiong Y, Mahmood A, Chopp M. Current understanding of neuroinflammation after traumatic brain injury and cell-based therapeutic opportunities. Chin J Traumatol 2018;21:137–51.

66. Coughlin JM, Wang Y, Minn I, et al. Imaging of glial cell activation and white matter integrity in brains of active and recently retired National Football League players. JAMA Neurol 2017;74:67–74.

67. Simon E, Obst J, Gomez-Nicola D. The evolving dialogue of microglia and neurons in Alzheimer's disease: microglia as necessary transducers of pathology. Neuroscience 2017;405:24–34.

68. Cherry JD, Tripodis Y, Alvarez VE, et al. Microglial neuroinflammation contributes to tau accumulation in chronic traumatic encephalopathy. Acta Neuropathol Commun 2016;4:112.

69. Alluri H, Wiggins-Dohlvik K, Davis ML, et al. Blood-brain barrier dysfunction following traumatic brain injury. Metab Brain Dis 2015;30:1093–104.

70. Doherty CP, O'Keefe E, Wallace E, et al. Blood-brain barrier dysfunction as a hallmark pathology in chronic traumatic encephalopathy. J Neuropathol Exp Neurol 2016;75:656–62.

71. Hay JR, Johnson VE, Young AM, et al. Blood-brain barrier disruption is an early event that may persist for many years after traumatic brain injury in humans. J Neuropathol Exp Neurol 2015;74:1147e1157.

72. Corps KN, Roth TL, McGavern DB. Inflammation and neuroprotection in traumatic brain injury. JAMA Neurol 2015;72:355e362.

73. Farrell M, Aherne S, O'Riordan S, et al. Blood-brain barrier dysfunction in a boxer with chronic traumatic encephalopathy and schizophrenia. Clin Neuropathol 2019;38:51–8.

74. Marques F, Sousa JC, Sousa N, et al. Blood-brain-barriers in aging and in Alzheimer's disease. Mol Neurodegener 2013;8:38.

75. Blair LJ, Frauen HD, Zhang BO, et al. Tau depletion prevents progressive blood-brain barrier damage in a mouse model of tauopathy. Acta Neuropathol Commun 2015;3:8.

76. Blyth BJ, Farahvar A, Gee CA, et al. 223: serum S-100b concentrations are an accurate indicator of blood brain barrier integrity. Ann Emerg Med 2008;51: 538–9.

77. Graham MR, Myers T, Evans P, et al. Direct hits to the head during amateur boxing is associated with a rise in serum biomarkers for brain injury. Int J Immunopathol Pharmacol 2011;24:119–25.

78. Puvenna V, Brennan C, Shaw G, et al. Significance of ubiquitin carboxy-terminal hydrolase L1 elevations in athletes after sub-concussive head hits. PLoS One 2014;9:e96296.

79. Marchi N, Bazarian JJ, Puvenna V, et al. Consequences of repeated blood-brain barrier disruption in football players. PLoS One 2013;8:e56805.

80. O'Keeffe E, Kelly E, Liu Y, et al. Dynamic blood-brain barrier regulation in mild traumatic brain injury. J Neurotrauma 2019;36:1–10.

81. Cubon VA, Putukian M, Boyer C, et al. A diffusion tensor imaging study on the white matter skeleton in individuals with sports-related concussion. J Neurotrauma 2011;28:189–201.

82. Mayinger MC, Merchant-Borna K, Hufschmidt J, et al. White matter alterations in college football players: a longitudinal diffusion tensor imaging study. Brain Imaging Behav 2018;12:44–53.

83. Koerte IK, Ertl-Wagner B, Reiser M, et al. White matter integrity in the brains of professional soccer players without symptomatic concussion. JAMA 2012;308: 1859–61.

84. Kuzminski SJ, Clark MD, Fraser MA, et al. White matter changes related to sub-concussive impact frequency during a single season of high school football. Am J Neuroradiol 2018;39:245–51.

85. Briggs DI, Angoa-Pérez M, Kuhn DM. Prolonged repetitive head trauma induces a singular chronic traumatic encephalopathy-like pathology in white matter despite transient behavioral abnormalities. Am J Pathol 2016;86:2869–86.

86. Stamm JM, Koerte IK, Muehlmann M, et al. Age of first exposure to football is associated with altered corpus callosum white matter microstructure in former professional football players. J Neurotrauma 2015;32:1–9.

87. McAllister TW, Flashman LA, McDonald BC, et al. Mechanisms of working memory dysfunction after mild and moderate TBI: evidence from functional MRI and neurogenetics. J Neurotrauma 2006;23:1450–67.

88. Smits M, Dippel DWJ, Houston GC, et al. Postconcussion syndrome after minor head injury: brain activation of working memory and attention. Hum Brain Mapp 2009;30:2789–803.

89. Mayer AR, Mannell MV, Ling J, et al. Auditory orienting and inhibition of return in mild traumatic brain injury: a FMRI study. Hum Brain Mapp 2009;30:4152–66.

90. Breedlove KM, Breedlove EL, Robinson M, et al. Detecting neurocognitive and neurophysiological changes as a result of subconcussive blows among high school football athletes. Athl Train Sports Health Care 2014;6:119–27.

91. Witol AD, Webbe FM. Soccer heading frequency predicts neuropsychological deficits. Arch Clin Neuropsychol 2003;18:397–417.

92. Hampshire A, MacDonald A, Owen AM. Hypoconnectivity and hyperfrontality in retired American football players. Sci Rep 2013;3:2972.

93. Zetterberg H, Smith DH, Blennow K. Biomarkers of mild traumatic brain injury in cerebrospinal fluid and blood. Nat Rev Neurol 2013;9:201–10.

94. Shahim P, Tegner Y, Gustafsson B, et al. Neurochemical aftermath of repetitive mild traumatic brain injury. JAMA Neurol 2016;73:1308–15.

95. Kondo A, Shahpasand K, Mannix R, et al. Antibody against early driver of neuro-degeneration cis P-tau blocks brain injury and tauopathy. Nature 2015;523: 431–6.

96. Neselius S, Brisby H, Theodorsson A, et al. CSF – biomarkers in olympic boxing: diagnosis and effects of repetitive head trauma. PLoS One 2012;7:e33606.

97. Wallace C, Smirl JD, Zetterberg H, et al. Heading in soccer increases serum neurofilament light protein and SCAT3 symptoms metrics. BMJ Open Sport Exerc Med 2018;4:e000433.

98. Di Battista AP, Rhind SG, Richards D, et al. Altered blood biomarker profiles in athletes with a history of repetitive head impacts. PLoS One 2016;11:e0164912.

99. Stålnacke BM, Ohlsson A, Tegner Y, et al. Serum concentrations of two biochemical markers of brain tissue damage S-100B and neurone specific enolase are increased in elite female soccer players after a competitive game. Br J Sports Med 2006;40:313–6.

100. Alosco ML, Tripodis Y, Jarnagin J, et al. Repetitive head impact exposure and later-life plasma total tau in former National Football League players. Alzheimers Dement (Amst) 2017;7:33–40.

101. Stern RA, Tripodis Y, Baugh CM, et al. Preliminary study of plasma exosomal tau as a potential biomarker for chronic traumatic encephalopathy. J Alzheimers Dis 2016;51:1099–109.

102. Iliff JJ, Chen MJ, Plog BA, et al. Impairment of glymphatic function promotes tau pathology after traumatic brain injury. J Neurosci 2014;34:16180–93.
103. Jessen NA, Munk ASF, Lundgaard I, et al. The glymphatic system: a beginner's guide. Neurochem Res 2015;40:2583–99.
104. Abbott NJ, Pizzo ME, Preston JE, et al. The role of brain barriers in fluid movement in the CNS: is there a 'glymphatic' system? Acta Neuropathol 2018;135: 387–407.
105. Prusiner SB. Biology and genetics of prions causing neurodegeneration. Annu Rev Genet 2013;47:601–23.
106. Bernick C, Banks SJ, Shin W, et al. Repeated head trauma is associated with smaller thalamic volumes and slower processing speed: the Professional Fighters' Brain Health Study. Br J Sports Med 2015;49:1007–11.
107. Roberts AH. Brain damage in boxers. London: Pitman Publishing; 1969.
108. Koerte IK, Mayinger M, Muehlmann M, et al. Cortical thinning in former professional soccer players. Brain Imaging Behav 2016;10:792–8.
109. Jordan BD. Chronic traumatic brain injury associated with boxing. Semin Neurol 2000;20:179–85.
110. Urban JE, Davenport EM, Golman AJ, et al. Head impact exposure in youth football: high school ages 14 to 18 years and cumulative impact analysis. Ann Biomed Eng 2013;41:2474–87.
111. Munce TA, Dorman JC, Thompson PA, et al. Head impact exposure and neurologic function of youth football players. Med Sci Sports Exerc 2015;47:1567–76.
112. Kendall M. Comparison and characterization of different concussive brain injury events. Canada: Doctorate Thesis. University of Ottawa; 2016.
113. Crisco JJ, Wilcox BJ, Beckwith JG, et al. Head impact exposure in collegiate football players. J Biomech 2011;44:2673–8.
114. Wilcox BJ, Beckwith JG, Greenwald RM, et al. Head impact exposure in male and female collegiate ice hockey players. J Biomech 2014;47:109–14.
115. King D, Hume PA, Brughelli M, et al. Instrumented mouthguard acceleration analysis for head impacts in amateur rugby union players over a season of matches. Am J Sports Med 2015;43:614–24.
116. McCuen E, Svaldi D, Breedlove K, et al. Collegiate women's soccer players suffer greater cumulative head impacts than their high school counterparts. J Biomech 2015;43:3720–3.
117. Broglio SP, Lapointe A, O'Connor KL, et al. Head impact density: a model to explain the elusive concussion threshold. J Neurotrauma 2017;34:2675–83.
118. Mihalik JP, Greenwald RM, Blackburn JT, et al. Effect of infraction type on head impact severity in youth ice hockey. Med Sci Sports Exerc 2010;42:1431–8.
119. Swartz EE, Myers JL, Cook SB, et al. A helmetless-tackling intervention in American football for decreasing head impact exposure: A randomized controlled trial. J Sci Med Sport 2019;22:1102–7.
120. Jadischke R, Viano DC, Dau N, et al. On the accuracy of the head impact telemetry (HIT) system used in football helmets. J Biomech 2013;46:2310–5.
121. Allison MA, Kang YS, Bolte JHIV, et al. Validation of a helmet-based system to measure head impact biomechanics in ice hockey. Med Sci Sports Exerc 2014;46:115–23.
122. Post A, Hoshizaki TB. Mechanisms of brain impact injuries and their prediction: a review. Trauma 2012;14:327–49.
123. Karton C, Hoshizaki TB. Concussive and subconcussive brain trauma: the complexity of impact biomechanics and injury risk in contact sport. In:

Hainline B, Stern RA, editors. Handbook of clinical neurology, vol. 158. Oxford (UK): Elsevier; 2018. p. 39–49.

124. Chen W. A comparison between peewee and bantam youth ice hockey brain trauma profiles. Canada: Master's thesis, University of Ottawa; 2018.

125. Paiement B. A comparison of brain trauma profiles between elite men's rugby union 15s and rugby union 7s game play. Master's thesis. Canada: University of Ottawa; 2020.

126. Khatib A. Comparison of brain trauma characteristics from head impacts for lightweight and heavyweight fighters in professional mixed martial arts. Canada: Master's thesis, University of Ottawa; 2019.

127. Nathanson JT, Connolly JG, Yuk F, et al. Concussion incidence in professional football: position-specific analysis with use of a novel metric. Orthop J Sports Med 2016;4(1):1–6.

128. Robidoux MA, Kendall M, Laflamme Y, et al. Comparing concussion rates as reported by hockey canada with head contact events as observed across minor ice-hockey age categories. J Concussion 2020. https://doi.org/10.1177/2059700220911285.

The Molecular Pathophysiology of Concussion

David R. Howell, PhD, ATC[a,b,*], Julia Southard, BS[a,c]

KEYWORDS

- Concussion • Mild traumatic brain injury • Pathophysiology • Molecular mechanisms

KEY POINTS

- After a concussive event, a complex set of processes occur that disrupt neuronal functioning and result in different signs and symptoms.
- Pathophysiologic processes after concussion include ionic shifts, neuronal architecture damage, increased neuroinflammation, increased release of excitatory neurotransmitters, and altered cerebral blood flow control.
- The inability to deliver energy to the brain after a concussion, paired with a high demand for energy to restore damaged functions, results in an energy mismatch.

INTRODUCTION

Concussion, a type of mild traumatic brain injury, has been defined through expert consensus as a complex pathophysiologic process that is the result of head trauma, and produces an onset of nonspecific signs or symptoms and/or changes in mental function.[1] For clinicians who diagnose and manage concussions, decision making can be challenging and imprecise owing to the limited clinical tools available to understand postinjury deficits, and the translation of knowledge from the underlying pathophysiologic processes responsible for signs and symptoms to clinical care.[2] Although concussion incidence increased from the early 2000s to mid 2010s,[3,4] more recent research indicates that sport-related concussions sustained during practice have decreased, as well as recurrent concussion rates from 2013 to 2018.[5] These results suggest that perhaps medical management of concussion has evolved, and the use of updated practice approaches and preventative strategies may be helping to

[a] Sports Medicine Center, Children's Hospital Colorado, 13123 East 16th Avenue, B060, Aurora, CO 80045, USA; [b] Department of Orthopedics, University of Colorado School of Medicine, Aurora, CO, USA; [c] Department of Psychology and Neuroscience, Regis University, 3333 Regis Boulevard, Denver, CO 80221, USA
* Corresponding author. Sports Medicine Center, Children's Hospital Colorado, 13123 East 16th Avenue, B060, Aurora, CO 80045.
E-mail address: David.Howell@cuanschutz.edu
Twitter: @HowellDR (D.R.H.)

Clin Sports Med 40 (2021) 39–51
https://doi.org/10.1016/j.csm.2020.08.001
0278-5919/21/© 2020 Elsevier Inc. All rights reserved.
sportsmed.theclinics.com

decrease the incidence of concussion. Despite these advancements, the physiologic processes that underlie the signs and symptoms of concussion, accurate methods to reliably diagnose concussion, and the time course of physiologic recovery remain difficult to discern.[6]

Currently, concussion remains a clinical diagnosis with few objective and widely used assessments that measure physiologic functions,[7] in part owing to the lack of paradigms available to assess pathophysiologic responses to injury in a feasible clinically viable manner. Some approaches such as advanced neuroimaging, cerebral blood flow assessment, or fluid biomarker analysis allow for the detection of persistent biological disruptions after clinically observed recovery,[6] but the usefulness of these techniques within widespread clinical practice is low. As a result, concussion diagnosis is less precise than other injuries, such as musculoskeletal sport injuries, which may alter the perception of recovery.[7] Despite this challenge, concussion management guidelines have evolved considerably over the past 2 decades.[1,2,8,9] Assessment methods such as the Sport Concussion Assessment Tool, and each subsequent version are intended for sideline use, and have a high positive predictive value for concussion identification.[10–15] According to the most recent guidelines from various medical associations and expert consensus groups, a critical aspect of concussion management is a multifaceted measurement approach intended to examine the various physiologic functions that are disrupted by a concussion. These metrics include, but are not limited to, assessments of symptoms, mental status, neurologic function, vision, gait, balance, and sleep–wake disturbances.[1,2,9] These approaches, however, have demonstrated a less than optimal level of reliability across time.[16] Furthermore, recovery as identified by these measures may not truly reflect the physiologic restoration of the brain, leading to further complications after clearance to return to preinjury activities, such as sports.[6,17] Studies using neuroimaging or animal models have also shown that physiologic restoration of the brain takes longer than symptoms.[18] Therefore, a thorough understanding of the physiologic disruption that occurs after a concussion may provide a translational link between impaired cell biology and appropriate clinical methods to consider when diagnosing and developing rehabilitation strategies for individuals with a concussion.

Although many clinical studies focus on the diagnostic accuracy of different assessments for concussion or track the trajectory of recovery,[19–21] the interpretation of changes across time continue to suffer from the difficulty of disentangling the effects of recovery compared with practice or learning effects. Furthermore, many assessment approaches are subjective in nature,[13] mitigating the ability to address causality within an investigation. As such, experimental models of concussion, primarily among rodents, have been used to better understand the mechanisms that underlie clinical signs and symptoms apparent after a concussion.[22] Among the more common models that have been used to this point, closed-skull weight decrease,[23,24] lateral fluid percussion,[25–28] controlled cortical impact,[29,30] and closed-skull controlled impact[31–33] models have each been developed to explore molecular alterations, ion fluxes, the role of excitatory neurotransmitters in dysfunction, and glucose metabolism. Therefore, the purpose of this review article is to discuss the molecular pathophysiology of concussion by examining each of the aforementioned aspects as they relate to concussion and their potential clinical implications. An emphasis on the translational aspects of the work done in this area is provided so that clinicians who diagnose, manage, and treat individuals with concussion can approach decision making with an understanding of mechanisms responsible for clinical observations.

NEUROMETABOLIC CASCADE OF CONCUSSION

An understanding of the acute pathophysiology of concussion has been laid out by many different researchers, led primarily by the work of Giza and Hovda.[34,35] In response to a concussive event, a cascade of pathophysiologic events occur simultaneously, leading to potential changes in mental status, symptoms, cognitive function, or motor control. Although a complex set of processes are responsible for each of these dysfunctional outcomes, researchers hypothesize that these changes are primarily the result of an abrupt neuronal depolarization, glucose metabolism changes, excitatory neurotransmitter release, altered cerebral blood flow, and disrupted axonal function, each occurring concurrently at different stages after the concussive event.[34] At the cellular level, potassium flows out of the neuron, and sodium and calcium flow in. These altered ionic flux processes then trigger voltage- or ligand-gated ion channels throughout the brain, and the result is a "widespread neuronal depression" state, priming the cell for barrier dysfunction as well as the inability to clear debris, resolve inflammation, and release trophic factors to repair neuronal connections.[36]

Owing to the ionic shifts after injury, the cell attempts to restore homeostasis via membrane ionic pumps. These pumps require energy, which is quickly exhausted.[37] The ability to deliver energy, via ATP, to the cell is also impaired after a concussion, resulting in an energy crisis.[35] In essence, there is a high demand for energy to restore homeostasis (ie, ionic pumps) paired with the simultaneous decreased ability to deliver energy (ie, altered cerebral blood flow). Furthermore, mitochondrial dysfunction may also occur owing to the increased calcium present with the cell, worsening the mismatch between demand for energy and the ability to produce or deliver energy. This state of mismatched energy demands may last for up to 10 days in adult animal models, and relates to behavioral impairments,[35,37] but the duration of recovery for these processes are not known in humans. This time period likely varies owing to cellular, individual, and environmental differences between people, although further investigations in humans are needed to determine which factors affect postconcussion cellular restoration.

The damage that occurs after a concussion can also affect the neuronal architecture. The integrity of microstructural features such as axons and microtubules collapse as a result of the calcium influx and subsequent phosphorylation, or axonal stretch.[35,38] Owing to the shear and/or tensile forces present during the traumatic insult, cellular transportation disruptions and axonal swelling have been observed.[38,39] In the pediatric population specifically, axonal myelination may affect the degree of disruption. Given the ongoing myelination that occurs during brain development, the axonal fibers and associated microstructures may be more vulnerable to traumatic injury in childhood relative to adulthood.[40] Advanced neuroimaging approaches may yield insights into disrupted axonal structure: diffusion tensor imaging has been used to measure the diffusion properties of water, thus providing a detailed view of how microstructural tissue functions.[41] However, the current widespread use of advanced neuroimaging approaches for clinical purposes does not occur. Recent research is encouraging related to its potential in the future.[42,43]

In addition to the energy crisis and neuromechanical deformation of cells leading to cellular disruption, neuroinflammation may occur and lead to functional changes. In rodent models, inflammatory genes have been reported to be upregulated,[44] and acute neuroinflammatory responses were seen such as greater microglia and macrophage presence, as well as reactive astrogliosis.[45] Thus, inflammation may be a source of neuronal disruption after a concussive event. Greater concentrations of inflammatory markers in the brain may reduce behavioral responses, and metabolites such as myo-Inositol (an osmolyte) has been used as a marker of neuroinflammation.[46] Myo-Inositol is a marker of astrocytes, which become hypertrophic during inflammatory responses to injury,[47] and increases after a concussion owing to membrane damage.[48,49] Given that traditional neuroimaging cannot adequately identify postconcussion alterations, magnetic resonance spectroscopy allows for the detection of subtle abnormalities by measuring brain metabolites.[49–51] A quantitative, noninvasive measurement apparatus, magnetic resonance spectroscopy has been used for diagnosis and prognosis in severe traumatic brain injury,[52] mild traumatic brain injury,[53,54] and among former collision sport athletes.[51,55–59] These studies indicate that magnetic resonance spectroscopy can identify otherwise unnoticed deficits after concussion or repetitive head trauma and point to pathophysiologic changes such as neuroinflammation.[60]

EXCITATORY NEUROTRANSMITTERS AND ION FLUX

Within the neurometabolic cascade of events that occurs after a concussion, an acute increase in excitatory neurotransmitters release likely causes alterations to glutamate, ion channels and N-methyl-D-aspartate(NMDA) receptor function.[34] After acute trauma, damage-associated molecular patterns (DAMPs), glutamate, glutamine, sodium, potassium, and calcium reach elevated levels for prolonged periods, altering cell function. DAMPs are proteins, nucleic acids, and other molecules that are present in cells before an injury[61] that remain dormant until an injury occurs and an immune response is elicited.[62] Although investigated within the context of cancer and rheumatoid arthritis, researchers are now investigating a possible connection between DAMPs and neuroinflammation after a concussion in and around the extracellular space.[63] Adenosine 5′-triphosphoate (ATP) acts as an important type of DAMP with both intracellular and extracellular roles after a concussive event.[64] ATP is mediated by purinergic receptors, but the mechanisms of these receptors after a traumatic neuronal insult are not well-established.[61] ATP and high mobility group box 1 (HMGB1) are secreted passively from dead cells and actively secreted by stressed cells[64] to recruit immune cells, stem cells, and neighboring cells to clear debris and generate new tissue growth.[65] HMGB1, another type of DAMP, has been identified as the proangiogenic factor that stimulates endothelial cells and macrophages, allowing for blood vessel repair and growth in damaged tissue.[65–67] The release of ATP and HMGB1 precedes microglia activation and other immune signals.[68] Microglia are the immune cells of the central nervous system, and are among the first responders after damage.[68,69] Microglia appear as early as 6 hours after a concussion, with noticeable morphologic changes within 72 hours after injury.[70] The release of DAMPs and microglia activation occur rapidly in extracellular space after injury, and are associated with poor outcomes after trauma.[68,71,72] Related to behavioral changes, outcomes among rodent models include decreased memory,[32,73,74] altered motor coordination,[75] and cognitive impairments.[74,76]

In addition to damaged cells releasing DAMPs after a concussion or traumatic brain injury, cells also release an increased concentration of glutamine and glutamate.[77–79] Glutamate receptors are ligand-gated ion channels that allow the passage of sodium and potassium, and in some cases small amounts of calcium.[80] Glutamate receptors produce postsynaptic excitatory responses, perpetuating the release of glutamate and allowing for an increased ionic flow rate. This process leads to the synapses becoming toxic and increasing the risk of neuronal death. A toxic environment then activates protective mechanisms, where astrocytes mediate extracellular toxicity. Glutamate transporter 1 and glutamate aspartate transporter are high-affinity sodium-dependent glial transporters that mediate the bulk of glutamate transport. In astrocytes, glutamate is converted to glutamine by glutamine synthase and shuttled back to the presynaptic neuron to be used.[81] However, a glutamate overload affects shuttling capabilities, leading to further damage owing to altered sodium concentrations. Rao and colleagues[82] reported that excitotoxic neuronal death may occur as a result of traumatic brain injury generating a transient downregulation of transporter proteins (glutamate transporter-1 and glutamate aspartate transporter) within the injured side of the cortex.[82] Without these transporters working efficiently, the toxicity of the cell cannot be mediated, resulting in cell death. Greater glutamate concentrations may also cause overstimulation of NMDA receptors, resulting in increased potassium and calcium concentration and flux through the neuronal membrane.[83,84] Accumulations have been identified during a concussive event in animal models,[85] but return to homeostatic levels may occur as soon as 3 hours in mild to moderately injured cells.[83,86]

Although existing research primarily focuses on increased intracellular and extracellular concentrations of calcium perpetuating cell death, Zander and colleagues[87] suggest that sodium should also receive consideration. Calcium influx increases into the cell after potassium efflux and sodium influx, which creates dysregulation that overwhelms glutamate and NMDA receptors and results in cellular damage. Therefore, it is possible that sodium is one source of ion dysregulation, although further experimental evidence is required. In a study by Paiva and colleagues,[88] sodium serum disorders were investigated in stable patients in the intensive care unit with a moderate to severe traumatic brain injury. Sodium serum disorders are not well-understood in the realm of neurologic disorders and even less well-understood in connection with neurologic trauma. The results suggest that sodium disorder incidence is higher among patients with diffuse traumatic brain injury relative to focal lesions. Thus, sodium regulation may play a central role in cellular dysregulation. Furthermore, sodium concentrations have been shown to become altered and persist for years after concussion symptom recovery, increasing the risk of negative outcomes, such as impaired memory.[89]

ALTERED BEHAVIORAL CHANGES

In addition to the neurometabolic alterations that occur after a concussion, researchers have investigated altered brain function and behavioral changes following concussion in humans. Although most patients recover quickly, recent work suggests that 43% of athletes may experience symptoms for more than 7 days after the injury.[90] However, concussion symptoms may arise owing to many different factors and, as such, they contain a low specificity for postconcussion problems, making it difficult to discern the mechanism by which they occur. Headache is one of the most common postconcussion symptoms reported, occurring in about 85% of patients.[91,92] External factors such as sleep dysregulation, emotional stress, and dehydration can increase the severity of headaches in patients with a concussion.[2,93] Approximately 30% to 85% of patients complain of sleep disturbances, with most resolving 3 months after injury.[94–96] Other cognitive alterations can occur after a concussion, including complications with verbal and visual memory, processing speed, impulse control, orientation, attention, and executive function.[74,97–99] With a variety of symptoms and the lack of effective and quick diagnosis techniques, multidisciplinary investigation into treatment options is needed to help combat patient discomfort and decrease the amount of time out of work, school, and exercise.[100,101] Although these behavioral changes are apparent upon clinical presentation, determining their causes and subsequently identifying appropriate therapeutic targets for interventions among individuals with concussion remains challenging. To prevent long-term problems and initiate appropriate treatments, determining the extent and the factors and mechanisms of the problem must first occur.[102]

TREATMENT

Many treatments have been proposed over the past decade. Although pharmacologic, nutritional, and therapy-based interventions have been tested, the most widely studied form of concussion treatment is subthreshold aerobic exercise.[103] Traditionally, complete physical and cognitive rest has been prescribed until symptom resolution.[104] However, researchers demonstrated that this strategy may actually have a negative effect on symptom recovery.[105] More recent work has observed that, relative to a nonaerobic form of exercise (ie, stretching), a tailored exercise program below the level of symptom exacerbation can actually help to shorten symptom recovery times among adolescents.[106] The physiologic mechanisms underlying this positive result have yet to be delineated. It is logical that a long period of rest, particularly among athletes, may lead to deconditioning that results in cerebrovascular control changes, and that these changes contribute to development of additional symptoms independent of the initial injury.[107] The addition of regular exercise after an injury may, therefore, require the integration of multiple mechanism that relate to cerebrovascular function. After a brief rest period after injury, physical and cognitive rest seems to be an ineffective strategy to facilitate healing. Additional work examining the mechanisms by which symptom improvement occurs as a result of exercise after concussion are needed.

Other non–exercise-based treatments have been proposed to affect brain healing after a concussion. However, evidence is sparse and mixed to this point. Currently, we are unaware of any human-based studies that have investigated the role of supplement or vitamin-based intervention for concussion recovery.[108] Furthermore, there is limited evidence to support the use of pharmacologic approaches to concussion treatment.[109] Thus, multisite and prospective studies of concussion treatments and their mechanistic effects are required.[110]

SUMMARY

Concussion results in a cascade of complex, overlapping, and disruptive processes to the brain. These disruptions occur owing to many different pathophysiologic processes, including ionic shifts, neuronal architecture damage, increased neuroinflammation, increased release of excitatory neurotransmitters, and altered cerebral blood flow control. Collectively, a subsequent energy crisis ensues, given the mismatch between the need for energy to restore these disruptions in the brain, and a reduced ability to deliver energy to, or produce energy within, the brain. Although human-based studies have recently shed light on the restoration of these processes, recovery of each may occur within a distinct timeline and is likely affected by many individual factors. Treatments have focused on the use of aerobic exercise that does not worsen symptoms, and this approach shows promise to alleviate many of the pathophysiologic disruptions present after injury. Currently, adequate time for recovery should occur (ie, not returning to unrestricted activities) so as to not worsen ongoing disruptions, but early integration into regular physical activity that does not worsen outcomes after a concussion should be considered to facilitate a proper healing environment.

CLINICS CARE POINTS

- Clinical evaluation of pathophysiological disruption is currently difficult within typical clinical concussion evaluations.
- Emerging techniques, such as advanced neuroimaging may eventually provide useful clinical information about neuropathology after concussion.
- To understand how treatment affects pathophysiological functioning after concussion, further clinical studies are needed.

DISCLOSURE

Dr D.R. Howell receives research support not related to this study from the Eunice Kennedy Shriver National Institute of Child Health & Human Development (R03HD094560), the National Institute of Neurological Disorders and Stroke (R01NS100952, R41NS103698, R43NS108823), and MINDSOURCE Colorado Brain Injury Network. The remaining author has nothing to disclose.

REFERENCES

1. McCrory P, Meeuwisse W, Dvorak J, et al. Consensus statement on concussion in sport—the 5th international conference on concussion in sport held in Berlin, October 2016. Br J Sports Med 2017;51(11):838–47.
2. Harmon KG, Clugston JR, Dec K, et al. American Medical Society for Sports Medicine position statement on concussion in sport. Br J Sports Med 2019; 53(4):213–25.
3. Lincoln AE, Caswell SV, Almquist JL, et al. Trends in concussion incidence in high school sports: a prospective 11-year study. Am J Sports Med 2011; 39(5):958–63.
4. Rosenthal JA, Foraker RE, Collins CL, et al. National high school athlete concussion rates from 2005-2006 to 2011-2012. Am J Sports Med 2014;42(7):1710–5.
5. Kerr ZY, Chandran A, Nedimyer AK, et al. Concussion Incidence and Trends in 20 High School Sports. Pediatrics 2019;e20192180. https://doi.org/10.1542/peds.2019-2180.
6. Kamins J, Bigler E, Covassin T, et al. What is the physiological time to recovery after concussion? A systematic review. Br J Sports Med 2017;51(12):935–40.
7. Anderson MN, Womble MN, Mohler SA, et al. Preliminary Study of Fear of Re-Injury following Sport-Related Concussion in High School Athletes. Dev Neuropsychol 2019;1–9. https://doi.org/10.1080/87565641.2019.1667995.
8. Aubry M, Cantu R, Dvorak J, et al. Summary and agreement statement of the first International Conference on Concussion in Sport, Vienna 2001. Br J Sports Med 2002;36(1):6–7.
9. Lumba-Brown A, Yeates KO, Sarmiento K, et al. Centers for Disease Control and Prevention Guideline on the Diagnosis and Management of Mild Traumatic Brain Injury Among Children. JAMA Pediatr 2018;e182853. https://doi.org/10.1001/jamapediatrics.2018.2853.
10. McCrory P, Johnston K, Meeuwisse W, et al. Summary and agreement statement of the 2nd international conference on concussion in Sport, Prague 2004. Br J Sports Med 2005;39(4):196–204.
11. Chin EY, Nelson LD, Barr WB, et al. Reliability and validity of the sport concussion assessment tool-3 (SCAT3) in high school and collegiate athletes. Am J Sports Med 2016;44(9):2276–85.

12. Chan M, Vielleuse JV, Vokaty S, et al. Test-retest reliability of the sport concussion assessment tool 2 (SCAT2) for uninjured children and young adults. Br J Sports Med 2013;47(5):e1.

13. Echemendia RJ, Meeuwisse W, McCrory P, et al. The Sport Concussion Assessment Tool 5th Edition (SCAT5). Br J Sports Med 2017;51:848–50.

14. Echemendia RJ, Broglio SP, Davis GA, et al. What tests and measures should be added to the SCAT3 and related tests to improve their reliability, sensitivity and/or specificity in sideline concussion diagnosis? A systematic review. Br J Sports Med 2017;51(11):895–901.

15. Guskiewicz KM, Register-Mihalik J, McCrory P, et al. Evidence-based approach to revising the SCAT2: introducing the SCAT3. Br J Sports Med 2013;47(5): 289–93.

16. Broglio SP, Katz BP, Zhao S, et al. CARE Consortium Investigators. Test-retest reliability and interpretation of common concussion assessment tools: findings from the NCAA-DoD CARE Consortium. Sports Med 2017. https://doi.org/10.1007/s40279-017-0813-0.

17. McPherson AL, Nagai T, Webster KE, et al. Musculoskeletal injury risk after sport-related concussion: a systematic review and meta-analysis. Am J Sports Med 2018. https://doi.org/10.1177/0363546518785901.

18. Kamins J, Giza CC. Concussion - mild TBI: recoverable injury with potential for serious sequelae. Neurosurg Clin N Am 2016;27(4):441–52.

19. Iverson GL, Gardner AJ, Terry DP, et al. Predictors of clinical recovery from concussion: a systematic review. Br J Sports Med 2017;51(12):941–8.

20. McCrory P, Meeuwisse WH, Echemendia RJ, et al. What is the lowest threshold to make a diagnosis of concussion? Br J Sports Med 2013;47(5):268–71.

21. McCrory P, Feddermann-Demont N, Dvořák J, et al. What is the definition of sports-related concussion: a systematic review. Br J Sports Med 2017;51(11): 877–87.

22. Barkhoudarian G, Hovda DA, Giza CC. The molecular pathophysiology of concussive brain injury. Clin Sports Med 2011;30(1):33–48, vii–iii.

23. Vagnozzi R, Signoretti S, Tavazzi B, et al. Hypothesis of the postconcussive vulnerable brain: experimental evidence of its metabolic occurrence. Neurosurgery 2005;57(1):164–71 [discussion: 164–71].

24. Vagnozzi R, Tavazzi B, Signoretti S, et al. Temporal window of metabolic brain vulnerability to concussions: mitochondrial-related impairment–part I. Neurosurgery 2007;61(2):379–88 [discussion: 388–9].

25. Shultz SR, Bao F, Omana V, et al. Repeated mild lateral fluid percussion brain injury in the rat causes cumulative long-term behavioral impairments, neuroinflammation, and cortical loss in an animal model of repeated concussion. J Neurotrauma 2011;29(2):281–94.

26. Lyeth BG. Historical Review of the Fluid-Percussion TBI Model. Front Neurol 2016;7. https://doi.org/10.3389/fneur.2016.00217.

27. Katz PS, Molina PE. A lateral fluid percussion injury model for studying traumatic brain injury in rats. In: Tharakan B, editor. Traumatic and ischemic injury: methods and protocols. Methods in molecular biology. New York: Springer; 2018. p. 27–36. https://doi.org/10.1007/978-1-4939-7526-6_3.

28. Lifshitz J, Rowe RK, Griffiths DR, et al. Clinical relevance of midline fluid percussion brain injury: acute deficits, chronic morbidities and the utility of biomarkers. Brain Inj 2016;30(11):1293–301.

29. Robinson S, Winer JL, Chan LAS, et al. Extended erythropoietin treatment prevents chronic executive functional and microstructural deficits following early severe traumatic brain injury in rats. Front Neurol 2018;9:451.
30. Osier N, Dixon CE. Controlled cortical impact for modeling traumatic brain injury in animals. In: Srivastava AK, Cox CS, editors. Pre-clinical and clinical methods in brain trauma research. Neuromethods. New York: Springer; 2018. p. 81–95. https://doi.org/10.1007/978-1-4939-8564-7_5.
31. Hoogenboom WS, Branch CA, Lipton ML. Animal models of closed-skull, repetitive mild traumatic brain injury. Pharmacol Ther 2019;198:109–22.
32. Deng-Bryant Y, Leung LY, Madathil S, et al. Chronic Cognitive Deficits and Associated Histopathology Following Closed-Head Concussive Injury in Rats. Front Neurol 2019;10. https://doi.org/10.3389/fneur.2019.00699.
33. Fehily B, Bartlett CA, Lydiard S, et al. Differential responses to increasing numbers of mild traumatic brain injury in a rodent closed-head injury model. J Neurochem 2019;149(5):660–78.
34. Giza CC, Hovda DA. The Neurometabolic Cascade of Concussion. J Athl Train 2001;36(3):228.
35. Giza CC, Hovda DA. The new neurometabolic cascade of concussion. Neurosurgery 2014;75(Suppl 4):S24–33.
36. Jassam YN, Izzy S, Whalen M, et al. Neuroimmunology of traumatic brain injury: time for a paradigm shift. Neuron 2017;95(6):1246–65.
37. Yoshino A, Hovda DA, Kawamata T, et al. Dynamic changes in local cerebral glucose utilization following cerebral conclusion in rats: evidence of a hyper- and subsequent hypometabolic state. Brain Res 1991;561(1):106–19.
38. Yuen TJ, Browne KD, Iwata A, et al. Sodium channelopathy induced by mild axonal trauma worsens outcome after a repeat injury. J Neurosci Res 2009; 87(16):3620–5.
39. Tang-Schomer MD, Johnson VE, Baas PW, et al. Partial interruption of axonal transport due to microtubule breakage accounts for the formation of periodic varicosities after traumatic axonal injury. Exp Neurol 2012;233(1):364–72.
40. Choe MC, Babikian T, DiFiori J, et al. A pediatric perspective on concussion pathophysiology. Curr Opin Pediatr 2012;24(6):689–95.
41. Shenton M, Hamoda H, Schneiderman J, et al. A review of magnetic resonance imaging and diffusion tensor imaging findings in mild traumatic brain injury. Brain Imaging Behav 2012;6(2):137–92.
42. Koerte IK, Hufschmidt J, Muehlmann M, et al. Advanced neuroimaging of mild traumatic brain injury. In: Laskowitz D, Grant G, editors. Translational research in traumatic brain injury. Frontiers in neuroscience. Boca Raton (FL): CRC Press/Taylor and Francis Group; 2016. Available at: http://www.ncbi.nlm.nih.gov/books/NBK326714/. Accessed January 22, 2016.
43. Jurick SM, Bangen KJ, Evangelista ND, et al. Advanced neuroimaging to quantify myelin in vivo: application to mild TBI. Brain Inj 2016;30(12):1452–7.
44. Li HH, Lee SM, Cai Y, et al. Differential gene expression in hippocampus following experimental brain trauma reveals distinct features of moderate and severe injuries. J Neurotrauma 2004;21(9):1141–53.
45. Shultz SR, MacFabe DF, Foley KA, et al. Sub-concussive brain injury in the Long-Evans rat induces acute neuroinflammation in the absence of behavioral impairments. Behav Brain Res 2012;229(1):145–52.
46. Chang L, Munsaka SM, Kraft-Terry S, et al. Magnetic resonance spectroscopy to assess neuroinflammation and neuropathic pain. J Neuroimmune Pharmacol 2013;8(3):576–93.

47. Albrecht DS, Granziera C, Hooker JM, et al. In Vivo Imaging of Human Neuro-inflammation. ACS Chem Neurosci 2016;7(4):470–83.

48. Henry LC, Tremblay S, Boulanger Y, et al. Neurometabolic Changes in the Acute Phase after Sports Concussions Correlate with Symptom Severity. J Neurotrauma 2010;27(1):65–76.

49. Lin AP, Liao HJ, Merugumala SK, et al. Metabolic imaging of mild traumatic brain injury. Brain Imaging Behav 2012;6(2):208–23.

50. Alosco ML, Jarnagin J, Rowland B, et al. Magnetic Resonance Spectroscopy as a Biomarker for Chronic Traumatic Encephalopathy. Semin Neurol 2017;37(5): 503–9.

51. Lin AP, Ramadan S, Stern RA, et al. Changes in the neurochemistry of athletes with repetitive brain trauma: preliminary results using localized correlated spectroscopy. Alzheimers Res Ther 2015;7(1):13.

52. Ross BD, Ernst T, Kreis R, et al. 1H MRS in acute traumatic brain injury. J Magn Reson Imaging 1998;8(4):829–40.

53. Vagnozzi R, Signoretti S, Cristofori L, et al. Assessment of metabolic brain damage and recovery following mild traumatic brain injury: a multicentre, proton magnetic resonance spectroscopic study in concussed patients. Brain 2010; 133(11):3232–42.

54. Vagnozzi R, Signoretti S, Tavazzi B, et al. Temporal window of metabolic brain vulnerability to concussion: a pilot 1H-magnetic resonance spectroscopic study in concussed athletes–part III. Neurosurgery 2008;62(6):1286–95 [discussion: 1295–6].

55. Poole VN, Abbas K, Shenk TE, et al. MR spectroscopic evidence of brain injury in the non-diagnosed collision sport athlete. Dev Neuropsychol 2014;39(6): 459–73.

56. Panchal H, Sollmann N, Pasternak O, et al. Neuro-Metabolite Changes in a Single Season of University Ice Hockey Using Magnetic Resonance Spectroscopy. Front Neurol 2018;9:616.

57. Chamard E, Théoret H, Skopelja EN, et al. A prospective study of physician-observed concussion during a varsity university hockey season: metabolic changes in ice hockey players. Part 4 of 4. Neurosurg Focus 2012;33(6):E4.

58. Gardner AJ, Iverson GL, Wojtowicz M, et al. MR spectroscopy findings in retired professional rugby league players. Int J Sports Med 2017;38(3):241–52.

59. Koerte IK, Lin AP, Muehlmann M, et al. Altered neurochemistry in former professional soccer players without a history of concussion. J Neurotrauma 2015; 32(17):1287–93.

60. Koerte IK, Lin AP, Willems A, et al. A review of neuroimaging findings in repetitive brain trauma. Brain Pathol 2015;25(3):318–49.

61. Braun M, Vaibhav K, Saad NM, et al. White matter damage after traumatic brain injury: a role for damage associated molecular patterns. Biochim Biophys Acta 2017;1863(10 Pt B):2614–26.

62. Foell D, Wittkowski H, Roth J. Mechanisms of disease: a "DAMP" view of inflammatory arthritis. Nat Clin Pract Rheumatol 2007;3(7):382–90.

63. Russo MV, McGavern DB. Immune surveillance of the CNS following infection and injury. Trends Immunol 2015;36(10):637–50.

64. Vénéreau E, Ceriotti C, Bianchi ME. DAMPs from cell death to new life. Front Immunol 2015;6. https://doi.org/10.3389/fimmu.2015.00422.

65. Yang S, Xu L, Yang T, et al. High-mobility group box-1 and its role in angiogenesis. J Leukoc Biol 2014;95(4):563–74.

66. van Beijnum JR, Nowak-Sliwinska P, van den Boezem E, et al. Tumor angiogenesis is enforced by autocrine regulation of high-mobility group box 1. Oncogene 2013;32(3):363–74.

67. Mitola S, Belleri M, Urbinati C, et al. Cutting edge: extracellular high mobility group box-1 protein is a proangiogenic cytokine. J Immunol 2006;176(1):12–5.

68. Davalos D, Grutzendler J, Yang G, et al. ATP mediates rapid microglial response to local brain injury in vivo. Nat Neurosci 2005;8(6):752–8.

69. Fourgeaud L, Través PG, Tufail Y, et al. TAM receptors regulate multiple features of microglial physiology. Nature 2016;532(7598):240–4.

70. Madathil SK, Wilfred BS, Urankar SE, et al. Early microglial activation following closed-head concussive injury is dominated by pro-inflammatory M-1 type. Front Neurol 2018;9:964.

71. Cristofori L, Tavazzi B, Gambin R, et al. Biochemical analysis of the cerebrospinal fluid: evidence for catastrophic energy failure and oxidative damage preceding brain death in severe head injury: a case report. Clin Biochem 2005; 38(1):97–100.

72. Mouzon BC, Bachmeier C, Ferro A, et al. Chronic neuropathological and neurobehavioral changes in a repetitive mild traumatic brain injury model. Ann Neurol 2014;75(2):241–54.

73. Cheng JS, Craft R, Yu G-Q, et al. Tau reduction diminishes spatial learning and memory deficits after mild repetitive traumatic brain injury in mice. PLoS One 2014;9(12):e115765.

74. Broussard JI, Acion L, De Jesús-Cortés H, et al. Repeated mild traumatic brain injury produces neuroinflammation, anxiety-like behaviour and impaired spatial memory in mice. Brain Inj 2018;32(1):113–22.

75. Mychasiuk R, Hehar H, Candy S, et al. The direction of the acceleration and rotational forces associated with mild traumatic brain injury in rodents effect behavioural and molecular outcomes. J Neurosci Methods 2016;257:168–78.

76. Petraglia AL, Plog BA, Dayawansa S, et al. The spectrum of neurobehavioral sequelae after repetitive mild traumatic brain injury: a novel mouse model of chronic traumatic encephalopathy. J Neurotrauma 2014;31(13):1211–24.

77. Kierans AS, Kirov II, Gonen O, et al. Myoinositol and glutamate complex neurometabolite abnormality after mild traumatic brain injury. Neurology 2014;82(6): 521–8.

78. Shutter L, Tong KA, Holshouser BA. Proton MRS in acute traumatic brain injury: role for glutamate/glutamine and choline for outcome prediction. J Neurotrauma 2004;21(12):1693–705.

79. Ashwal S, Holshouser B, Tong K, et al. Proton MR spectroscopy detected glutamate/glutamine is increased in children with traumatic brain injury. J Neurotrauma 2004;21(11):1539–52.

80. Purves D, Augustine GJ, Fitzpatrick D, et al. Glutamate Receptors. Neuroscience 2nd edition. 2001. Available at: https://www.ncbi.nlm.nih.gov/books/NBK10802/. Accessed January 14, 2020.

81. Guerriero RM, Giza CC, Rotenberg A. Glutamate and GABA imbalance following traumatic brain injury. Curr Neurol Neurosci Rep 2015;15(5):27.

82. Rao VL, Başkaya MK, Doğan A, et al. Traumatic brain injury down-regulates glial glutamate transporter (GLT-1 and GLAST) proteins in rat brain. J Neurochem 1998;70(5):2020–7.

83. Fineman I, Hovda DA, Smith M, et al. Concussive brain injury is associated with a prolonged accumulation of calcium: a 45Ca autoradiographic study. Brain Res 1993;624(1–2):94–102.

84. Nilsson P, Hillered L, Olsson Y, et al. Regional changes in interstitial K+ and Ca2+ levels following cortical compression contusion trauma in rats. J Cereb Blood Flow Metab 1993;13(2):183–92.

85. Büki A, Povlishock JT. All roads lead to disconnection?–Traumatic axonal injury revisited. Acta Neurochir (Wien) 2006;148(2):181–93 [discussion: 193–4].

86. Weber JT, Rzigalinski BA, Willoughby KA, et al. Alterations in calcium-mediated signal transduction after traumatic injury of cortical neurons. Cell Calcium 1999; 26(6):289–99.

87. Zander NE, Piehler T, Banton R, et al. Effects of repetitive low-pressure explosive blast on primary neurons and mixed cultures. J Neurosci Res 2016;94(9): 827–36.

88. Paiva WS, Bezerra DAF, Amorim RLO, et al. Serum sodium disorders in patients with traumatic brain injury. Ther Clin Risk Manag 2011;7:345–9.

89. Grover H, Qian Y, Boada FE, et al. MRI Evidence of Altered Callosal Sodium in Mild Traumatic Brain Injury. AJNR Am J Neuroradiol 2018;39(12):2200–4.

90. McCrea M, Broglio S, McAllister T, et al. Return to play and risk of repeat concussion in collegiate football players: comparative analysis from the NCAA Concussion Study (1999-2001) and CARE Consortium (2014-2017). Br J Sports Med 2019. https://doi.org/10.1136/bjsports-2019-100579.

91. Gladstone J. From psychoneurosis to ICHD-2: an overview of the state of the art in post-traumatic headache. Headache 2009;49(7):1097–111.

92. Bramley H, Heverley S, Lewis MM, et al. Demographics and treatment of adolescent posttraumatic headache in a regional concussion clinic. Pediatr Neurol 2015;52(5):493–8.

93. Wicklund AH, Gaviria M. Multidisciplinary approach to psychiatric symptoms in mild traumatic brain injury: complex sequelae necessitate a cadre of treatment providers. Surg Neurol Int 2013;4. https://doi.org/10.4103/2152-7806.110150.

94. Wickwire EM, Schnyer DM, Germain A, et al. Sleep, sleep disorders, and circadian health following mild traumatic brain injury in adults: review and research agenda. J Neurotrauma 2018;35(22):2615–31.

95. Bramley H, Henson A, Lewis MM, et al. Sleep disturbance following concussion is a risk factor for a prolonged recovery. Clin Pediatr (Phila) 2017;56(14):1280–5.

96. Howell DR, Oldham JR, Brilliant AN, et al. Trouble falling asleep after concussion is associated with higher symptom burden among children and adolescents. J Child Neurol 2019;34(5):256–61.

97. Mayers LB, Redick TS, Chiffriller SH, et al. Working memory capacity among collegiate student athletes: effects of sport-related head contacts, concussions, and working memory demands. J Clin Exp Neuropsychol 2011;33(5):532–7.

98. Broglio SP, Puetz TW. The effect of sport concussion on neurocognitive function, self-report symptoms and postural control: a meta-analysis. Sports Med 2008; 38(1):53–67.

99. Howell DR, Osternig L, van Donkelaar P, et al. Effects of concussion on attention and executive function in adolescents. Med Sci Sports Exerc 2013;45(6): 1030–7.

100. Knollman Porter K, Constantinidou F, Hutchinson Marron K. Speech-language pathology and concussion management in intercollegiate athletics: the Miami University Concussion Management Program. Am J Speech Lang Pathol 2014;23(4):507–19.

101. Zuckerman SL, Yengo-Kahn AM, Buckley TA, et al. Predictors of postconcussion syndrome in collegiate student-athletes. Neurosurg Focus 2016;40(4):E13.

102. van Mechelen W, Hlobil H, Kemper HC. Incidence, severity, aetiology and prevention of sports injuries. A review of concepts. Sports Med 1992;14(2):82–99.
103. Leddy J, Hinds A, Sirica D, et al. The Role of Controlled Exercise in Concussion Management. PM R 2016;8(3 Suppl):S91–100.
104. McCrory P, Meeuwisse WH, Aubry M, et al. Consensus statement on concussion in sport: the 4th International Conference on Concussion in Sport held in Zurich, November 2012. Br J Sports Med 2013;47(5):250–8.
105. Thomas DG, Apps JN, Hoffmann RG, et al. Benefits of strict rest after acute concussion: a randomized controlled trial. Pediatrics 2015;135(2):213–23.
106. Leddy JJ, Haider MN, Ellis MJ, et al. Early subthreshold aerobic exercise for sport-related concussion: a randomized clinical trial. JAMA Pediatr 2019; 173(4):319–25.
107. Tan CO, Meehan WP, Iverson GL, et al. Cerebrovascular regulation, exercise, and mild traumatic brain injury. Neurology 2014;83(18):1665–72.
108. Ashbaugh A, McGrew C. The Role of Nutritional Supplements in Sports Concussion Treatment. Curr Sports Med Rep 2016;15(1):16–9.
109. Schneider KJ, Leddy JJ, Guskiewicz KM, et al. Rest and treatment/rehabilitation following sport-related concussion: a systematic review. Br J Sports Med 2017; 51(12):930–94.
110. Collins MW, Kontos AP, Okonkwo DO, et al. Statements of agreement from the Targeted Evaluation and Active Management (TEAM) approaches to treating concussion meeting held in Pittsburgh, October 15-16, 2015. Neurosurgery 2016;79(6):912–29.

Diagnosis and Sideline Management of Sport-Related Concussion

Andrew Gregory, MD[a],*, Sourav Poddar, MD[b]

KEYWORDS

• Concussion • Sports • Diagnosis • Sideline • Evaluation

KEY POINTS

- "When in doubt, sit them out" If a concussion is suspected by anyone, then the athlete should be removed from play until evaluation by a medical professional.
- History and physical examination are the gold standard for the diagnosis of concussion. Use of a standardized history and examination form with a graded symptom checklist is recommended.
- There are no proven tests that can diagnose a concussion, and so tests should never be used in isolation.
- An athlete that is on the sideline for a suspected concussion should be monitored for deterioration.
- Any athlete exhibiting red-flag signs or symptoms should be sent to an Emergency Department via Emergency Medical Services.

DIAGNOSIS OF SPORT-RELATED CONCUSSION

Sport-related concussion is a clinical diagnosis. History and physical examination are the cornerstones to identification. Several challenges exist, including a lack of a validated binary objective test, reliance on self-report, and symptoms that may overlap with other common conditions. Sometimes symptoms do not present initially and evolve over time, making serial checks of the affected athlete important. Despite this, synthesizing a combination of history, self-reported symptoms, balance testing, and vestibular, oculomotor, and other available testing can provide a foundation for appropriate diagnosis.

[a] Vanderbilt University Medical Center, Vanderbilt Sports Medicine, Medical Center East, Suite 3200, Nashville, TN 37232, USA; [b] Family Medicine and Orthopedics, University of Colorado School of Medicine, CU Sports Medicine Center, 2000 South Colorado Boulevard, The Colorado Center Tower One, Suite 4500, Denver, CO 80222, USA
* Corresponding author.
E-mail address: andrew.gregory@vumc.org

Clin Sports Med 40 (2021) 53–63
https://doi.org/10.1016/j.csm.2020.08.011
0278-5919/21/© 2020 Elsevier Inc. All rights reserved.
sportsmed.theclinics.com

Key initial elements of the history include sport, age, and education. Younger athletes and children should be evaluated with a heightened sensitivity. Past concussion history, including number, how recent, and length of time to recovery, can help risk-stratify for diagnosis. Additional information regarding confounding variables, such as history of hospitalization for a head injury, history of headache disorder or migraines, attention deficit disorder/attention-deficit/hyperactivity disorder, learning disability, dyslexia, or depression/anxiety or other psychiatric disorder, can provide additional insight during evaluation.

An additional important component of history intake includes determining mechanism of action. Concussion is typically produced by a direct or indirect blow to the head or body that produces transient neurologic disruption. Initial presentation can range from an athlete whose coaches and teammates notice that they are "not acting right" to a downed competitor on the field. In the latter scenario, emergent evaluation for catastrophic injury is primary and paramount. In the more common former situation, an athlete may exhibit symptoms such as dizziness, disorientation, headaches, mood changes, balance problems and visual disturbance. The most common presenting symptom is headache, followed by dizziness.[1] Immediate-onset dizziness correlates with greater than 6-fold risk for prolonged recovery.[2] As mentioned, these and other concussion-related symptoms may also arise from other causes. Another challenge in diagnosis is underreporting of symptoms by an athlete in an attempt to prevent removal from competition. Despite this, taking a symptom inventory is a cornerstone of diagnostic evaluation of a concussion and has good sensitivity and internal reliability (**Box 1**).

CONCUSSION TESTS

With the known challenges of concussion symptom intake (eg, underreporting), tests to provoke physical examination findings in different domains can provide added diagnostic insight (**Table 1**). In addition to clinical examination to screen for catastrophic injury, sideline/locker room tests, such as the Modified Balance Error Scoring System (mBESS), Sports Concussion Assessment Tool 5 (SCAT5),[3] King-Devick (KD), and vestibular/ocular motor screen (VOMS), can be helpful in this setting.

The SCAT5 is a comprehensive and rigorously developed instrument published in 2017 after the Berlin Concussion in Sports Consensus meeting. Components include a brief neurologic examination, symptom checklist, and cognitive and balance assessment. Cognitive screening is a key component of the SCAT5, and the standardized assessment of concussion (SAC) measures orientation, immediate memory, concentration, and delayed recall. Comparison to preinjury baseline provides a constructive component for diagnosis. The SAC in the SCAT5 includes an option for a 10-word

Box 1 Concussion-related symptoms		
Headache	"Pressure in head"	Neck pain
Nausea or vomiting	Dizziness	Blurred vision
Balance problems	Sensitivity to light	Sensitivity to noise
Feeling slowed down	Feeling like "in a fog"	"Don't feel right"
Difficulty concentrating	Difficulty remembering	Fatigue or low energy
Confusion	Drowsiness	More emotional
Irritability	Sadness	Nervous or anxious
Trouble falling asleep (if applicable)		

Table 1
Psychometric properties of sideline assessment tests[a]

Author	Type of Athletes	Athletes (n)	Concussed	Controls	Test and/or Criterion	Sensitivity (%)	Specificity (%)	Test-Retest Reliability	AUC
Symptoms									
McCrea et al[19]	College football	1631	94	56		89	100		
Putukian et al[22]	College athletes	263	32	23	SCAT2	84	100		
Chin et al[23]	High-school and college athletes	2018	166	164					0.88
Resch et al[120]	College athletes		40	40	Revised Head Injury Scale	98	100		
Garcia et al[40]	College athletes		733		SCAT3	93	97		0.98
Broglio et al[33]	College athletes	4360						0.40[b]	
Total		3192	1065	283					
Standardized assessment of concussion									
Barr and McCrea[15]	High-school and college football	1313	50	68	3-point decline	72	94	0.55[c]	
McCrea et al[19]	High-school and college football	1325	63	55	3-point decline	78	95	0.48[d]	
McCrea et al[17]	High-school and college football	2385	91		<10th percentile of normative	79			
McCrea et al[19]	College football	1631	94	56	?	80	91		
Echlin et al[121]	Ice hockey (age 16–21)	67	21	—	1-point decline	54			
Barr et al,[16] 2019	High-school and college football	823	59	31	?	46	87		
Marinides et al[20]	College athletes	217	30		2-point decline	52	82		
Galetta et al[21]	Hockey/lacrosse youth/college	332	12	14	2-point decline	20	21		0.68
Putukian et al[22]	College athletes	263	32	23	<10th percentile of normative	41	91		
Chin et al[23]	High-school and college athletes	2018	166	164				0.39[b]	0.56
Broglio et al[33]	College athletes	4874						0.39[b]	

(continued on next page)

Table 1
(continued)

Author	Type of Athletes	Athletes (n)	Concussed	Controls	Test and/or Criterion	Sensitivity (%)	Specificity (%)	Test-Retest Reliability	AUC
Total		15,284	618	411					
BESS									
McCrea et al[19]	College football	1631	94	56	Modified BESS	36	95		
Broglio et al[122]	Young adults	48			BESS			0.60[e]	
Barr et al,[16] 2019	High-school and college football	823	59	31	Modified BESS	31	71		
Putukian et al[22]	College athletes	263	32	23	Modified BESS	25	100		
Chin et al[23]	High-school and college athletes	2018	166	164	Modified BESS			0.54[b]	0.56
Broglio et al[33]	College athletes	2894			BESS			0.41[b]	
Total		4735	351	274					
Oculomotor (KD)									
Galetta et al[21]	Football men's/women's basketball	219	10		Worsening of KD time	100			
Leong et al[123]	Boxing				Worsening of KD >5 s	100	100	0.9[b]	
Galetta et al[21]	Hockey/lacrosse youth/college	332	12	14	Worsening of KD time	75	93		0.92
Leong et al[28]	College football, men's/women's basketball	127	11		Worsening of KD time	89		0.95[b]	
King et al[124]	Amateur rugby			94	Worsening of KD time	100		0.92[b]	
Marinides et al[20]	Football women's lacrosse, soccer	217	30		Worsening of KD time	79			
Seidman et al[24]	High-school football	343	9		Worsening of KD time	100	100		

Dhawan et al[29]	Youth hockey	141	20	Worsening of KD >5 s	100	91	0.51
Fuller et al[125]	Elite English rugby	145		Worsening of KD time	60	39	
Hecimovich et al[126]	Australian football	22	22	Worsening of KD time	98	96	0.91[b]
	Professional football	1223	84	Worsening of KD	84	62	0.88[b]
Broglio et al[33]	College athletes	755					0.74[b]
Eddy et al[127]	Recreational college athletes	63					0.90[b]
Total		2041	310		99		
Clinical reaction time (dropped weighted stick)							
Eckner[128]	College football, wrestling, women's soccer	102					0.65[b]
Eckner et al[47]	High-school and college athletes	28	28	90% CI	50	86	
Broglio etai[33]	College athletes	261					0.32[b]
Total							

Abbreviations: AUC, area under the curve; CI, confidence interval.

Test-retest reliability:

a Study selection criteria: athletes competing at any level of sport using any sideline screening assessment or studies with test-retest reliability of included assessments. All studies were of high risk of bias as assessed using Quality Assessment of Diagnostic Accuracy Studies, 2, except for Fuller et al,[125] which was of low risk of bias.

b Intraclass correlation coefficient.

c Reliable change index.

d Pearson's correlation coefficient.

e Generalizability coefficient.

From Harmon KG, Clugston JR, Dec K, Herring S, Hainline B, Kane SF, Kontos AP, Leddy JJ, McCrea M, Poddar SK, Putukian M, Wilson JC, Roberts WO. American Medical Society for Sports Medicine position statement on concussion in sport. Br J Sports Med. 2019 Feb;53(4):213-225; with permission.

immediate and delayed memory testing option as well as a longer reverse digit-span evaluation to minimize the ceiling effect that was considered a weakness of the SCAT3.[4]

Neurologic examination is a fundamental part of evaluation for concussion. In addition to comprehensive strength, sensation, and reflex assessment, evaluation of balance is an important component. The mBESS is a validated method of doing this and is included as part of the SCAT5.[5] Errors are counted in 20-second trials in double-leg, single-leg (nondominant), and tandem stance (dominant leg in the back). The mBESS score is calculated by adding 1 error point for each error during the three 20-second tests. The maximum number of errors for any single condition is 10. A complete second series of tests using the same 3 stances on a foam surface can be performed for additional diagnostic testing (balance error scoring system).[5] Comparing this to a pre-injury baseline can be a component of concussion detection and ongoing management. Tandem gait, finger-to-nose coordination, and cranial nerve function evaluations are additional useful tests.

Vestibular and oculomotor assessment is another cornerstone of diagnostic evaluation of concussion. A brief VOMS has been described to assess the integration of vision, balance, and movement.[6] The test array seeks to provoke symptoms by stressing the oculomotor and vestibular systems. The 5 components include smooth pursuit, vertical and horizontal saccades, horizontal and vertical vestibular-ocular reflex, visual motion sensitivity, and near point convergence. Subjects are asked the extent of headache, dizziness, nausea, and fogginess symptoms on a scale of 0 to 10 before administration of each element of the test. An increase of 2 points posttest may indicate oculovestibular dysfunction. For near point convergence testing, seeing double outside of 5 cm is considered abnormal.

The KD is a proprietary, rapid, number-naming, saccadic eye movement test sensitive to oculovestibular dysfunction in concussion.[7] The test gauges integration of oculomotor coordination, attention, and language function and typically can be completed within 2 minutes. This brevity and sensitivity lend feasibility as a diagnostic sideline tool. The KD has shown a modest inherent learning effect with repetitive administration but has demonstrated good internal reliability.[8] Given potential limitations of its psychometric properties, like other components of evaluation of concussion, it should not be used in isolation for diagnosis.[9]

Imaging tests for concussion are an evolving frontier. Head computed tomography is not useful in concussion diagnosis but has utility if there is concern for intracranial bleed or skull fracture. Conventional MRI has no clear role in acute assessment in concussion. Advanced multimodal MRI techniques (diffusion tensor imaging, resting-state functional MRI, quantitative susceptibility imaging, magnetic resonance spectroscopy, arterial spin labeling) are part of current ongoing research protocols.[10] Further work is needed to determine the role of these imaging modalities in diagnosis and management of concussion.

Body fluid biomarkers are another developing field of concussion research. Certain serum markers have shown promise in the setting of more severe neurotrauma, but there is no definitive evidence currently of any that have value in the diagnosis of sports-related concussion.[10] Additional research is also needed to determine the role of genetic factors in the evaluation and management of concussion.

SIDELINE MANAGEMENT OF SPORT-RELATED CONCUSSION

The sideline management of sport-related concussion is based on recognition, diagnosis, and initial treatment. Any athlete with a suspected concussion should immediately be removed from play and evaluated on the sideline.[1] If, after history and physical examination, a concussion is still suspected, then the athlete should not be allowed to return to the field of play and should be monitored on the sideline. Any athlete exhibiting red-flag signs or symptoms should be sent to an Emergency Department (ED) via Emergency Medical Services.

RECOGNITION

Immediate recognition of concussion signs and symptoms is imperative because failure to do so could result in repeat injury or worsening of symptoms. All players, coaches, staff, and referees should be trained in the signs and symptoms of concussion so that they can act accordingly if they are observed. Some professional and college leagues have turned to using spotters remotely who are watching on TV specifically for these signs and symptoms.[11] Realistically, most teams will not have access to spotters, and so everyone should be on the lookout. Video review may prove to be a useful tool in the immediate recognition and sideline evaluation.[12]

Some observable signs for possible concussion that are being used by spotters after a blow to the head or chest include lying motionless, posturing, seizure-like activity, ataxia, head shaking, bloody nose, and blank stare (**Box 2**). If a player is observed to be lying motionless, seizing, or posturing, then an emergency action plan should be initiated. After cervical spine immobilization, then evaluation of the airway, breathing, and circulation should follow. If loss of consciousness persists, then the spine should be immobilized with a cervical collar and spine board, and the patient should be transported immediately to an ED.

Often these observable signs are brief and may be missed by sideline observers. This is again where video review can be helpful. If the player comes to after a brief loss of consciousness or did not have loss of consciousness and does not complain of neck pain, weakness, or paresthesia, then they can be taken to the sideline for a complete assessment. Otherwise, a cervical spine assessment should be done while maintaining stabilization. If the conscious athlete with neck pain exhibits midline neck tenderness, exhibits neurologic abnormality, has altered consciousness, or has a distracting injury, then the cervical spine should be immobilized in a collar and referred for imaging according to the NEXUS (National Emergency X-radiography Utilization Study) criteria (**Box 3**).[13]

If the athlete exhibits any of the red-flag signs and symptoms at any time, they should be referred to an ED for advanced imaging. These red flags include prolonged loss of consciousness (>1 minute), vomiting, neurologic abnormality, seizure, severe headache, or signs of skull fracture (hemotympanum, racoon eyes, or battle sign) (**Box 4**).[3]

Box 2
Signs for possible concussion during play

1. Lying motionless

2. Posturing

3. Seizure-like activity

4. Ataxia/staggering

5. Head shaking

6. Bloody nose/facial laceration

7. Blank or vacant stare

> **Box 3**
> **NEXUS criteria**
>
> 1. Midline neck tenderness
> 2. Focal neurologic deficit
> 3. Altered consciousness
> 4. Distracting injury
> 5. Intoxication

The initial screening assessment should include questions that assess the athlete's orientation and memory.[14] Frequently, these questions can be asked while on the field or while walking with the athlete to the sideline. The Maddocks questions are useful to assess orientation and memory (**Box 5**).[15] They were designed for Australian Rules Football and so should be modified for specific sports. They have been modified for use in the SCAT5.[3]

SIDELINE EVALUATION

A complete sideline evaluation at minimum should consist of a graded symptom checklist, a cognition evaluation, neurologic examination, and balance testing. The cognitive evaluation should include testing orientation, immediate and delayed memory, new learning, and concentration. A sideline assessment tool that contains all of these elements is recommend even though none have been scientifically validated to date.[12]

Even though the athlete needs to be validated further, use of a sideline assessment tool like the SCAT5 is recommended. The SCAT5 is a free tool that was published in 2017 by the Concussion in Sport Group and is a modification of previous versions.[3] There is a separate version (Child SCAT5) for young athletes under the age of 12. Both versions contain all the important elements listed previously.

The evaluation should be conducted by a medical professional who is trained in the diagnosis and management of concussion in athletes. Individual states have laws that determine which professionals are allowed to perform the concussion evaluation. This

> **Box 4**
> **Red-flag symptoms for intracranial/cervical injury (from Sports Concussion Assessment Tool 5)**
>
> 1. Neck pain or tenderness
> 2. Double vision
> 3. Weakness, burning or tingling in the extremities
> 4. Severe or increasing headache
> 5. Seizure
> 6. Loss of consciousness
> 7. Deteriorating condition
> 8. Vomiting
> 9. Increasing restless, agitated, or combative

Box 5
Maddock's questions
1. What is your name?
2. What is your date of birth?
3. How old are you?
4. What is the year?
5. What is the month?
6. What is the day of the week?
7. What is the date?
8. What time of day is it? Morning, afternoon, or evening?
9. At which ground are we?
10. Which quarter is it?
11. How far into the quarter is it?
12. Which side kicked the last goal?
13. Which team did we play last week?
14. Did we win last week?

evaluation should not be performed by professionals for whom this is out of their scope of practice.

After the evaluation is complete, a determination must be made if a concussion is diagnosed, or unknown, or not diagnosed. Only if a concussion is not diagnosed should the athlete be allowed to return to play on the same day. If the diagnosis is still unclear, then it is prudent to continue to treat the athlete as if the concussion has been diagnosed.

MONITORING

Any athlete who has been removed from play should be monitored continuously on the sideline. Specifically, they should not be sent back to the locker room or showers unless they are accompanied by a responsible adult. If the athlete shows signs of deterioration or worsening symptoms, then they should be reevaluated. After the practice or competition is over, the athlete should be monitored by family or roommates and should not go home alone. Athletes should be allowed to sleep and should not be woken up periodically.

INITIAL CARE AND FOLLOW-UP

A concussed athlete and their family should be educated about what the evaluation showed, what a concussion is, and what the natural history entails.[16] They should be counseled on what care is appropriate and inappropriate. In addition to physical and mental rest, sleep hygiene should be discussed. Any activities (triggers) that make symptoms worse should be discontinued. Acetaminophen is appropriate for initial treatment of headaches. Narcotics should not be used because they can cause confusing symptoms, such as vomiting, drowsiness, or disorientation. Most providers recommend avoiding nonsteroidal anti-inflammatory drug use within the first 24 hours of injury because of the theoretic risk of bleeding. An athlete who has been diagnosed with a concussion should have a follow-up appointment scheduled with their primary care provider or sports medicine physician within 2 to 3 days.

CLINICS CARE POINTS

- When in doubt sit them out.
- Use a standardized history and examination form with a graded symptom checklist.
- Do not use concussion tests in isolation.
- Monitor the athlete for deterioration.
- Send the athlete to an Emergency Department if any red flags are present.

DISCLOSURE

A. Gregory: Dr A. Gregory is an editor for *UpToDate* and receives royalties. S. Poddar: The author has nothing to disclose.

REFERENCES

1. Harmon KG, Drezner JA, Gammons M, et al. American Medical Society for Sports Medicine position statement: concussion in sport. Br J Sports Med 2013;47(1): 15–26.

2. Mucha A, Collins MW, Elbin RJ, et al. A brief Vestibular/Ocular Motor Screening (VOMS) assessment to evaluate concussions: preliminary findings. Am J Sports Med 2014;42(10):2479–86.

3. Echemendia RJ, Meeuwisse W, McCrory P, et al. The Sport Concussion Assessment Tool 5th Edition (SCAT5): background and rationale. Br J Sports Med 2017;1–3. https://doi.org/10.1136/bjsports-2017-097506.

4. Norheim N, Kissinger-Knox A, Cheatham M, et al. Performance of college athletes on the 10-item word list of SCAT5. BMJ Open Sport Exerc Med 2018;4(1): e000412.

5. Guskiewicz KM. Assessment of postural stability following sport-related concussion. Curr Sports Med Rep 2003;2(1):24–30.

6. Whitney SL, Eagle SR, Marchetti G, et al. Association of acute vestibular/ocular motor screening scores to prolonged recovery in collegiate athletes following sport-related concussion. Brain Inj 2020;34(6):840–5.

7. Leong DF, Balcer LJ, Galetta SL, et al. The King-Devick test for sideline concussion screening in collegiate football. J Optom 2015;8:131–9.

8. Breedlove KM, Ortega JD, Kaminski TW, et al. King-Devick test reliability in National Collegiate Athletic Association Athletes: a National Collegiate Athletic Association–Department of Defense Concussion Assessment, Research and Education Report. J Athl Train 2019;54(12):1241–6.

9. Legaretta AD, Mummareddy N, Yengo-Kahn AM, et al. On-field assessment of concussion: clinical utility of the King-Devick test. Open Access J Sports Med 2019;10:115–21.

10. McCrea M, Meier T, Huber D, et al. Role of advanced neuroimaging, fluid biomarkers and genetic testing in the assessment of sport-related concussion: a systematic review. Br J Sports Med 2017;51(12):919–29.

11. Mack C, Myers E, Barnes R, et al. Engaging athletic trainers in concussion detection: overview of the National Football League ATC Spotter Program, 2011-2017. J Athl Train 2019;54(8):852–7.

12. Patricios J, Fuller GW, Ellenbogen R, et al. What are the critical elements of sideline screening that can be used to establish the diagnosis of concussion? A systematic review. Br J Sports Med 2017;51(11):888–94.
13. Hoffman JR, Mower WR, Wolfson AB, et al. Validity of a set of clinical criteria to rule out injury to the cervical spine in patients with blunt trauma. National Emergency X-Radiography Utilization Study Group. N Engl J Med 2000;343(2):94–9.
14. Putukian M. Clinical evaluation of the concussed athlete: a view from the sideline. J Athl Train 2017;52(3):236–44.
15. Maddocks DL, Dicker GD, Saling MM. The assessment of orientation following concussion in athletes. Clin J Sport Med 1995;5(1):32–3.
16. Doperak J, Anderson K, Collins M, et al. Sport-related concussion evaluation and management. Clin Sports Med 2019;38(4):497–511.

Outpatient Management of Sport-Related Concussion, Return to Learn, Return to Play

Peter K. Kriz, MD[a,b,1], James P. MacDonald, MD, MPH[c,]*

KEYWORDS

- Concussion • Evaluation • Management

KEY POINTS

- Outpatient management of sports-related concussion (SRC) has undergone a paradigm shift from strict cognitive and physical rest to active rehabilitation, because emerging evidence supports a multidisciplinary approach to the clinical assessment of SRC.
- SRC symptoms are typically clustered into five specific domains: somatic, cognitive, affective, vestibular, and sleep/wake disturbances. Domain-based therapy is now recommended and should be individualized.
- Although computerized neurocognitive testing (CNT) remains a frequently used assessment tool in clinical practice, the role of baseline CNT in SRC management has recently been questioned, because cost, age-related differences in test performance, and uncertain retesting intervals are factors that affect its utility.
- As additional diagnostic tools become available and are supported by evidence, published guidelines for SRC care should take into consideration time and resource constraints of clinicians who perform clinical assessments of athletes with SRC.

INTRODUCTION

Expert opinion and limited evidence suggest that sports-related concussion (SRC) is a self-limited condition with expected symptom duration less than 2 weeks in adults, and less than 4 weeks in children and adolescents.[1,2] However, 10% to 30% of adult athletes experience symptoms beyond 10 to 14 days, and when comprehensive

[a] Division of Sports Medicine, Department of Pediatrics, Warren Alpert Medical School, Brown University, Rhode Island Hospital/Hasbro Children's Hospital, Providence, RI, USA; [b] Division of Sports Medicine, Department of Orthopedics, Warren Alpert Medical School, Brown University, Rhode Island Hospital/Hasbro Children's Hospital, Providence, RI, USA; [c] Division of Sports Medicine, Department of Pediatrics, Ohio State University, College of Medicine, Nationwide Children's Hospital, Columbus, OH, USA
[1] Present address: 1 Kettle Point Drive, Suite 300, East Providence, RI 02915.
* Corresponding author. 584 County Line Road, West, Westerville, OH 43082.
E-mail address: James.MacDonald@nationwidechildrens.org
Twitter: @DrPKrizBrownU (P.K.K.); @sportingjim (J.P.M.)

Clin Sports Med 40 (2021) 65–79
https://doi.org/10.1016/j.csm.2020.08.015
0278-5919/21/© 2020 Elsevier Inc. All rights reserved.

assessment approaches (eg, postconcussion symptom scales, cognitive, vestibular-oculomotor) are used, concussion recovery may extend up to 21 to 28 days in high school and collegiate athletes.[2,3] Recent literature suggests that adolescent and young adult patients who receive clinical care within 7 days of SRC recover faster and are less likely to have prolonged (≥30-day) recoveries compared with those initiating care between 1 and 3 weeks after their SRC.[4] Given this information, a clinician who is well-versed in contemporary SRC management strategies has the potential to expedite the recovery and return to academics and sports for patients who report their symptoms and are evaluated in a timely fashion.

Outpatient management of SRC has evolved significantly over the past few decades, as evidence emerges supporting a multidisciplinary approach to the clinical assessment of SRC[2,3,5] and an adoption of active rehabilitation rather than strict, sustained cognitive and physical rest, otherwise known as "cocoon therapy."[6,7] With this paradigm shift in SRC management, pragmatic approaches are highly sought after by clinicians in busy outpatient settings who may not have the same spectrum of resources available to manage SRC as a provider practicing in a tertiary or quaternary care facility.

In this article, we review the office-based approach to SRC management, including the recommended tools for clinical evaluation, prescribed cognitive and physical activity, adjunctive therapies, and future directions of outpatient SRC management.

OFFICE-BASED EVALUATION: RECOMMENDED TOOLS FOR CLINICAL ASSESSMENT
Overview

SRC is a challenging diagnosis to make and relies to a great degree on history, physical examination, and clinical judgment. Because there does not currently exist an accurate, objective diagnostic measure for SRC, the treating clinician typically supports their judgment with a variety of assessment tools. The more common tools used when evaluating SRC are discussed, but the reader should note that all current tools have less than optimal reliability.[8] The development of more reliable clinical tools and a gold standard diagnostic measure are among the more active issues in SRC research.

History

As with any clinical scenario, obtaining a detailed history is vitally important when assessing an individual for a possible SRC. Defined by the 2016 Consensus Statement on Concussion in Sport drafted by the Concussion in Sport Group (CISG), SRC is an injury that can result from either a direct blow to the head or an impulsive force delivered elsewhere to the body and transmitted to the head, resulting in transient neurologic deficits.[1] Therefore, the treating clinician should assess whether the presenting individual had a plausible mechanism of injury either by direct query of the patient and/or of witnesses. The latter group of potential historians is especially important when assessing pediatric patients or in an instance where the individual themselves has had either loss of consciousness (LOC) or amnesia around the time of the injury. The assessment of the transient neurologic deficits expected with this injury includes assessing for expected signs and symptoms (discussed later).

The past medical history is of importance primarily for two reasons. First, a history of any previous concussion is needed. A recent concussion temporally close to the current injury, or a litany of having had multiple previous concussions, might alert the treating clinician to the possibilities of a prolonged recovery or a need to discuss the possibility of an extended break from the sport of concern. Second, comorbidities must be assessed because they can affect the expected progression of concussion. It is important to inquire specifically about preexisting neurologic (history of migraines), psychological (anxiety, depression), or cognitive (attention-deficit/hyperactivity disorder, other learning disorders) conditions because these can affect the longitudinal evaluation of recovery and modify prognosis.[9]

Regarding the social history, it is important to ask about other sports or activities where the individual participates, including work and school. Driving status should be obtained when relevant, bearing in mind that even preadolescents may in some circumstances be operating motor vehicles (eg, a farming child using a tractor). Finally, when relevant an alcohol/substance use history should be obtained.

Symptom Evaluation

SRC is a challenging diagnosis because the clinical evaluation relies heavily on self-reported symptoms, many of which are nonspecific to concussion. Moreover, these same symptoms may evolve over time and the diagnosis may only become clear sometime after the injury itself (hours to days postinjury).

Given this, the serial evaluation of symptoms is a cornerstone of the diagnosis and management of SRC. The potential symptoms are various and cluster into five specific domains:

- Somatic (headache, neck pain, nausea/vomiting, photophobia, phonophobia)
- Cognitive (confusion, amnesia, difficulty concentrating)
- Affective (emotional, irritable, sad, anxious/depressed)
- Vestibular (balance problems, dizziness, blurred vision)
- Sleep/wake disturbance (drowsiness, fatigue/low energy, difficulty falling asleep)

The most universally used tools for clinical evaluation in SRC are an adult and pediatric version of the Sport Concussion Assessment Tool (SCAT), 5th edition (SCAT5)[10] and the Child SCAT5.[11] These are iterative versions released in 2017 by the CISG and represent an evolution from previous tools known as the SCAT3 and Child SCAT3. The Child SCAT5 is designed for use in children aged 5 to 12 and the SCAT5 for individuals 13 and older. The two tools are used for sideline evaluation and serial, postinjury assessments in the training room or clinic; are widely available; free of cost; and provide a standardized approach to the care of SRC.

These two tools include a standardized symptom checklist in addition to a guided physical examination (discussed next). The SCAT5 includes a 22-item, seven-point Likert scale (0–6) symptom checklist incorporating the five domains in which SRC symptoms cluster. The Child SCAT5 is modified to address the unique concerns associated with pediatric patients ages 5 to 12. In these individuals, the symptom checklist is filled out by parent and patient. The wording for the 21-item symptom checklist is different and more child-friendly than the wording used in the SCAT5 checklist. A four-point Likert scale (0–3) is used in the Child SCAT5.

Physical Examination

An SRC is a traumatic brain injury (TBI). A brief period of LOC is associated with many SRCs, but it is unlikely to last longer than 30 to 60 seconds and once resolved the patient's LOC should be full. Once possible LOC has resolved, the clinician should expect the 15-point Glasgow Coma Scale to be greater than 13 at all times in the acute and subacute settings of this injury. If the GCS is 13 or lower, a more severe TBI is present and emergency medical care should be initiated, the details of which are beyond the scope of this article.

In the setting of a TBI, the evaluating clinician must be aware of the possibility of associated trauma to the body and perform a pertinent secondary survey of the patient as one would do with all trauma patients. Given the mechanism of injury and presenting symptoms, this is a limited, focused examination to assess for possible injury sustained concurrent with the concussion itself and typically constitutes a thorough HEENT and cervical spine examination. The cranium must be examined for possible soft tissue injury (lacerations) or bony injury (eg, fractures of the basilar skull, frontal bone and sinus, orbit, and maxillae). The ear and nasal canals should be examined to rule out tympanic membrane or auricular injury or a nasal septal hematoma. It may be necessary to evaluate the oropharynx, dentition, and temporomandibular joint based on presenting complaints and do a thorough ophthalmologic examination if a primary eye injury is suspected. Finally, the cervical spine must not be overlooked because cervical sprains and vertebral fracture/dislocations are frequently seen in conjunction with concussions. The specifics of evaluation and treatment of these comorbidities are beyond the scope of this article, but each of these injuries may require evaluation (eg, imaging) and treatment separate from concussion care.

The core of the neurologic assessment of the SRC patient includes:

- A mental status assessment
- Oculomotor function
- Gross sensorimotor function
- Coordination, gait, balance, and vestibular assessment

These components are part of the previously referenced SCAT5 and Child SCAT5 tools, which in addition to a symptom checklist include a brief cognitive assessment (the Standardized Assessment of Concussion), a brief neurologic examination checklist, and a balance assessment (the modified Balance Error Scoring System [mBESS]).

Assessment of Vestibuloocular, Vestibulospinal Pathways

Vestibular and oculomotor impairments have been increasingly recognized as common following SRC. Vestibular symptoms include dizziness, nausea, vertigo, blurred or unstable vision, and discomfort in busy environments.[12,13] Oculomotor symptoms include headaches, dizziness, nausea, eye strain, difficulty reading or tracking moving targets, blurred vision, convergence insufficiency, diplopia, and problems scanning for visual information.[13,14] Dizziness is reported by 50% of concussed athletes[15] and is associated with a greater than six-fold increased risk of protracted (>21 days) recovery compared with any other on-field symptom.[16] Delayed recognition of these symptoms can lead to a protracted recovery.[17,18]

The vestibular system is a complex network connecting the inner ear to the brainstem, cerebellum, cerebral cortex, ocular system, and muscles responsible for postural stability. Functionally, it is divided into two pathways: the vestibuloocular pathway and the vestibulospinal pathway (**Fig. 1**). These pathways do not share identical circuitry. The vestibuloocular pathway is responsible for maintaining visual stability during head movements. Vestibular/Ocular Motor Screening (VOMS) and King-Devick Test are screening tools that assess components of the vestibuloocular pathway; King-Devick Test is primarily used as a sideline screen and is discussed in detail in Andrew Gregory and Sourav Poddar's article, "Diagnosis and Sideline Management of Sport Related Concussion," elsewhere in this issue. The vestibulospinal pathway is responsible for postural control. Disrupted balance is the primary symptom associated with vestibulospinal pathway impairment. Until recently, standard assessments of SRC only assessed the vestibulospinal pathway. Balance Error Scoring System (BESS), mBESS, and tandem gait testing are tests designed to assess postural stability and the vestibulospinal pathway. Because most balance impairments in SRC patients recover within 3 to 5 days of injury,[19,20] using postural stability

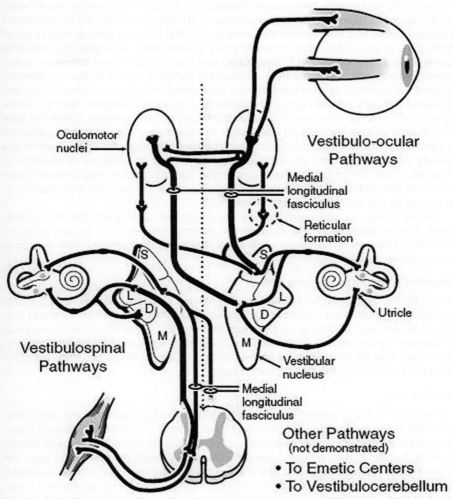

Oculomotor
nuclei

Vestibulo-ocular
Pathways

Medial
longitudinal
fasciculus

Reticular
formation

Utricle

Vestibulospinal
Pathways

Vestibular
nucleus

Medial
longitudinal
fasciculus

Other Pathways
(not demonstrated)

• To Emetic Centers
• To Vestibulocerebellum

Fig. 1. Schematic representation of the vestibular system and its pathways. (*From* Young Kim H. Reciprocal Causal Relationship between Laryngopharyngeal Reflux and Eustachian Tube Obstruction. J Otolaryngol ENT Res 2015 2(6): 00046; with permission.)

tests alone as a measure of a vestibular system injury inadequately assesses vestibuloocular impairment. It is critical for clinicians to use tools that assess for vestibuloocular and vestibulospinal impairment to identify vestibular system involvement related to SRC.

Vestibular/Ocular Motor Screening

The VOMS is a valid clinical tool that is used in patients older than 10 years of age. VOMS measures symptom provocation in SRC patients after assessment of each of the following domains: (1) smooth pursuit, (2) horizontal and vertical saccades, (3) near point convergence (NPC), (4) horizontal vestibuloocular reflex, and (5) visual motion sensitivity. Convergence is evaluated based on the average measurement of three trials of NPC distance in centimeters. Patients are asked to rate symptoms of headache, dizziness, nausea, and fogginess (scale 0–10, with 0 representing no symptoms present) before and after provocative testing. An NPC distance greater than or equal to 5 cm and any VOMS item symptom score greater than two higher than baseline constitutes a positive screen.[21] The VOMS tool has strong internal consistency and significant correlation with the Post-Concussion Symptom Scale. It has also demonstrated the ability to differentiate between concussed individuals and healthy control subjects.[21] VOMS typically takes 10 minutes to administer. Clinicians need to decide whether to perform universal or targeted screening of SRC patients. Given the time constraints placed on busy clinicians and the pressures of productivity, universal screening of SRC patients may be challenging for health care providers outside of a tertiary center to perform, and a targeted screen based on presence or absence of vestibuloocular symptoms on Post-Concussion Symptom Scale may be more pragmatic. Additionally, the optimal timing of VOMS screening (eg, initial evaluation, 2-week follow-up) has yet to be determined.

Current consensus statements on SRC recognize that although oculomotor assessment may be indicated in SRC assessment, the most valid method for assessing oculomotor function is not clear. Therefore, oculomotor screening has not been incorporated into the SCAT5.[22]

Modified Balance Error Scoring System

The mBESS, developed by Guskiewicz,[23] provides a rapid assessment of postural stability in an outpatient clinic setting. The athlete stands on a firm surface and performs double leg, single leg, and tandem stances. Each trial/stance is 20 seconds in duration. Errors (eg, hands lifted off iliac crest, opening eyes, stumbling, hip movement, foot/heel lift, remaining out of test position >5 seconds) are counted, one point for each error, during the six 20-second tests.[10]

Tandem Gait

Timed tandem gait is an alternative test of postural stability in patients with SRC. Athletes are instructed to stand with their feet together, and then walk in a forward direction as quickly and accurately as possible, preferably along a 3-m long piece of athletic tape on the floor, using a heel-to-toe gait. Once they reach the end of the tape, the athlete turns 180° and returns to the starting point along the tape. Time is recorded, and a total of four trials are performed. Tandem gait should be completed in 14 seconds or less.[10,24] Howell and colleagues[25] recently showed that tandem gait testing demonstrates high test-retest reliability in a cohort of healthy, uninjured pediatric and adolescent patients, although a moderate practice effect was noted.

Neurocognitive Testing

Neuropsychological (NP) assessment is recommended as a cornerstone of a multidisciplinary approach to the management of SRC by the CISG.[1] The CISG also notes the significant limitation that NP is in many cases not readily accessible to clinicians and patients.

In lieu of formal NP assessment, computerized neurocognitive testing (CNT) is frequently used in the clinic. The CISG notes that CNT is not a substitute for complete NP assessment, but in practice CNT is frequently more accessible and can be rapidly administered in the clinic, schools, and training rooms. The different CNTs are proprietary products (**Table 1**), which have variable psychometric properties.[26,27]

There is considerable controversy associated with many of the aspects of CNT use in SRC management. The standard of care for how CNT is administered and how the

Table 1
Computerized neurocognitive testing products available to clinicians managing sports-related concussion

Trade Name Product	Manufacturer
ANAM[a]	Vista LifeSciences, Parker, CO
Axon Sports CogState	CogState Ltd, Melbourne, Australia
Concussion Vital Signs (CNS-VS)	CNS Vital Signs, LLC, Morrisville, NC
Headminder Concussion Resolution Index	Headminder Inc, New York, NY
ImPACT[b]	ImPACT Applications, Inc, Pittsburgh, PA

[a] Automated Neuropsychological Assessment Metrics.
[b] Immediate Post-Concussion Assessment and Cognitive Testing.

results are interpreted are evolving.[28] There are questions not fully answered surrounding the importance of so-called "baseline testing," with some making the case for the importance of preseason testing to establish an individual's performance in a noninjured state.[29] Others note the limitations of baseline testing and prefer to compare an individual's CNT testing with normative data.[30] There are potential significant limitations, however, with a reliance on this approach.[31]

The American Medical Society for Sports Medicine (AMSSM) in its 2019 position statement on SRC notes that baseline CNT testing is associated with a cost, the ideal interval for retesting has not been established, and age-related differences in test performance remain unknown.[32,33] The statement concludes "baseline testing may be useful in some cases but is not necessary, required, or an accepted standard of care for the appropriate management of SRC." Whether using a baseline or normative data comparative approach, CNT testing may be a useful adjunct in SRC care when formal NP is unavailable, but it is not an indispensable tool.

SPORT-RELATED CONCUSSION: RETURN TO ACTIVITY

The hallmark of the treatment of SRC historically has consisted of a period of complete cognitive and physical rest.[24] It is thought that a period of rest post-SRC is beneficial because it frees up energy for the brain's significantly increased metabolic needs postinjury. Recently, however, it has been found that strict rest may be maladaptive, most especially in adolescents, potentially slowing recovery and iatrogenically worsening symptoms.[6] There has been a paradigm shift moving toward the direction of earlier return to some cognitive and physical activity if symptom exacerbation and the chance for reinjury are avoided.

The current recommendations are to endorse a brief period of cognitive and physical rest after injury (24–48 hours) followed by a gradual and progressive introduction of school/work and physical activity.[1] The progression of return to cognitive activity should be paced to avoid symptom exacerbation. Athletes who tolerate exercise should (1) begin with noncontact, aerobic exercise; (2) take care to avoid symptom exacerbation; and (3) avoid the possibility of head injury (eg, an errant ball hitting the patient's head). The athlete should progress to more intense activity only under guidance.[34] To avoid a prolonged recovery or secondary morbidity event, including second-impact syndrome, a full return to contact or collision sport must be delayed until a clinician is convinced the athlete has fully recovered from the current injury.

Return to Learn

The CISG recommends a graduated return to school strategy after a brief period of rest.[1] The strategy should be tailored to the individual's needs and often relies on a coordinated assessment by the clinician, teachers, parents, and injured individual. There is little evidence to guide a clinician on the specifics of such a tailored strategy and much that still relies on clinician judgment. Such decisions as how much school (half-days vs full days), classroom activity (use of computers or not), and participation in nonsport extracurricular activity (band, theater) are made by balancing findings on an objective assessment of the individual state with a frank discussion with the stakeholders involved (**Table 2**). There is wide geographic variability in the understanding and application of academic accommodations for concussed students.[35] However, in the authors' experience, the nation-wide adoption of concussion laws has paralleled an increased understanding of the need for academic accommodations in the setting of concussion care.

Return to Play

Although a gradual increase in low-risk physical activity can be coordinated with a return to school, as a general principle it is recommended that a return to full, unrestricted school precede a return to play (RTP), or sport.[36] The following stepwise, graduated RTP progression is used commonly when guiding the injured athlete back to full, unrestricted activity: Step 1, light aerobic activity (eg, walking) for 5–20 min; Step 2, moderate aerobic activity (eg, jogging) for 15–20 min; Step 3, noncontact practice, including sport-specific drills, sprinting, and light resistance training; Step 4, full contact practice; Step 5, full game. Although there is some variability in the specifics of what this RTP progression looks like, there is an evolving standard of care. Please see **Box 1** for notes and principles related to this standard of care.[37,38]

Other modifying factors, such as a prolonged recovery, a history of multiple concussions, or a series of recent concussions need to be factored into a final RTP decision,

Table 2
Return to learn following sports-related concussion: suggested accommodations

Possible Accommodations	Noted Signs/Symptoms	Other Considerations
Half-days at school	All[a]	Complicating factor may be family need for latchkey care
Extension of assignments	All[a]	
Rest periods during school	All[a]	
Untimed tests/delayed tests	All[a]	May be difficult to arrange for standardized testing
Reduced classwork/makeup work	All[a]	
No physical education	Exercise intolerance	Concern for inadvertent injury in setting of physical education
Preprinted materials	Visual symptoms, photophobia	
Sunglasses in class	Visual symptoms, photophobia	
Avoid band, music class	Phonophobia/headache	

[a] Denotes any concussion symptom may prompt the accommodation.

Box 1
Notes and principles on the stepwise gradual return to play following sports-related concussion

Notes and Principles
1. Ideally this progression should be done under supervision.
2. Moving from one step to the next must be accomplished without symptom exacerbation.
3. A minimum of 24 hours is spent at each step; at clinician discretion a longer period at each step may be prescribed.
4. Pediatric (<13 years) patients should spend a minimum of 48 hours at each step.
5. Certain sports with high vestibular demands, such as swimming, dance, gymnastics, and figure skating, may need to spend more time at Step 3 when sport-specific activity is initiated.

---

even when an individual has successfully completed an RTP progression, most especially in the contact or collision sport athlete. A more conservative approach and delayed return (eg, taking the season off entirely) is often prescribed for an athlete with one or more of these concerns. Supporting this approach is recent literature that suggests that the physiologic recovery time may outlast the clinical recovery time.[1] There is a growing body of clinical evidence suggesting a period of vulnerability exists after SRC, even after symptom resolution.[39]

Return to Drive

For adolescents and adults, it is important to ask about driving habits after concussion. Driving is an inherently dangerous activity and one that may be still more hazardous for the driver recovering from SRC. There is evidence to suggest that restricting driving in the first 24 to 48 hours postinjury is reasonable, but for time frames beyond 48 hours the evidence is inconclusive.[40] The clinician should exercise prudence in evaluating the individual for driving fitness beyond 48 hours and balance safety concerns with the implications of restricting what is for many an instrumental activity of daily living.[41]

ADJUNCTIVE THERAPIES FOR SPORTS-RELATED CONCUSSION: WHEN/WHAT TO PRESCRIBE

SRC rehabilitative and pharmacologic therapies are emerging treatments for SRC that are discussed in-depth in M. Nadir Haider and colleagues' article, "Rehabilitation of Sport Related Concussion"; and Jacob C. Jones and Michael J. O'Brien's article, "Medical Therapies for Concussion," elsewhere in this issue; therefore, the focus of this section is on the optimal timing and dosing of these adjunctive therapies. Deciding when to initiate these interventions in SRC management is challenging and such decisions are often individualized; health care providers must primarily rely on clinical judgment and local practice cultures to guide their decision-making, because limited evidence pertaining to timing/dosing exists.[42] Because most adults recover in 10 to 14 days, formal physical therapy (PT) interventions (progressive exercise training, manual therapy, and vestibuloocular therapy) and pharmacotherapy traditionally have not been initiated before 2 weeks of symptoms. However, researchers have begun to investigate the safety and outcomes of multimodal SRC therapeutic interventions in early phases of SRC recovery.

Leddy and colleagues[43] performed a prospective randomized clinical trial enrolling 103 male and female adolescent athletes (age 13–18 years) who presented within

10 days of SRC. Participants were randomized to aerobic exercise (Buffalo Concussion Treadmill Test at 80% of heart rate threshold) or a placebo-like stretching program; activities were performed approximately 20 minutes a day, and participants self-reported daily symptoms and compliance with the exercise prescription via a Web site. Athletes in the aerobic exercise arm recovered in a median of 13 days, whereas athletes in the stretching arm recovered in 17 days ($P = .009$).[43] This study demonstrates that prescribed submaximal threshold exercise during the first week after SRC safely expedites recovery in adolescent athletes with SRC, supporting the use of therapeutic intervention early in SRC recovery. Limitations of the study include self-reporting (dose of exercise therefore not measured objectively), and lack of generalizability because younger children, non-SRC patients, and patients with depression, anxiety, and attention-deficit/hyperactivity disorder were excluded.

Lennon and colleagues[42] performed a retrospective analysis of symptom recovery, safety, and preliminary outcomes of a multimodal PT program for 120 concussion patients 12 to 21 years of age (mean age, 14.77 years). Thirty-three patients initiated therapy 0 to 20 days following injury (early intervention), 39 patients began therapy 21 to 41 days postinjury (middle intervention), and 48 patients started therapy greater than or equal to 42 days postinjury (late intervention). Post-Concussion Symptom Inventory score from the beginning to end of PT care was the primary outcome. There were no statistical differences among the early, middle, or late intervention cohorts regarding symptom change on the Post-Concussion Symptom Inventory from beginning to end of PT care ($P > .05$), number of PT sessions ($P = .21$), or duration of PT care ($P = .19$), suggesting that early initiation of PT in adolescent and young adult patients may be safe and tolerable.[42] Limitations include a retrospective study design, which increases the likelihood for selection bias, and lack of a control group.

Schneider and colleagues[44] performed a single-blind randomized clinical trial evaluating the effect of combined vestibular rehabilitation and cervical spine physiotherapy on 31 patients (18 male, 13 female) ages 12 to 30 years (median age, 15 years) following an SRC. Inclusion criteria included dizziness, neck pain, and/or headaches for greater than 10 days reported on the SCAT2 in addition to a clinical examination suggesting vestibular and/or cervical spine involvement. The intervention group received an individually designed combination of vestibular rehabilitation and cervical spine physiotherapy, whereas both groups rested until symptom free and performed range of motion exercises, stretching, and postural education. Patients were seen once weekly by the study treatment physiotherapist for 8 weeks or until time of medical clearance to return to sport. The primary outcome was medical clearance to return to sport, evaluated by a study sports medicine physician blinded to the treatment group. Two control patients withdrew from the study. Time since SRC was median 53 days in the intervention group, 47 days in the control group. Seventy-three percent (11/15) of intervention group participants were medically cleared within 8 weeks of beginning treatment, compared with 7% (1/14) in the control group. Using an intention-to-treat analysis, treatment group participants were 3.91 (95% confidence interval, 1.34–11.34) times more likely to be medically cleared by 8 weeks.[44] Limitations include poor generalizability to other age groups, potential expectation, and differential misclassification bias.

Although there is limited evidence to support the use of pharmacologic treatments in SRC for somatic, emotional, cognitive, and sleep-related symptoms, researchers have begun to investigate the effect of pharmacologic agents on mitigating the secondary injury that shortly follows primary blunt-force injury with SRC and non-SRC. Specifically, delayed secondary injury caused by oxidative stress, inflammation, and glutamate toxicity could potentially be reduced by targeting biomechanical and molecular factors in the neurometabolic cascade of concussion.[45] Hoffer and colleagues[46] performed a randomized double-blind, placebo-controlled study on 81 US active duty service members who met criteria for mild TBI enrolled within 72 hours of blast exposure while deployed in Iraq. Following evaluation, patients were randomized to receive N-acetylcysteine, an effective neuroprotective agent with a long safety history, or placebo for 7 days. Subjects were re-evaluated at 3 and 7 days, and the following outcomes following mild TBI were measured: dizziness, hearing loss, headache, memory loss, sleep disturbances, and neurocognitive dysfunction. Main outcome was resolution of these symptoms 7 days after blast exposure. N-acetylcysteine treatment was significantly better than placebo regarding symptom resolution by Day 7 (odds ratio, 3.6; $P = .006$). Subjects receiving N-acetylcysteine within 24 hours (n = 29) of blast exposure had an 86% chance of symptom resolution with no untoward side effects compared with 42% of those subjects (n = 31) receiving placebo within 24 hours of blast exposure.[46] The study results may not be generalizable to females (1/81 enrollees was female), and further studies with a larger number of subjects are necessary to determine the effects of treatment on longer term outcomes.

SUMMARY/FUTURE DIRECTIONS

The outpatient management of SRC has changed over the past two decades. Such notions as cocoon therapy and the grading of injury as simple versus complex have been discarded.[47] New therapies, such as prescribed exercise, and new diagnostic tools, such as VOMS, have been introduced. The tools and terminology the clinician will use in another decade or two will surely be different than some of what has been reviewed in this article. Predicting the specifics of what SRC care may look like in the future is difficult. The authors conclude this article with some thoughts about possible future directions.

The evidence behind the introduction of prescribed activity at an early stage in recovery, and without symptom exacerbation, is likely to grow stronger. Despite consensus clinical guidelines that support this intervention, knowledge is still lacking about the specifics of what prescribed activity should look like. The precise timing of introduction of activity, the dosage and intensity, and the variability in response in different subpopulations (male, female, pediatric, adolescent) all need further elucidation.

Leddy and colleagues have conducted much of the research that investigates the specifics of the exercise prescription. This work relies on the Buffalo Concussion Treadmill Test, a supervised graded exercise protocol that is used to determine reliably the symptom exacerbation threshold in patients with SRC.[43,48,49] The Bruce and Balke exercise protocols have also been used in this research.[50] Although these exercise tests are useful, they require supervision, equipment, and time, and may not be easily accessible to many patients and clinicians. A potential alternative is the Karsch Pulse Recovery test, a simple and practical tool that is conducted in 3 minutes using a step. Preliminary evidence has found the Karsch Pulse Recovery test may be useful in determining when children and adolescents can safely begin graded exercise.[51] More work is needed to determine the ideal options for exercise testing in SRC, but the authors hope that such values as practicality and time efficiency are addressed and the all-important values of accuracy, safety, and validity.

The characteristic symptoms of SRC are clustered into domains: somatic, cognitive, affective, vestibular, and sleep/awake disorders. The AMSSM position statement on concussion in sport[32] explores the emerging concept that the degree to which an individual has symptoms clustering in one or more specific clinical domains or profiles may potentially influence prognosis and treatment. Furthermore, the AMSSM authors state "It is currently unknown at what post-injury time point these profiles become clinically important as most SRCs resolve with time. Thus, clinical profiles may be more applicable to athletes with persistent symptoms." The concept of clinical domains is likely to be of increasing importance in the future and warrants additional research.

Predicting which athletes with SRC will recover in the expected timeframe and which will go on to have a prolonged recovery is and will remain an important task. Currently, there is a reliance on the stated symptom profile and the history (including comorbidities and previous concussion history). Johnson and colleagues[52] published work that showed salivary microRNA changes in concussed patients ages 7 to 21 outperformed standard symptom survey measures in predicting individuals with prolonged recovery. It is an exciting prospect that point-of-care testing, such as salivary microRNA, may possibly be an important clinical aid in prognosis and diagnosis of SRCs for the clinician of the future.

Finally, as the evidence increases for the use of tools discussed in this article, or for yet-to-be-determined tools, attention must be paid to time and resource constraints. A comprehensive in-clinic assessment of the athlete with SRC stretches the limits of many busy clinical practices. Not all clinicians will have the luxury of referring patients to a nearby multidisciplinary concussion clinic, and they will consequently need to practice the best, most recent, evidence-based concussion care within the limits imposed by economics or geography. As experts in this field continue to publish iterative guidelines for SRC care, it is hoped that these potential constraints are included in the discussion of what constitutes best practice.

CLINICS CARE POINTS

- Persistent post-concussion symptoms (e.g., clinical symptoms persisting beyond expected time frames) differ for children (>4 weeks) and adults (>10-14 days).
- An elevated score on a standardized symptom checklist (e.g. Post-Concussion Symptom Scale, Step 2 of SCAT5) in the first/initial day of symptoms is the strongest, most consistent predictor of slower recovery from concussion.
- Risk factors for persistent post-concussion symptoms include pre-injury, subacute diagnoses of migraines and depression, but do NOT include histories of ADHD or learning disabilities.
- Recent literature suggests that a period of vulnerability may exist even after concussion symptom resolution, as physiological time of recovery may outlast clinical recovery time.

DISCLOSURE

The authors have nothing to disclose.

REFERENCES

1. McCrory P, Meeuwisse W, Dvořák J, et al. Consensus statement on concussion in sport—the 5th international conference on concussion in sport held in Berlin, October 2016. Br J Sports Med 2017;51(11):838–47.

2. Ellis MJ, Leddy J, Willer B. Multi-disciplinary management of athletes with post-concussion syndrome: an evolving pathophysiological approach. Front Neurol 2016;7:1–14.

3. Henry LC, Elbin RJ, Collins MW, et al. Examining recovery trajectories after sport-related concussion with a multimodal clinical assessment approach. Neurosurgery 2016;78(2):232–40.

4. Kontos AP, Jorgensen-wagers K, Trbovich AM, et al. Association of time since injury to the first clinic visit with recovery following concussion. JAMA Neurol 2020;77(4):435–40.

5. Collins MW, Kontos AP, Reynolds E, et al. A comprehensive, targeted approach to the clinical care of athletes following sport-related concussion. Knee Surg Sports Traumatol Arthrosc 2014;22(2):235–46.

6. Thomas DG, Apps JN, Hoffmann RG, et al. Benefits of strict rest after acute concussion: a randomized controlled trial. Pediatrics 2015;135(2):213–23.

7. Leddy J, Hinds A, Sirica D, et al. The role of controlled exercise in concussion management. PM R 2016;8(3):S91–100.

8. Broglio SP, Katz BP, Zhao S, et al. Test-retest reliability and interpretation of common concussion assessment tools: findings from the NCAA-DoD CARE Consortium. Sports Med 2018;48(5):1255–68.

9. Kutcher JS, Eckner JT. At-risk populations in sports-related concussion. Curr Sports Med Rep 2010;9(1):16–20.

10. Echemendia RJ, Meeuwisse W, McCrory P, et al. The Sport Concussion Assessment Tool 5th Edition (SCAT5). Br J Sports Med 2017. https://doi.org/10.1136/bjsports-2017-097506. bjsports-2017-097506.

11. Davis GA, Purcell L, Schneider KJ, et al. The Child Sport Concussion Assessment Tool 5th edition (child SCAT5): background and rationale. Br J Sports Med 2017;51(11):859–61.

12. Kontos AP, Ortega J. Future directions in sport neuropsychology. In: Webbe F, editor. The handbook of sport neuropsychology. New York: Springer Publishing; 2011. p. 383–93.

13. Kontos AP, Deitrick JMA, Collins MW, et al. Review of vestibular and oculomotor screening and concussion rehabilitation. J Athl Train 2017;52(3):256–61.

14. Kapoor N, Ciuffreda KJ. Vision disturbances following traumatic brain injury. Curr Treat Options Neurol 2002;4(4):271–80.

15. Kontos AP, Elbin RJ, Schatz P, et al. A revised factor structure for the post-concussion symptom scale: baseline and postconcussion factors. Am J Sports Med 2012;40(10):2375–84.

16. Lau BC, Kontos AP, Collins MW, et al. Which on-field signs/symptoms predict protracted recovery from sport-related concussion among high school football players? Am J Sports Med 2011;39(11):2311–8.

17. Hoffer ME, Gottshall KR, Moore R, et al. Characterizing and treating dizziness after mild head trauma. Otol Neurotol 2004;25(2):135–8.

18. Naguib MB, Madian Y, Refaat M, et al. Characterisation and objective monitoring of balance disorders following head trauma, using videonystagmography. J Laryngol Otol 2012;126(1):26–33.

19. Guskiewicz KM, Ross SE, Marshall SW. Postural stability and neuropsychological deficits after concussion in collegiate athletes. J Athl Train 2001;36(3):263–73.

20. Riemann BL, Guskiewicz KM. Effects of mild head injury on postural stability as measured through clinical balance testing. J Athl Train 2000;35(1):19–25.

21. Mucha A, Collins MW, Elbin RJ, et al. A brief vestibular/ocular motor screening (VOMS) assessment to evaluate concussions: preliminary findings. Am J Sports Med 2014;42(10):2479–86.

22. Echemendia RJ, Broglio SP, Davis GA, et al. What tests and measures should be added to the SCAT3 and related tests to improve their reliability, sensitivity and/or specificity in sideline concussion diagnosis? A systematic review. Br J Sports Med 2017;51(11):895–901.

23. Guskiewicz KM. Assessment of postural stability following sport-related concussion. Curr Sports Med Rep 2003;2(1):24–30.

24. McCrory P, Meeuwisse WH, Aubry M, et al. Consensus statement on concussion in sport: the 4th international conference on concussion in sport, Zurich, November 2012. J Athl Train 2013;48(4):554–75.

25. Howell DR, Brilliant AN, Meehan WP. Tandem gait test-retest reliability among healthy child and adolescent athletes. J Athl Train 2019. https://doi.org/10.4085/1062-6050-525-18.

26. Farnsworth JL, Dargo L, Ragan BG, et al. Reliability of computerized neurocognitive tests for concussion assessment: a meta-Analysis. J Athl Train 2017;52(9):826–33.

27. MacDonald J, Duerson D. Reliability of a computerized neurocognitive test in baseline concussion testing of high school athletes. Clin J Sport Med 2015;25(4):367–72.

28. Moser RS, Schatz P, Lichtenstein JD. The importance of proper administration and interpretation of neuropsychological baseline and postconcussion computerized testing. Appl Neuropsychol Child 2015;4(1):41–8.

29. Herring SA, Cantu RC, Guskiewicz KM, et al. Concussion (mild traumatic brain injury) and the team physician: a consensus statement-2011 update. Med Sci Sports Exerc 2011;43(12):2412–22.

30. Abeare CA, Messa I, Zuccato BG, et al. Prevalence of invalid performance on baseline testing for sport-related concussion by age and validity indicator. JAMA Neurol 2018;75(6):697–703.

31. Schatz P, Robertshaw S. Comparing post-concussive neurocognitive test data to normative data presents risks for under-classifying "above average" athletes. Arch Clin Neuropsychol 2014;29(7):625–32.

32. Harmon KG, Clugston JR, Dec K, et al. American Medical Society for Sports Medicine position statement on concussion in sport. Clin J Sport Med 2019;29(2):87–100.

33. American Medical Society for Sports Medicine position statement on concussion in sport: erratum. Clin J Sports Med 2019;29(3):256.

34. Silverberg ND, Duhaime AC, Iaccarino MA. Mild traumatic brain injury in 2019-2020. JAMA 2019. https://doi.org/10.1001/jama.2019.18134.

35. Olympia RP, Ritter JT, Brady J, et al. Return to learning after a concussion and compliance with recommendations for cognitive rest. Clin J Sport Med 2016;26(2):115–9.

36. Frémont P, Schneider K. New recommendations on sport-related concussions: stronger methodology, practical messages, and remaining challenges. Clin J Sport Med 2019;29(6):439–41.

37. Wallace J, Covassin T, Lafevor M. Use of the stepwise progression return-to-play protocol following concussion among practicing athletic trainers. J Sport Health Sci 2018;7(2):204–9.

38. Suggested guidelines for management of concussion in sports. National Federation of State High School Associations (NFHS) Sports Medicine Advisory

Committee (SMAC). Available at: https://www.nfhs.org/media/1018446/ suggested_guidelines__management_concussion_april_2017.pdf. Accessed January 30, 2020.

39. Maugans TA, Farley C, Altaye M, et al. Pediatric sports-related concussion produces cerebral blood flow alterations. Pediatrics 2012;129(1):28–37.

40. Christensen J, McGrew CA. When is it safe to drive after mild traumatic brain injury/sports-related concussion? Curr Sports Med Rep 2019;18(1):17–9.

41. MacDonald J, Patel N, Young J, et al. Returning adolescents to driving after sports-related concussions: what influences physician decision-making. J Pediatr 2018;194:177–81.

42. Lennon A, Hugentobler JA, Sroka MC, et al. An exploration of the impact of initial timing of physical therapy on safety and outcomes after concussion in adolescents. J Neurol Phys Ther 2018;42(3):123–31.

43. Leddy JJ, Haider MN, Ellis MJ, et al. Early subthreshold aerobic exercise for sport-related concussion: a randomized clinical trial. JAMA Pediatr 2019; 173(4):319–25.

44. Schneider KJ, Meeuwisse WH, Nettel-Aguirre A, et al. Cervicovestibular rehabilitation in sport-related concussion: a randomised controlled trial. Br J Sports Med 2014;48(17):1294–8.

45. Giza CC, Hovda DA. The neurometabolic cascade of concussion. J Athl Train 2001;36(3):228–35.

46. Hoffer ME, Balaban C, Slade MD, et al. Amelioration of acute sequelae of blast induced mild traumatic brain injury by N-acetyl cysteine: a double-blind, placebo controlled study. PLoS One 2013;8(1):1–10.

47. Iverson G. Predicting slow recovery from sport-related concussion: the new simple-complex distinction. Clin J Sport Med 2007;17(1):31–7.

48. Leddy JJ, Willer B. Use of graded exercise testing in concussion and return-to-activity management. Curr Sports Med Rep 2013;12(6):370–6.

49. Leddy JJ, Haider MN, Hinds AL, et al. A preliminary study of the effect of early aerobic exercise treatment for sport-related concussion in males. Clin J Sport Med 2019;29(5):353–60.

50. Leddy JJ, Baker JG, Kozlowski K, et al. Reliability of a graded exercise test for assessing recovery from concussion. Clin J Sport Med 2011;21(2):89–94.

51. Fyffe A, Bogg T, Orr R, et al. Association of simple step test with readiness for exercise in youth after concussion. J Head Trauma Rehabil 2019. https://doi.org/10. 1097/HTR.0000000000000512.

52. Johnson JJ, Loeffert AC, Stokes J, et al. Association of salivary microRNA changes with prolonged concussion symptoms. JAMA Pediatr 2018;172(1): 65–73.

Neuropsychological Assessment of Sport-Related Concussion

Sabrina Jennings, PhD[a],*, Michael W. Collins, PhD[a],
Alex M. Taylor, PsyD[b]

KEYWORDS

- Neuropsychological • Assessment • Concussion • Sports • Treatment • Cognitive

KEY POINTS

- Neuropsychological assessment is an integral component in the treatment and management of a sport-related concussion (SRC).
- Neurocognitive testing is not a stand-alone measure for diagnosing and management, but instead is used as a valuable tool in a comprehensive evaluation.
- Computerized neurocognitive tests batteries are the most widely used modality of neurocognitive assessment for SRC.
- Clinical neuropsychologists are the most uniquely qualified professionals to interpret, assess, and incorporate the data in the treatment and management of SRC.

INTRODUCTION

Neuropsychological assessment has a long history of being one of the key components in a comprehensive evaluation of a head injury.[1] A sport-related concussion (SRC) has been labeled one of the most complex injuries in sports medicine to diagnose, assess, and manage.[1] An SRC is understood to be a complex pathophysiological rather than neurostructural process, induced by a biomechanical force.[2,3] As such, changes are not readily observed with traditional neuroimaging and for some, deficits can still be present even when physical symptoms have resolved.[4–6] Therefore, neuropsychological testing plays an integral role in providing a standardized, methodological approach in a comprehensive evaluation. This article reviews the history of neuropsychological assessment in SRC, as well as the role of neuropsychologists in a multifaceted assessment. This article also includes a case study demonstrating the practical use of computerized neurocognitive testing in a comprehensive neuropsychological assessment of an SRC.

[a] Department of Orthopedics, UPMC Sport Medicine Concussion Program, 3200 South Water Street, Pittsburgh 15203, PA, USA; [b] Brain Injury Center, Boston's Children Center, 300 Longwood Avenue, Boston, MA 02115, USA
* Corresponding author.
E-mail address: skjenn24@gmail.com

Clin Sports Med 40 (2021) 81–91
https://doi.org/10.1016/j.csm.2020.08.002
0278-5919/21/© 2020 Elsevier Inc. All rights reserved.
sportsmed.theclinics.com

HISTORY OF NEUROPSYCHOLOGICAL ASSESSMENT AND CONCUSSION

Clinical neuropsychology as a field emerged during the beginning of the twentieth century, with the growing interest in the behavioral expression of brain dysfunction.[7–9] Clinical neuropsychologists have used neuropsychological assessment as a means by which to detect and characterize neurocognitive impairment.[10] Initially, most of the field focused on assessing moderate to severe brain injuries. It was not until 1974, in New Zealand, with the work of Gronwall and Wrightson on mild head injuries,[11] that the subspecialty of Sport Neuropsychology emerged.[9]

In the 1980s research from Barth and colleagues,[12] along with studies from the University of Virginia,[13] served as springboards for others to supply empirical evidence of the neurocognitive impact after an SRC and the timeframe for resolution of cognitive symptoms.[12] Neurocognitive characteristic deficits following an SRC are typically seen in the areas of memory, attentional processes, reaction time, and processing speed.[14–16] Barth and colleagues[12] introduced the Sports Laboratory Assessment Model approach where athletes complete a neuropsychological assessment before their competitive seasons and test again following concussion with the same assessment to compare baseline scores to postinjury scores.[17] This approach not only provided a starting point for research and generalizations regarding concussions but allowed for clinicians to take an individualistic approach with treatment management.

The modality of neurocognitive assessments has transformed over the years. In the early 1980s, assessments used traditional neuropsychological measures. The development of computerized assessment in the 1990s has guided a shift in neurocognitive assessments. It has now become standard practice for neuropsychologists to use computerized neurocognitive test protocols as part of the evaluation and for baselines.[18] Each approach has its strengths and weaknesses. Traditional paper-pencil testing is reasonably reliable and valid[19–21]; however, it lacks feasibility in a sport setting, particularly when there is a need to acquire large numbers of baseline assessments.[22] Computerized testing on the other hand allows for efficient administration, storage, and access to large numbers of baseline assessments. Computerized testing also has minimal practice effects, given that it allows for multiple versions and randomization of stimuli.[23] Furthermore, computerized testing allows for better accuracy and increased validity when assessing reaction time to within one-hundredth of a second and changes or deficits in cognitive speed.[23] This approach is not without its limitations in that it does not allow for direct observation, only provides a brief snapshot of limited cognitive domains, and if not interpreted by the appropriate individuals may be used incorrectly.[14] Taking these strengths and limitations into consideration, there is support for a hybrid approach of using both paper-pencil and computerized modalities. However, there is a paucity of research regarding the clinical utility of this approach. Regardless of the modality of administration, a comprehensive neuropsychological assessment of SRC is multifaceted in nature. Currently, a complete neuropsychological evaluation of SRC not only includes neurocognitive testing but also a clinical evaluation, symptom inventory, postural/vestibular screen, as well as assessment of emotional functioning.[24–27]

BASELINE TESTING

As previously discussed, the seminal study by Barth and colleagues[12] set the stage for including baseline testing in SRC management. SRC is a clinical diagnosis that has been primarily based on the subjective assessment of a variety of symptoms including somatic, cognitive, emotional, and/or sleep disturbances. It is often evaluated in the absence of loss of consciousness or other neurologic markers. Therefore, using preinjury baseline assessments helps to control for individual differences such as ADHD, various learning delays, cultural/linguistic differences, age, education, and the possible influence of psychiatric issues,[20,28–33] by increasing diagnostic accuracy.[22] There is no universal or standard clinical profile, trajectory of recovery, or type of dysfunction that is always observed.[12,34,35] Each injury is unique to the individual considering preexisting history. Opponents of baseline testing contend that it does not provide any added value beyond normative data and raise concerns related to invalid administration.[36] Baseline assessments are currently instituted as part of a concussion management program in professional sports, colleges, and high schools.[22] However, when baseline data are unavailable, neuropsychologists typically rely on normative-based comparison scores corrected for age, sex, and education to determine any declines.[37]

SYMPTOM INVENTORIES

The assessment and measurement of symptoms is an important component in a comprehensive neuropsychological evaluation of SRC. Perhaps the most commonly used symptom inventory is the Postconcussion Symptom Scale (PCSS).[38] The PCSS is a battery of concussion-related symptoms rated on a severity scale from 0 to 6 with 0 being none and 6 being severe.[39] It has a reported sensitivity of 40.81%, specificity of 79.31%, a positive predictive value of 62.50%, and a negative predictive value of 61.33%.[40] Limitations of the PCSS include the intrinsic subjective nature of a self-reported questionnaire, as well as research revealing a wide range of variability among concussed individuals.[38]

A recently developed symptom inventory, the Concussion Clinical Profile Screening tool (CP Screen), was developed to evaluate concussion-specific symptoms that may reflect established concussion profiles and minimize overlap with other health conditions.[41] A preliminary analysis of the CP Screen revealed high internal consistency of the CP Screen in the control (Cronbach's alpha = .87) and concussed (Cronbach's alpha = .93).[41] Moderate to high correlations among the CP Screen factors and PCSS factors and Vestibular/Ocular Motor Screening (VOMS) items, support concurrent validity. The receiver operating characteristic curve analysis for identifying concussed from controls was also significant ($P<.001$) for all CP Screen factor and modifier scores with excellent areas under the curve (AUCs) for migraine (.93), ocular (.88), vestibular (.85), and cognitive (.81) factors, demonstrating predictive validity.[41] More research is needed to demonstrate the generalizability of these findings.

COMPUTERIZED NEUROPSYCHOLOGICAL ASSESSMENT

A vast amount of studies has found that both traditional and computerized versions of neuropsychological batteries are sensitive to the acute effects of a concussion.[4,23,42–47] Computerized assessments have gained increasing popularity given that they allow for group administration, are scored automatically, and limit the effects of human variability.[18,48]

The Immediate Post-concussion Assessment and Cognitive Test (ImPACT) is a 20- to 25-minute computerized baseline and postconcussion testing battery that has well established reliability and validity for the assessment of symptoms and cognitive functions associated with SRC.[37,49,50] It is regarded as the most commonly used measure in the neurocognitive assessment of SRC.[9] ImPACT is composed of 6 modules, which produce 4 output scores, including verbal memory, reaction time, visual-motor speed, and visual-memory composites.[39] ImPACT has been found to be sensitive to the acute effects of concussion, revealing substantial changes in functioning in the first few days postinjury.[4,51] Pearson test-retest correlation coefficients for the verbal memory, visual memory, reaction time, and processing speed composite scores ranged from 0.65 to 0.86.[4] These coefficients are comparable to or even higher than many other paper-pencil neuropsychological measures.[38] The battery also contains criteria that identifies invalid performances,[52] and the overall sensitivity and specificity have been determined to be 81.9% to 91.4% and 69.1% to 89.4%, respectively.[46] Currently, ImPACT is the most widely used computerized neurocognitive assessment[38]; it is the only neurocognitive assessment that has garnered Food and Drug Administration approval for marketing and is commonly used in high school, collegiate (NCAA), and professional sports (NFL, NBA, MLB, Auto-Racing & USOC) nationally.[51,53]

Other less-widely used computerized neurocognitive assessments for SRC and their limitations include:

HeadMinder, Inc.'s Concussion Resolution Index (CRI) is an online neurocognitive and neurobehavioral assessment tool.[38] The test includes 6 subtests that evaluate the speed of information processing, visual recognition, and reaction time. Past research has observed it to be sensitive (88%) in identifying postconcussion symptoms and resistant to retest effects.[39,54] Limitations include false positives recorded in the protracted phases of recovery[39,54] and no explicit assessment for memory impairment.

CogSport/Axon is composed of series of 7 card tasks measuring 5 composite cognitive domains. These domains are reaction time, decision-making, matching, working memory, and attention. Collie and colleagues[55] found that CogSport reliably measures psychomotor function, decision-making, working memory, and learning. Despite high correlations to paper-pencil neuropsychological tests, there has been considerable variability reported in the specificity and sensitivity of the composite scores.[56]

C3 Logix is composed of 4 neuropsychological tests: Simple Reaction Time, Choice Reaction Time, Trail-Making Difference (Trails A subtracted from Trails B), and Symbol-Digit Modalities.[57] Throughout the literature there has been considerable debate surrounding the tests used in this assessment.[57] Research is limited regarding the psychometric properties of this assessment, and test-retest reliability has only been founded in 2 of the neuropsychological tests used.[58]

Central Nervous System Vital Signs (CNS-VS), initially developed as a routine clinical screening instrument, is composed of 7 tests: visual and verbal memory, finger-tapping, symbol digit coding, the Stroop, continuous performance test, and a test of shifting attention.[59] Its psychometric characteristics are similar to the paper-pencil version of the neurocognitive measures that it is composed of.[59] However, one limitation of CNS-VS is the practice effects, as it has been proved that individuals score significantly better on the second and/or third session when compared with the first on 6 out of the 9 domains.[60]

BRIEF SIDELINE COGNITIVE ASSESSMENTS

Apart from the aforementioned neuropsychological measures, rapid cognitive screening tests have been developed to assess the immediate effects of a head injury.[22,61] One example of a rapid cognitive screening test is the Standardized Assessment of Concussion (SAC).[16] The SAC is a tool developed to identify the effects of mild traumatic brain injury on the sideline and does not require specific training in neuropsychology for the purposes of administration or interpretation. The test assesses orientation, immediate recall, concentration, and delayed recall.[16] The SAC has been shown to have a sensitivity and specificity of 80% to 94% and 76%–91%, respectively.[62] This measure is embedded in the Sport Concussion Assessment Tool (SCAT-5),[63] the most recent revision of a sideline evaluation screening tool. The SCAT-5 includes indications for emergent management, signs of concussion, Glasgow Coma Score, Maddocks questions, rapid neurologic screen, medical health history questions, symptom evaluation, cognitive screen, neck evaluation, balance evaluation, coordination evaluation, and considerations for management and advice.[1] These abbreviated testing paradigms are not to be in replacement of a comprehensive neuropsychological evaluation or used as a standalone measure, it is more appropriately used as a rapid screen for SRC on the sidelines.

NEUROPSYCHOLOGICAL ASSESSMENT OF YOUTH SPORT–RELATED CONCUSSION

There are unique challenges present when assessing and managing SRC in children. When considering neuropsychological assessment in a younger population, children's cognitive, emotional, and physical development must be regarded.[64] Three computerized batteries used in children, are CogSport, The Pediatric ImPACT, and CNS-VS.[22] This modality of assessment works well with this age group, but each test has its strengths and weaknesses.

The Pediatric ImPACT is a computerized assessment battery used in children aged 5 to 12 years. It is one of the few that incorporates developmentally appropriate stimuli and task instructions, factor-derived composite scores, empirically based clinical algorithms, and comprehensive normative data sets. The 6 Pediatric ImPACT neurocognitive subtests are consistent with the original measure with adaptations of instructions, cognitive demands, and stimuli, made to be more appropriate for a younger age range.[53]

ASSESSING VISUAL-MOTOR DEFICITS

A comprehensive neuropsychological assessment of symptoms often includes the evaluation of visual-motor and vestibular deficits. Dysfunction of the vestibular system, including dizziness, balance difficulties, and visual deficits, is commonly seen after concussion.[65] In fact, poor oculomotor function has been reported as one of the most robust discriminators for the identification of mild traumatic brain injury.[66] The visual-motor deficits often reported by such patients include difficulty with saccades, accommodation, smooth pursuit, fixation, reading, and photosensitivity.

The VOMS assessment consists of 5 domains: (1) smooth pursuit, (2) horizontal and vertical saccades, (3) convergence (NPC), (4) horizontal vestibular ocular reflex (VOR), and (5) visual motion sensitivity (VMS).[65] The VOMS has demonstrated internal consistency in identifying concussed patients with a high predicated probability of AUC (0.89) with VOR, VMS, and NPC distance.[65]

Another measure, the King-Devick test, was initially created in 1976 to evaluate horizontal-saccade performance and reading performance and in 2011 became adapted in concussion screening.[67] The assessment takes approximately 2 minutes to administer and is sensitive to vestibulo-ocular changes secondary to concussion (sensitivity = 86%; specificity = 90%).[67,68]

ROLE OF NEUROPSYCHOLOGISTS

Neuropsychologists are key members in a multidisciplinary team in the treatment and management of SRCs. Interpretation of test scores following a neuropsychological evaluation is intricate and requires specialized knowledge about the psychometric properties of assessment (eg, validity, reliability, normative data, base rates, and reliable change).[9,14,22] Additional factors such as culture, preexisting (eg, LD or ADHD), or co-occurring diagnoses (eg, mood symptoms) can influence test performance and the interpretive process of any neuropsychological assessment. Furthermore, the most recent consensus statement highlights the growing body of literature reporting that psychological factors play a significant role in symptom recovery and presentation.[1] A clinical neuropsychologist is specifically trained in conceptualizing the psychological, cognitive, behavioral, physiologic as well as neurologic principals when treating and managing SRCs.[14] Given these multiple factors, it is clear that neuropsychologists are uniquely qualified to interpret assessments and incorporate the data in the treatment and management of concussions.[14,69–71]

CASE STUDY

John Smith is a 15-year-old high school male football player running back that sustained a frontal, helmet-to-helmet hit during the third quarter of a regular season game. Acutely, the athlete reported experiencing dizziness, blurred vision, and an immediate headache. He got up independently, and while attempting to return to the huddle, displayed balance difficulties and confusion (ie, did not comprehend the plays that were being called). He was immediately pulled off the field by the certified athletic trainer (ATC), where the SCAT-5 was completed on the sideline. The rapid screener identified a high likelihood of an SRC. John Smith was removed from the game and recommended to follow with a sport neuropsychologist.

John Smith presented to his initial neuropsychological clinic visit 2 days after the injury. A clinical interview was completed that revealed no prior history of concussion, a personal and family history of motion sickness, as well as a family history of migraines. During this initial visit the athlete reported experiencing constant, daily headaches that worsened during the bus ride to and from school. He also reported dizziness with quick movements, photosensitivity, and mild nausea. During school, he experienced cognitive difficulties particularly with attention, processing speed, and short-term memory. Emotionally, the athlete and his parents endorsed increased irritability. Neurocognitive testing with ImPACT revealed statistically significant deficits in memory (visual and verbal), reaction time, and visual motor speed in comparison to his baseline performance (**Table 1**). The neuropsychologist also completed the VOMS, which revealed deficits; specifically, it was provocative for dizziness. His clinical profile was primarily a vestibular and secondarily a posttraumatic migraine profile.[72]

Table 1
Sample output from computerized neurocognitive testing

Examination	Baseline		Postinjury #1		Postinjury #2		Postinjury #3	
Date Tested	06/30/2018		08/16/2018		08/23/2018		08/31/2018	
Composite Scores (Raw score/Percentile)								
Verbal Memory	99	99%	**62**	**2%**	83	53%	94	88%
Visual Memory	83	75%	**66**	**25%**	61	17%	81	69%
Visual Motor Speed	34.73	43%	**27.03**	**5%**	32.83	32%	44.05	89%
Reaction Time	0.73	9%	**0.81**	**2%**	0.76	6%	0.55	75%
Total Symptom Score	0		**37**		**11**		0	

Values in bold indicate scores that are statistically different from baseline performance.

The overall results of John Smith's initial neuropsychological interview revealed postconcussive symptomatology including physical, emotional, and cognitive symptoms. Given his presentation, it was recommended that he modify his level of physical exertion to include light noncontact, nonrisk exertion (ie, walking, or stationary bike). It was also recommended that he reduce his cognitive activities by providing light accommodations throughout the school day to help manage his symptoms (ie, structured breaks throughout the day and extra time on tests if needed). In addition, John Smith was referred for a formal vestibular evaluation to determine if additional therapy was warranted. In addition, John Smith was introduced to behavioral management strategies to assist with overall recovery and regulation (ie, regulated sleep, diet, hydration, and stress management skills).

The neuropsychologist followed John Smith 1 week after his initial assessment, and he demonstrated improvements in frequency, severity, and duration of his physical symptoms (ie, headache and dizziness), as well as improvement in neurocognitive testing (see **Table 1**). Specifically, ImPACT data revealed 2 out of the 4 domains were below baseline performance and they were both memory composites. He completed one session of vestibular therapy and was performing his provided home exercise plan daily. During this second appointment the neuropsychologist recommended increasing his physical activity from light to moderate levels of noncontact, nonrisk physical exertion (ie, running, weight-training, and independent skills and drills). He was instructed to continue to increase to heavy levels with his ATC throughout the week.

Again, after a 1-week interval John Smith followed with his neuropsychologist for a third and final evaluation. He reported that he was asymptomatic at rest and with graduated physical activity over the past 3 days. Before this final neuropsychological evaluation, John Smith successfully completed an exertion evaluation composed of aerobic activities that both elevated his heart rate and assessed his response to dynamic movements. In addition, he reported that his academic performance in school returned to his baseline and that he was no longer experiencing any difficulties or in need of any accommodations. His neurocognitive performance on ImPACT did not reveal any deficits and all scores were within reliable change of his baseline performance (see **Table 1**). At this evaluation John Smith was cleared to return to full physical and academic activities.

This case study illustrates several key points in the neuropsychological assessment of SRCs. First, it demonstrates how accurate identification and evaluation of symptoms is a crucial initial component of concussion management. Secondly, the utility of baseline neurocognitive assessments and how they are used in a neuropsychological evaluation is demonstrated. Thirdly, the case example illustrates the vital role of the neuropsychologist and neuropsychological assessment in SRC management. Particularly, the computerized neurocognitive testing tools such as ImPACT can help clinicians to appropriately implement individualized treatment plans for the patient to return to school. Neuropsychological evaluation encompasses more than an interpretation of cognitive scores; it involves incorporating preexisting risk factors and postinjury presentation. This multifaceted approach best allows for certainty that the individual has returned to preinjury status before returning to play.

CLINICS CARE POINTS

- Neuropsychological assessment is a valuable component of a comprehensive evaluation of SRC that provides specific and sensitive information regarding the neurobehavioral and neurocognitive functioning of the individual.

- Neuropsychological instruments, whether computerized or paper-pencil, should not be used as a stand-alone method in guiding treatment.
- The interpretation of neurocognitive assessments is complex and should be interpreted by a neuropsychologist who can appropriately incorporate it in an individualized treatment plan.

DISCLOSURE

Dr S. Jennings has nothing to disclose. Dr M.W. Collins does not currently have a conflict of interest with ImPACT but was a board member and co-owner until Dec 16, 2019.

REFERENCES

1. McCrory P, Meeuwisse W, Dvorak J, et al. Consensus statement on concussion in sport—the 5th international conference on concussion in sport held in Berlin, October 2016. Br J Sports Med 2017;51(11):838–47.
2. Giza CC, Hovda DA. The neurometabolic cascade of concussion. J Athl Train 2001;36(3):228.
3. Lovell MR, Iverson GL, Collins MW, et al. Measurement of symptoms following sports-related concussion: reliability and normative data for the post-concussion scale. Appl Neuropsychol 2006;13(3):166–74.
4. Iverson GL, Lovell MR, Collins MW. Interpreting change on ImPACT following sport concussion. Clin Neuropsychol 2003;17(4):460–7.
5. Lovell MR, Collins MW, Iverson GL, et al. Recovery from mild concussion in high school athletes. J Neurosurg 2003;98(2):296–301.
6. Lovell MR, Pardini JE, Welling J, et al. Functional brain abnormalities are related to clinical recovery and time to returnâ€Stoâ€Splay in athletes. Neurosurgery 2007;61(2):352–60.
7. Lezak MD, Howieson DB, Loring DW, et al. Neuropsychological assessment. Oxford University Press; 2004.
8. Webbe FM, Zimmer A. History of neuropsychological study of sport-related concussion. Brain Inj 2014;29(2):129–38.
9. Echemendia RJ, Bruce JM, Meeuwisse W, et al. Can visible signs predict concussion diagnosis in the National Hockey League? Br J Sports Med 2018;52(17): 1149–54.
10. Barr WB, McCrea M. Sensitivity and specificity of standardized neurocognitive testing immediately following sports concussion. J Int Neuropsychol Soc 2001; 7(06):693–702.
11. Gronwall D, Wrightson P. Delayed recovery of intellectual function after minor head injury. Lancet 1974;304(7881):605–9.
12. Barth JT, Alves WM, Ryan TV, et al. Mild head injury in sports: neuropsychological sequelae and recovery of function. Mild Head Injury 1989;257–75.
13. Rimel RW, Giordani B, Barth JT, et al. Disability caused by minor head injury. Neurosurgery 1981;9(3):221–8.
14. Echemendia RJ, Herring S, Bailes J. Who should conduct and interpret the neuropsychological assessment in sports-related concussion? Br J Sports Med 2009;43(Suppl 1):i32–5.
15. Lovell MR, Iverson GL, Collins MW, et al. Does loss of consciousness predict neuropsychological decrements after concussion? Clin J Sport Med 1999;9(4): 193–8.

16. McCrea M. Standardized mental status testing on the sideline after sport-related concussion. J Athl Train 2001;36(3):274.
17. Comper P, Hutchison M, Magrys S, et al. Evaluating the methodological quality of sports neuropsychology concussion research: a systematic review. Brain Inj 2010;24(11):1257–71.
18. Meyer JE, Arnett PA. Changes in Symptoms in concussed and non-concussed athletes following neuropsychological assessment. Dev Neuropsychol 2015; 40(1):24–8.
19. Macciocchi SN, Barth JT, Alves W, et al. Neuropsychological functioning and recovery after mild head injury in collegiate athletes. Neurosurgery 1996;39(3): 510–4.
20. Randolph C. Baseline neuropsychological testing in managing sport-related concussion: does it modify risk? Curr Sports Med Rep 2011;10(1):21–6.
21. Echemendia RJ, Putukian M, Mackin RS, et al. Neuropsychological test performance prior to and following sports-related mild traumatic brain injury. Clin J Sport Med 2001;11(1):23–31.
22. Echemendia RJ, Iverson GL, McCrea M, et al. Advances in neuropsychological assessment of sport-related concussion. Br J Sports Med 2013;47(5):294–8.
23. Johnson EW, Kegel NE, Collins MW. Neuropsychological assessment of sport-related concussion. Clin Sports Med 2011;30(1):73–88.
24. Covassin T, Stearne D, Elbin R III. Concussion history and postconcussion neurocognitive performance and symptoms in collegiate athletes. J Athl Train 2008; 43(2):119–24.
25. Elbin R, Covassin T, Gallion C, et al. Factors influencing risk and recovery from sport-related concussion: reviewing the evidence. SIG 2 Perspectives on Neurophysiology and Neurogenic Speech and Language Disorders 2015;25(1):4–16.
26. Kontos AP, Elbin R, Schatz P, et al. A revised factor structure for the postconcussion symptom scale baseline and postconcussion factors. Am J Sports Med 2012;40(10):2375–84.
27. Moran RN, Covassin T, Elbin R, et al. Reliability and normative reference values for the vestibular/ocular motor screening (VOMS) tool in youth athletes. Am J Sports Med 2018;46(6):1475–80.
28. Arnett P, Meyer J, Merritt V, et al. Neuropsychological testing in mild traumatic brain injury: what to do when baseline testing is not available. Sports Med Arthrosc Rev 2016;24(3):116–22.
29. Benedict C, Parker TM. Baseline concussion testing: a comparison between collision, contact, and non-contact sports. 2014. Honors Projects. 319.
30. Covassin T, Elbin RJ III, Larson E, et al. Sex and age differences in depression and baseline sport-related concussion neurocognitive performance and symptoms. Clin J Sport Med 2012;22(2):98–104.
31. Lichtenstein JD, Moser RS, Schatz P. Age and test setting affect the prevalence of invalid baseline scores on neurocognitive tests. Am J Sports Med 2014;42(2). 0363546513509225.
32. McClure DJ, Zuckerman SL, Kutscher SJ, et al. Baseline neurocognitive testing in sports-related concussions the importance of a prior night's sleep. Am J Sports Med 2014;42(2):472–8.
33. Zuckerman SL, Lee YM, Odom MJ, et al. Baseline neurocognitive scores in athletes with attention deficit–spectrum disorders and/or learning disability: clinical article. J Neurosurg Pediatr 2013;12(2):103–9.
34. Iverson G, Brooks B, Lovell M, et al. No cumulative effects for one or two previous concussions. Br J Sports Med 2006;40(1):72–5.

35. Collins M, Lovell MR, Iverson GL, et al. Examining concussion rates and return to play in high school football players wearing newer helmet technology: a three-year prospective cohort study. Neurosurgery 2006;58(2):275–86.

36. Kontos AP, Sufrinko A, Womble M, et al. Neuropsychological assessment following concussion: an evidence-based review of the role of neuropsychological assessment pre-and post-concussion. Curr Pain Headache Rep 2016; 20(6):38.

37. Covassin T, Elbin R, Nakayama Y. Tracking neurocognitive performance following concussion in high school athletes. Phys sportsmed 2010;38(4):87–93.

38. Dessy AM, Yuk FJ, Maniya AY, et al. Review of assessment scales for diagnosing and monitoring sports-related concussion. Cureus 2017;9(12):e1922.

39. Broglio SP, Ferrara MS, Macciocchi SN, et al. Test-retest reliability of computerized concussion assessment programs. J Athl Train 2007;42(4):509.

40. Lau BC, Collins MW, Lovell MR. Sensitivity and specificity of subacute computerized neurocognitive testing and symptom evaluation in predicting outcomes after sports-related concussion. Am J Sports Med 2011;39(6):1209–16.

41. Kontos AP, Elbin R, Trbovich A, et al. Concussion clinical profiles screening (CP Screen) tool: preliminary evidence to inform a multidisciplinary approach. Neurosurgery 2020;87(2):348–56.

42. Alsalaheen BA, Whitney SL, Marchetti GF, et al. Relationship between cognitive assessment and balance measures in adolescents referred for vestibular physical therapy after concussion. Clin J Sport Med 2015;26(1):46–52.

43. Collins MW, Grindel SH, Lovell MR, et al. Relationship between concussion and neuropsychological performance in college football players. JAMA 1999; 282(10):964–70.

44. Collins MW, Iverson GL, Lovell MR, et al. On-field predictors of neuropsychological and symptom deficit following sports-related concussion. Clin J Sport Med 2003;13(4):222–9.

45. Iverson GL, Gaetz M, Lovell MR, et al. Relation between subjective fogginess and neuropsychological testing following concussion. J Int Neuropsychol Soc 2004; 10(06):904–6.

46. Schatz P, Pardini JE, Lovell MR, et al. Sensitivity and specificity of the ImPACT test battery for concussion in athletes. Arch Clin Neuropsychol 2006;21(1):91–9.

47. Van Kampen DA, Lovell MR, Pardini JE, et al. The 'value added' of neurocognitive testing after sports-related concussion. Am J Sports Med 2006;34(10):1630–5.

48. Collie A, McCrory P, Makdissi M. Does history of concussion affect current cognitive status? Br J Sports Med 2006;40(6):550–1.

49. Anderson M, Elbin R, Dobbs E, Schatz P. Baseline normative data and test-retest reliability of the Vestibular/Ocular Motor Screening (VOMS) Assessment for High School Athletes. Paper presented at: International Journal of Exercise Science: Conference Proceedings (2015Vol. 11, No. 3, p. 30).

50. Elbin R, Kontos AP, Kegel N, et al. Individual and combined effects of LD and ADHD on computerized neurocognitive concussion test performance: evidence for separate norms. Arch Clin Neuropsychol 2013;28(5):476–84.

51. Iverson GL, Schatz P. Advanced topics in neuropsychological assessment following sport-related concussion. Brain Inj 2014;29(2):263–75.

52. Allen BJ, Gfeller JD. The immediate post-concussion assessment and cognitive testing battery and traditional neuropsychological measures: a construct and concurrent validity study. Brain Inj 2011;25(2):179–91.

53. Schatz P, Sandel N. Sensitivity and specificity of the online version of ImPACT in high school and collegiate athletes. Am J Sports Med 2013;41(2):321–6.

54. Broglio SP, Macciocchi SN, Ferrara MS. Sensitivity of the concussion assessment battery. Neurosurgery 2007;60(6):1050–8.
55. Collie A, Maruff P, Makdissi M, et al. CogSport: reliability and correlation with conventional cognitive tests used in postconcussion medical evaluations. Clin J Sport Med 2003;13(1):28–32.
56. Gardner A, Shores EA, Batchelor J, et al. Diagnostic efficiency of ImPACT and CogSport in concussed rugby union players who have not undergone baseline neurocognitive testing. Appl Neuropsychol Adult 2012;19(2):90–7.
57. Masterson CJ, Tuttle J, Maerlender A. Confirmatory factor analysis of two computerized neuropsychological test batteries: immediate post-concussion assessment and cognitive test (ImPACT) and C3 logix. J Clin Exp Neuropsychol 2019; 41(9):925–32.
58. Simon M, Maerlender A, Metzger K, et al. Reliability and concurrent validity of select C3 logix test components. Dev Neuropsychol 2017;42(7–8):446–59.
59. Gualtieri CT, Johnson LG. Reliability and validity of a computerized neurocognitive test battery, CNS Vital Signs. Arch Clin Neuropsychol 2006;21(7):623–43.
60. Littleton AC, Register-Mihalik JK, Guskiewicz KM. Test-retest reliability of a computerized concussion test: CNS vital signs. Sports health 2015;7(5):443–7.
61. McCrea M, Kelly JP, Randolph C, et al. Immediate neurocognitive effects of concussion. Neurosurgery 2002;50(5):1032–42.
62. Guskiewicz KM. Balance assessment in the management of sport-related concussion. Clin Sports Med 2011;30(1):89–102.
63. Echemendia RJ, Meeuwisse W, McCrory P, et al. The sport concussion assessment tool 5th edition (SCAT5): background and rationale. Br J Sports Med 2017;51(11):848–50.
64. Baillargeon A, Lassonde M, Leclerc S, et al. Neuropsychological and neurophysiological assessment of sport concussion in children, adolescents and adults. Brain Inj 2012;26(3):211–20.
65. Mucha A, Collins MW, Elbin R, et al. A brief vestibular/ocular motor screening (VOMS) assessment to evaluate concussions preliminary findings. Am J Sports Med 2014;42(10):2479–86, 0363546514543775.
66. Tjarks BJ, Dorman JC, Valentine VD, et al. Comparison and utility of King-Devick and ImPACT® composite scores in adolescent concussion patients. J Neurol Sci 2013;334(1–2):148–53.
67. Breedlove KM, Ortega JD, Kaminski TW, et al. King-Devick test reliability in national collegiate athletic association athletes: a national collegiate athletic association–department of defense concussion assessment, research and education report. J athl Train 2019;54(12):1241–6.
68. Vartiainen M, Holm A, Peltonen K, et al. King Devick test normative reference values for professional male ice hockey players. Scand J Med Sci Sports 2014; 25(3):e327–30.
69. Amin DJ, Coleman J, Herrington LC. The test-retest reliability and minimal detectable change of the balance error scoring system. J Sports Sci 2014;2:200–7.
70. Harmon KG, Clugston JR, Dec K, et al. American Medical Society for Sports Medicine position statement on concussion in sport. Br J Sports Med 2019;53(4):213–25.
71. Schneider KJ, Iverson GL, Emery CA, et al. The effects of rest and treatment following sport-related concussion: a systematic review of the literature. Br J Sports Med 2013;47(5):304–7.
72. Kontos AP, Sufrinko A, Sandel N, et al. Sport-related concussion clinical profiles: clinical characteristics, targeted treatments, and preliminary evidence. Curr Sports Med Rep 2019;18(3):82–92.

Rehabilitation of Sport-Related Concussion

Mohammad Nadir Haider, MD[a], Lenore Herget, PT, DPT, SCS, MEd, CSCS[b],
Ross D. Zafonte, DO[c], Adam G. Lamm, MD[c], Bonnie M. Wong, MD[c],
John J. Leddy, MD[a,*]

KEYWORDS

- Sport-related concussion • Rehabilitation • Exercise tolerance
- Sub–symptom threshold exercise prescription

KEY POINTS

- Older guidelines for sport-related concussion (SRC) recommended strict rest until symptom resolution. However, emerging research is identifying causes for many post-SRC symptoms based on the predominant symptom generators identified on physical examination.
- The most recent International Concussion in Sport Group guidelines recommend a multidisciplinary team approach to SRC treatment. This article introduces clinicians to a systematic approach to SRC assessment and treatment based on a pertinent physical examination.
- The physical examination assessment of SRC for the purposes of guided physical rehabilitation is focused on the autonomic, ocular, vestibular, and cervical subsystems and, where indicated, assessment of exercise tolerance. These clinical profiles rarely exist in isolation and often overlap.
- The approach to SRC assessment and treatment is undergoing a paradigm shift. This article presents the current evidence base to inform best practice by providers.

INTRODUCTION

Most adult patients with sport-related concussion (SRC) recover spontaneously within 7 to 14 days, whereas adolescents may require up to 4 weeks to recover; however, some take significantly longer.[1] SRC is a complex disorder that the most recent

[a] UBMD Orthopaedics and Sports Medicine, Concussion Management Clinic and Research Center, State University of New York at Buffalo, 160 Farber Hall, Buffalo, NY 14214, USA;
[b] Massachusetts General Hospital, MGH Sports Medicine, New England Patriots, Boston Bruins, Boston Celtics, New England Revolution and Boston Red Sox, 55 Fruit Street, Boston, MA 02114, USA; [c] Department of Physical Medicine and Rehabilitation, Spaulding Rehabilitation Hospital, Massachusetts General Hospital, Brigham and Women's Hospital, Harvard Medical School, 25 Shattuck Street, Boston, MA 02115, USA
* Corresponding author.
E-mail address: leddy@buffalo.edu

Clin Sports Med 40 (2021) 93–109
https://doi.org/10.1016/j.csm.2020.08.003
0278-5919/21/© 2020 Elsevier Inc. All rights reserved.

Concussion in Sport Group (CISG) international guidelines state is one of the most challenging diseases to diagnose and manage.[1] There is no gold-standard treatment of SRC so treatment modalities must be individualized based on the predominant symptom generators.[2] It is important to identify the cause for SRC symptoms because they can vary and evolve over different time frames.[3–5] Some investigators have categorized SRC into the following clinical profiles: physiologic, cervicogenic, vestibulo-ocular, and mood related.[6,7] Clinically, these profiles rarely exist in isolation and often overlap.[8] **Fig. 1** summarizes the nonpharmacologic treatment modalities for each SRC clinical profile, which are described in detail later. This article introduces clinicians to a systematic approach to SRC assessment and evidence-based, nonpharmacologic rehabilitation. Pharmacologic therapies are discussed (See article "Medical Therapies for Concussion" by Jacob C. Jones and Michael J. O'Brien) in this issue. There are no pathophysiologic findings specific to mood-related SRC.[8] The management of this clinical profile is challenging because of the extensive overlap with symptoms of preexisting primary mood disorders, and treatment involves symptom-specific pharmacologic and nonpharmacologic therapies. The CISG guidelines recommend a multidisciplinary team approach to treatment.[1] Assessment and treatment of the neuropsychological aspects of SRC is also discussed elsewhere in this issue. Posttraumatic headaches are also common after SRC; the medical management of these is discussed elsewhere in this issue.

ASSESSMENT

The physical examination assessment of SRC for the purposes of guided physical rehabilitation is focused on the ocular, vestibular, and cervical subsystems and, where indicated, assessment of exercise tolerance. A recent study showed that early

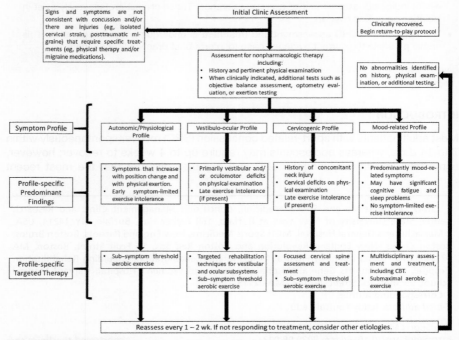

Fig. 1. Clinical management of concussion profiles. Symptom profiles frequently overlap after concussion and it is possible for patients to require more than 1 type of therapy. CBT, cognitive behavior therapy.

assessment and intervention for the clinical profiles of SRC resulted in better out-comes versus delayed evaluation.[9]

Assessment for Ocular Dysfunction

The incidence of oculomotor dysfunction after mild traumatic brain injury (mTBI) can be substantial, with some investigators estimating it to be present in up to 70% of pa-tients.[10] However, the incidence has been reported to vary from 9% to 90%.[11–13] The variability stems from the sensitivity of the measurement tools used to identify ocular dysfunction. Impairments in smooth pursuits, saccades, alignment, vergence (conver-gence and divergence), and accommodation have been reported, which can be detected using standard physical assessment techniques.[7] After taking a history, including mechanism of injury, a thorough binocular functional vision examination should be completed that highlights eye tracking skills (smooth pursuits and sac-cades) and eye teaming/focusing skills (vergence and accommodation).

Eye tracking smooth pursuits
Eye tracking smooth pursuits can be examined with a simple H, I, or X test where a target is moved slowly in the formation of the letter and the examiner observes for any sustained nystagmus (fatigable nystagmus is normal), difficulty with gaze holding, and accuracy.

Eye tracking saccades
The patient is asked to visually track an object moving slowly in the horizontal direction with the head stationary. Target movement should be limited to 30° from the midline to avoid eliciting end-gaze nystagmus. Abnormal is sustained nystagmus, staccatic (or jerking) eye motion, loss of conjugate vision, corrective (catch-up or backup) sac-cades, loss of visual fixation, or symptom provocation (dizziness, nausea, or headache).

Repetitive saccades
The examiner holds both index fingers 0.5 m apart at half an arm length from the pa-tient. The patient is instructed to move the eyes side to side in rapid succession in the horizontal plane, rapidly switching focus between the examiner's 2 index fingers. The test may be repeated in the vertical plane as well. Abnormal responses include delayed initiation of eye movement, slow velocity, or inaccurate movements such as overshooting/undershooting with greater than 1 refixation saccade.[14] Abnormal movements or symptom provocation qualify as abnormal responses. Patients are considered to have healthy function when they can do 20 repetitions with normal ve-locity and accuracy without eliciting symptoms of headache, dizziness, or nausea. This test in the healthy population can sometimes elicit eye strain but should not pro-voke symptoms of increased headache or dizziness.

Eye teaming/focusing
Eye teaming skills are necessary for depth perception to coordinate eye movements as objects move closer to or further away from the person. Vergence is the simulta-neous movement of both eyes in opposite directions to obtain or maintain single binocular vision as objects move toward (convergence) or away from the person (divergence). Near point convergence (NPC) can be measured by placing a standard accommodation ruler at the forehead just above the patient's nose. Starting at a point where the patient can easily focus on the target (20–30 cm from nose), the patient is asked to focus on the target as it is moved slowly toward the face. As soon as the pa-tient reports splitting of the target in 2, the NPC distance is recorded to the nearest

0.5 cm. Ideally, this should be performed 3 times and the better recording reported. This distance should be less than 10 cm in the general population,[15] and less than 6 cm in children and adolescents.[16] Note that the NPC is not taken where the target blurs but where it splits. Accommodation (monocular vision) is also measured to the nearest 0.5 cm using the same ruler and is acquired over 2 trials for each eye. The patient is instructed to cover 1 eye and, starting at the furthest distance away from the nose, the target is moved slowly toward the face. Accommodation distance is determined when the patient reports blurring (not doubling) of the image. A value of greater than or equal to 12 cm is considered to be abnormal.[16]

A more objective and thorough assessment of ocular function is possible using computerized eye tracking software.[17–19] This technology, which includes a combination of high-speed cameras and infrared sensors, evaluates predictive attention performance and synchronization in the spatial and temporal domains, both of which can be impaired after SRC.[20]

Assessment for Vestibular Dysfunction

SRC often produces symptoms of dizziness, headache, nausea, visual motion sensitivity, vertigo, feeling disconnected from the environment, and/or feeling off balance.[21] There is significant interaction of the vestibular and oculomotor systems; for example, intact binocular visual function is essential to normal vestibular function,[22] so the symptoms of injuries to both often overlap or reinforce one another. It is important to remember that dynamic vestibular examinations should not be performed until significant cervical dysfunction has first been ruled out or treated. It is thought that most vestibular dysfunction after SRC is central (brainstem or cerebellar), although peripheral injury can on occasion be observed.[23]

Vestibulo-ocular reflex

The vestibulo-ocular reflex (VOR) integrates the vestibular and oculomotor systems by testing the ability to keep an image centered on the fovea during horizontal and vertical head motion. The patient is asked to maintain visual fixation on the examiner's finger located directly in the frontal-central field of vison, held approximately 30 cm from the nose, while rotating the head as rapidly as possible for at least 10 complete turns. Inability to maintain visual fixation (ie, beating back to the center) and/or symptom provocation of headache, dizziness, or lightheadedness is abnormal. The VOR is often impaired after SRC so that head movement at speeds necessary ($\geq$2 Hz) for daily activities causes dizziness, nausea, or blurred vision.[7,24] The head thrust maneuver is another method to assess VOR dysfunction.[25] It involves a rapid twisting motion of the neck rather than active patient-initiated motion, so it should be performed only after a significant cervical injury has been ruled out by an experienced practitioner.

Dynamic visual acuity

Static visual acuity measured with a Snellen or handheld eye chart provides a baseline of visual acuity without head motion. Using the same eye chart, the patient is instructed to read the lowest line on the chart while performing horizontal head rotation at greater than or equal to 2 Hz. The difference in line numbers on the eye chart between stationary (static) versus head motion (dynamic) should be no more than 1 to 3 lines for the healthy population, and less than 2 lines in higher-level athletes.[26] Visually complex environments are more difficult to maintain a functioning VOR; therefore, the dynamic visual acuity (DVA) should be tested in a calm environment.

Static and dynamic balance

Static balance is assessed by tandem stance. The patient puts hands on the hips and 1 foot is planted directly in front of the other, attempting to hold it for 20 seconds with eyes closed. Dynamic balance is assessed using tandem gait, eyes open and closed. The patient is asked to walk in a straight line for 5 steps eyes open, heel to toe, hands at the side, while looking straight ahead at a fixed point on the wall. The patient then continues for 5 steps with eyes closed. The patient then walks backward with eyes open, toe to heel, along the same line for 5 steps. The patient then repeats this with eyes closed. Inability to walk the line, stumbling, or stepping out of line while walking forward, backward, or during tandem stance is abnormal.[27] More objective methods of assessing balance include adding a dynamic component as well as a cognitive dual task.[28] Balance and gait assessment technologies, which are more reliable than clinician-performed techniques, are also available but require specialized equipment and may be expensive.[29]

Less often, athletes injure the peripheral vestibular system when they sustain a concussion. In contrast, they may have an isolated vestibular injury without concussion, such as benign paroxysmal positional vertigo (BPPV).[30] BPPV is assessed through a variety of head and body positions, most commonly the Dix-Hallpike maneuver.[30] In addition, proper balance assessment must include a cervical examination (described later). The postural control system relies on multiple inputs from the somatosensory/proprioceptive organs in the extremities and the cervical muscles and joints, as well as from the vestibular and visual systems.[31] This complex interplay allows people to maintain head and body position, perceive motion, stabilize gaze, control eye movements, and orient themselves in space. Cervical injury affects cervical afferents and the proprioceptive system of mechanoreceptors, including muscle spindles, joint position receptors, and Golgi tendon organs,[31] which can cause dizziness of cervical origin, called cervicogenic dizziness.[32] Unlike vertigo, which is typically associated with a spinning or motion sensation, cervicogenic dizziness is commonly described as feelings of disorientation and unsteadiness exacerbated by neck motion. Injuries to the cervical spine and associated myofascial pain often cause restricted cervical motion, which can further cause feelings of unsteadiness.[33]

Assessment for Cervical Dysfunction

There are numerous structures in the neck that may generate pain following a concussive head injury, including the cervical zygapophyseal (facet) joints, bony structures, parascapular muscles, ligamentous structures, and nerve entrapments.[34] The C1 nerve (suboccipital nerve) provides innervation to the atlanto-occipital joint, with pain commonly referred to the posterior occiput.[35] The C2 nerve passes in close proximity to the atlantoaxial joint and innervates it and the C2-C3 zygapophyseal joint.[36] The C3 nerve also innervates the C2-C3 zygapophyseal joint, which can refer pain to the frontotemporal and periorbital regions of the head, and is thought to be involved in up to 70% of cervicogenic headaches.[37]

The evaluation of neck pain following SRC should include a comprehensive history and a physical examination. A detailed history of neck pain is important because different cervical disorders cause different patterns of pain specific to the particular muscles that are disrupted through the biomechanics of the injury.[38] These pain syndromes are treated with a combination of focused physical therapy strengthening exercises, manual therapy, myofascial release, and/or trigger point injections individualized to the disorder. Cervical physical examination includes palpation and range-of-motion assessment. A palpatory examination should evaluate the rhomboids, trapezii, infraspinatus, supraspinatus, and cervical paraspinal musculature, with a particular focus on the splenius cervicis and splenius capitis, because both are common myofascial pain generators.[39] Range of motion includes flexion, extension, lateral rotation, and lateral flexion of the neck. The strength of both the sternocleidomastoids and the shoulder elevators (trapezii) should be noted, because both reflect the integrity of the spinal accessory nerve (cranial nerve XI). Listening for carotid or cavernous bruits is warranted in some cases.

One of the primary objectives of cervical assessment is to screen for any red flag signs or symptoms that warrant further evaluation. These signs include myotomal weakness or sensory loss in a dermatomal pattern, change in bowel/bladder function, or the presence of the Spurling or Lhermitte sign, all of which may indicate the presence of a radiculopathy or myelopathy.[40] The Spurling test for cervical radiculopathy is best viewed as confirmatory rather than as a screening test because of its high specificity and low sensitivity.[41] In patients with cervical instability, these tests should be performed with caution because of the provocative stress required. The presence of the Hoffmann reflex may suggest an upper motor neuron lesion in the brain, brainstem, or cervical spinal cord, although it may be a normal finding in a subset of healthy patients who are generally diffusely hyper-reflexic.[42,43] A positive Wallenberg (vertebral artery test) test may indicate vertebrobasilar insufficiency and warrants further investigation.[44]

Cervical posttraumatic disorders

Injuries to the cervical spine may occur in patients who sustain head trauma, with or without a concussion. The same acceleration-deceleration forces that are transmitted to the brain can be transferred to the neck, causing excessive extension-flexion of the neck and concomitant whiplash injury. Injuries to the cervical spine include sprain-strain and joint injuries that can cause symptoms similar to those of SRC.[45]

Cervical strain and sprain injuries Cervical strain and sprain are the cause of most acute neck pain after whiplash injuries.[46] Cervical strain refers to injury to the muscles or tendons, whereas cervical sprain refers to overstretching or tearing of the spinal ligaments.[47] Acceleration-deceleration forces can cause the cervical spine to take on an S-shaped curvature. As the neck flexes forward, the posterior neck extensors are prone to injury as they eccentrically contract to decelerate the head.[48] This contraction can strain the levator scapulae, superior trapezius, sternocleidomastoid, scalene, and suboccipital muscles.[49] The anterior longitudinal ligament merges with the intervertebral disc, injury to which can be associated with injuries to the cervical disc. Patients with cervical strain and sprain injuries may have tension-type headaches typically described as a dull, pressure pain located on both sides of the head.[50] On examination, there may be pain to palpation of the muscles with limited range of motion and muscle guarding. When clinically warranted, radiographs of the cervical spine with flexion and extension views may be obtained to evaluate for bony abnormalities or to rule out acute instability before initiation of treatment.

Cervical myofascial pain syndrome Myofascial pain syndrome refers to pain generated from a palpable taut band of hypercontracted muscle fiber called a myofascial trigger point that causes referred pain.[38] Myofascial trigger points are categorized as active if they cause pain spontaneously, or latent if they are painful only on palpation. The underlying mechanism that causes myofascial trigger points is unknown but is thought to involve muscular overuse or overload. Pain is often described as dull, deep, diffuse, aching, or a soreness. As mentioned earlier, physical examination should focus on palpation of rhomboids, trapezii, infraspinatus, supraspinatus, and the cervical paraspinal musculature, particularly the splenius cervicis and splenius capitis, because these are all common myofascial pain generators.

Cervical-joint pain After a whiplash-type injury, the cervical zygapophyseal (facet) joints have been shown to be among the most common sources of pain.[51] Reports indicate that up to 60% of cases of posttraumatic neck pain involve the facet joints alone or in combination with injury to the cervical intervertebral discs.[52] Other studies have shown that 58% to 88% of patients with chronic facet joint pain complain of cervicogenic headaches.[53] Branches of the C1 and C2 ventral rami innervate the atlanto-occipital (C0-C1) and atlanto-axial joints (C1-C2), whereas medial branches from the cervical dorsal rami innervate the cervical facet joints. Injury to the facet joints during a whiplash injury is likely secondary to excessive compression of the facet joints and capsular ligament sprain.[54] Cervical facet joint–mediated pain is commonly described as dull and achy with particular referral patterns to the head, neck, and periscapular regions. Pain from the C1-C2 joint tends to refer to the occipital and suboccipital region but can also be referred to the vertex, orbit, and ear. Pain from C2-C3 facet joints refers to the occipital region, but can also spread to the parietal, frontal, and orbital regions. Pain from C3-C4 and C4-5 facet joints more commonly refers to the upper and lateral cervical region. The C5-6 facet joint produces pain over the supraspinatus fossa of the scapula, whereas C6-C7 facet joints typically produce pain over the scapula. However, there are no clinical examination findings that are diagnostic specifically for cervical facet joint pain.

Cervical disc pain Cervical intervertebral discs can be injured in conjunction with the facet joints. There can be internal disc disruption, which is damage of the internal nucleus pulposus or annular fibers without evidence of external deformation. More significant injury can lead to cervical disc herniation, which can be described as protrusion, extrusion, or sequestration.[55] Patients complain primarily of axial, bilateral paravertebral, occipital, or scapular pain that is exacerbated by activities that increase intradiscal pressure, such as prolonged sitting, coughing, sneezing, or lifting. When examining patients, it is always important to do a thorough neuromuscular examination to exclude myelopathy or radiculopathy. It is notable that many disc abnormalities seen on imaging are not associated with pain or physical examination findings; they reflect the normal aging process of the cervical spine.[56]

A 2016 Delphi study by Luedtke and colleagues[57] concluded that the most useful techniques used by physical therapists for patients with headache include the craniocervical flexion test, cervical flexion rotation test, active range of cervical movement, trigger point palpation, muscle tests of the shoulder girdle, passive physiologic intervertebral movements, thoracic spine screening, and combined movement tests. The cervical flexion rotation test, smooth-pursuit neck torsion test, and cervical-joint reposition error test have been shown to have high reliability and strong diagnostic accuracy for diagnosing cervicogenic headache, which is often a comorbid contributor or sole cause of headache in this patient population.[58–60] These tests attempt to minimize visual and vestibular factors while targeting cervical position and movement-sensory information to help isolate cervical disorder. The cervical-joint reposition error test identifies damage to muscle spindles in the neck, whereas the smooth-pursuit neck torsion test is used to identify cervico-ocular disturbances.[61] The right and left alar ligament tests assess the integrity of the upper cervical spine using lateral flexion, which has been validated to significantly increase the length of the contralateral alar ligament.[62] The transverse ligament integrity of the cervical spine is assessed using the Sharp Purser test.[63,64]

Assessment for Exercise Tolerance

Exercise intolerance, the inability to exercise to age-appropriate maximum because of exacerbation of concussion-like symptoms, is a characteristic of SRC.[65] This exacerbation is suspected to be caused by abnormalities in the autonomic nervous system that lead to abnormal cerebral blood flow (CBF) regulation.[65] Exercise intolerance is associated with symptoms such as cognitive fatigue, headaches, and balance problems.[66] The degree of exercise intolerance can assist in identifying symptom generators after SRC. Early exercise intolerance (defined as symptom exacerbation at <70% of age-appropriate maximum heart rate) is characteristic of autonomic/physiologic dysfunction in SRC, which is thought to reflect abnormal autonomic control of CBF during exercise.[67]

The safety of exercise tolerance testing after SRC has been assessed in several studies. The Bruce treadmill protocol was used to safely assess exercise tolerance within 5 to 7 days of SRC, and the degree of exercise intolerance was associated with increased recovery time.[68] Similarly, the McMaster All-Out Progressive Continuous Cycling Test was used to assess exercise tolerance after mTBI.[69] Although there was an increase in symptoms on the day of the test, patients improved significantly within 24 hours, and temporary symptom exacerbation was not associated with negative outcomes.[69] In addition, in a randomized controlled trial (RCT), Leddy and colleagues[70] assigned adolescents within 10 days of SRC to perform the Buffalo Concussion Treadmill Test (BCTT) or not and tracked symptoms daily for 2 weeks. There was no significant difference in daily symptoms or recovery duration between the 2 cohorts. Thus, exercise testing is safe to perform in the acute period after SRC provided the patient is not pushed past the point of significant symptom exacerbation. This study also showed that greater early exercise intolerance (ie, the lower the heart rate at symptom exacerbation on the BCTT) was associated with longer duration of recovery. This relationship was subsequently validated in 3 separate cohorts by Haider and colleagues,[71] providing further evidence for the usefulness of exercise tolerance testing. The BCTT is the preferred exercise tolerance assessment protocol because it has been designed for patients with concussion, and its safety and reliability have been validated in patients with SRC.[72] There is now a cycle ergometer version of the BCTT, the Buffalo Concussion Bike Test, which is recommended for patients with orthopedic injuries or significant balance dysfunction that may prevent safely walking on a treadmill.[73]

Considerations for exertion testing

Before ordering any exertion test, patients must be screened for contraindications to exercise, including significant orthopedic or cervical injury, balance problems, or cardiovascular issues. A complete list of contraindications to exertion testing is provided in the American Heart Association guideline for exercise testing.[74] Patients should wear a reliable heart rate monitor because it is important to know the threshold heart rate when symptoms increase. Any increase in concussion-like symptoms is abnormal, defining exercise intolerance. Significant exercise intolerance to terminate the test occurs when symptoms increase by 3 or more points from baseline (a point or more given for symptom increase or appearance of a new symptom).[75] Termination of the test because of voluntary exhaustion, or achievement of 85% to 90% of age-appropriate maximum heart rate, defines normal exercise tolerance. It is hypothesized that early exercise intolerance (test termination because of symptom exacerbation at <70% of age-predicted maximum) is characteristic of physiologic dysfunction from concussion and portends a worse prognosis.[70,71] Exercise cessation beyond 70% of age-predicted maximum heart rate is consistent with near or complete recovery from global metabolic dysfunction,[70] or with patients whose symptoms have been identified to emanate from a cervical or vestibulo-ocular disorder.[76]

REHABILITATION

Multimodal sub-system impairment-based therapies that are individualized to the patient, including oculomotor, vestibular, and cervical therapies, as well as sub–symptom threshold aerobic exercise, have been associated with a reduced incidence of persistent symptoms.[77,78] Most impairments in the vestibular and ocular systems recover spontaneously without treatment;[1] however, if these impairments do not resolve by 2 weeks in adults or by 3 to 4 weeks in adolescents, patients should be referred to an appropriate clinician for focused treatment.[79] Cervical injury or aerobic exercise intolerance can be treated as soon as possible because there is evidence that early intervention improves patient outcome.[61,80,81]

Ocular Rehabilitation

After identifying the presence and degree of impairments using physical examination techniques, specific treatments can be prescribed.

Repetitive saccades

Patients are instructed to put 2 targets (eg, Post-it notes) on the wall 0.5 m apart horizontally and vertically, and stand 0.5 m away. While keeping the head still, the patient looks back and forth from each target. Patients start with the number of repetitions that cause symptoms plus 3 more to increase task stamina, then take a brief rest and repeat until they have completed 1 minute of horizontal and vertical saccades each. Patients should advance by 3 to 5 repetitions every 1 to 2 days with an eventual goal of 120 Hz (1 Hz for moving from 1 target to the other) without symptom provocation.

Static fixation

For static fixation, patients are instructed to put 3 beads on a string (Brock string): 1 on the end, 1 in the middle, and 1 as close to the nose as possible but still in focus. Patients start by looking at the farthest, then the middle, then the closest. The goal is to keep each bead in focus (clear, not blurry or double). As patients improve with training, they move the closest bead closer to the nose while keeping it clear, with the goal of getting it within 6 cm from the nose without diplopia.

Dynamic fixation

Patients are instructed to perform pencil pushups. The patient holds a pen at an arm's length away and focuses on a single point (eg, some letters on the pen) while slowly (~1 cm/s) bringing the pen closer to the nose and attempting to keep it in focus. When the letters blur, the patient continues until the letters become double. The patient then brings the pen back out until it becomes single and clear again. This process is repeated for at least 1 minute until the patient is able to keep the letters in focus within 6 cm from the nose.

To increase compliance with these exercises, there are multiple smartphone/tablet app-based protocols, approved and recommended by the College of Optometrists in Vision Development, that are easily accessible with built-in parameters for progression.[82]

Vestibular Rehabilitation

In an RCT by Schneider and colleagues,[83] 25 patients with SRC were randomized to either manual cervical therapy (placebo) or manual cervical therapy plus vestibular rehabilitation. Patients in the manual cervical therapy plus vestibular rehabilitation group were medically cleared to return to sports at a much faster rate. Vestibular rehabilitation includes techniques to improve gaze stabilization and dynamic balance. Some patients have a concomitant BPPV after SRC and may require a physical therapist to supervise habituation and desensitization exercises and/or perform canalith repositioning maneuvers.

Gaze stabilization

Patients are instructed to practice focusing on a target while turning the head from side to side, then up and down. The goal is to improve until the head moves 20° to 30° in each direction at greater than or equal to 2 Hz with precise focus (no blurriness) or symptom provocation. Often this means starting at a lower level and making accommodations to achieve perfect visual focus without symptoms; for example, using a larger target in a visually simplistic environment and moving the head at a slower speed (using a metronome helps) until the desired level is achieved.

For patients with visual motion sensitivity or visual vertigo, habituation exercises to desensitize provocative visual environments are beneficial for symptom management and clear vision.[79] To improve balance, minimizing visual input and maximizing vestibular and somatosensory input with challenges to posture, center of gravity, base of support, and head/body movement has been shown to be effective.[83]

Cervical Rehabilitation

The management of cervical strain with cervicalgia is designed to reduce local inflammation and muscle spasm, restore range of motion, and recalibrate communication between the cervical spine and the vestibular and oculomotor systems. This outcome requires a tailored cervical spine rehabilitation program that includes manual therapy, passive and active range-of-motion exercises, low-velocity mobilizations, proprioceptive retraining, and exercises to strengthen the deep and superficial cervical musculature.[84] Empirical support for this approach is provided by the Schneider and colleagues[83] RCT (described earlier), as well as observational studies showing improved pain and sensorimotor outcomes in patients with whiplash treated with multimodal cervical spine rehabilitation.[85,86] In addition, a recent review concluded that rehabilitation programs that use cervical spine mobilization and manipulation techniques are effective for cervicogenic headaches.[87] Patients with severe whiplash-type injuries who develop persistent cervicogenic headaches and occipital neuralgia may benefit from pharmacologic management and occipital nerve injections.[88] Patients with predominantly cervical symptoms typically do not experience an early symptom-limited threshold on graded aerobic exercise testing and so may exercise to prevent aerobic deconditioning.

Sub–symptom Exercise Rehabilitation

The treatment of SRC has changed significantly in recent years. Emerging research has shown that mild symptom exacerbation does not damage the brain and may be essential to helping patients recover from SRC.[89] Prolonged rest causes physical deconditioning and impairs CBF regulation,[90] whereas regular exercise is known to improve CBF control.[91] Exercise is known to reduce concussion symptom burden,[92] and improves sleep problems[93] and mental alertness.[94] Several recent RCTs and well-designed experimental trials have shown the benefit of this approach.[80,95–98] Although subsymptomatic aerobic exercise seems to be beneficial for SRC, it is crucial to remember that patients should be cautioned that intense exercise performed soon after injury can increase symptoms and prolong recovery.[89,99] In an animal study by

Griesbach and colleagues,[100] rats with simulated concussion who were allowed to exercise voluntarily showed improved cognitive performance versus those that were forced to exercise. This study highlights the importance of a correct dose of exercise for SRC rehabilitation.

If exercise tolerance testing is available, an individualized sub–symptom threshold aerobic exercise prescription can be provided. Patients are instructed to exercise to symptom exacerbation or for at least 20 minutes a day at 80% to 90% of the heart rate achieved on the treadmill test. Patients typically return every 1 to 2 weeks to reassess exercise tolerance for a new heart rate prescription.[80] If exercise tolerance testing is not available, a more conservative approach for prescribing exercise should be used to not exacerbate symptoms beyond rehabilitative value. Patients with SRC can calculate their age-appropriate maximum heart rates using the Karvonen equation[101] (maximum heart rate = 220 − age in years) and begin exercising at 50% of their maximum using a heart rate monitor. If the patient is able to tolerate this intensity of exercise without worsening of symptoms, it may be possible to increase the target heart rate by 5 to 10 beats/min the subsequent day. If the patient begins to feel symptomatic, the patient should perform aerobic exercise below that level until able to tolerate higher intensities. It is of paramount importance to caution patients to avoid sustained exercise above the symptom-exacerbation threshold because it may be detrimental to recovery.[89,99]

Aerobic exercise is recommended rather than resistance exercise (eg, rowing and weight lifting) because the concussed brain is intolerant of wide swings in blood pressure. The authors recommend stationary biking to begin with because it is safe and minimizes head motion. If tolerated, the patient may advance to brisk walking or jogging, either on a treadmill or outside. Swimming is an ideal form of aerobic exercise but patients may find it hard to actively monitor heart rate, although water jogging with a flotation device would be acceptable. Similarly, outdoor biking is not recommended to begin with because patients with vestibular dysfunction may be at risk for high-velocity falls. Delayed recovery from SRC despite return of good exercise tolerance should prompt the clinician to evaluate other potential symptom generators (eg, oculomotor, vestibular, cervical, mood, or migraine disorders). In cases where the lowest exercise prescription elicits significant symptom exacerbation, physical rest is indicated.[1] Patients are encouraged to keep a daily diary of exercise performance and symptoms.

CLEARANCE AND RETURN TO PLAY

The 2016 Berlin CISG guideline defines clinical functional recovery as a return to normal activities, including school, work, and sport.[1] Operationally, this means that the athlete has returned to a baseline level of symptoms with a normal neurologic examination, including an assessment of oculomotor function and balance.[102] Athletes should have returned to normal school participation before returning to sport. As outlined in the Berlin CISG guideline, the recovery process and return to sport participation after SRC follows a graduated stepwise rehabilitation strategy of increasing tolerance to exercise and sport skills. The athlete proceeds to the next level when criteria (activity, heart rate, duration of exercise) are met without recurrence of concussion-related symptoms. In general, in younger and nonprofessional athletes, each step requires 24 hours so that it takes approximately 1 week to proceed through the full return-to-play (RTP) protocol once they have been declared recovered at rest.[1] However, in professional athletes, the rate of progression through the RTP protocol may be modified to the individual to speed recovery and may progress through more than 1 stage a day.[103] The time frame for RTP varies with player age, concussion history, and level of sport.

DISCLOSURE

The authors have nothing to disclose.

REFERENCES

1. McCrory P, Meeuwisse W, Dvorak J, et al. Consensus statement on concussion in sport—the 5th international conference on concussion in sport held in Berlin, October 2016. Br J Sports Med 2017;51(11):838–47.
2. Haider MN, Willer B, Leddy J, et al. Multidisciplinary assessment and treatment. In: Silver JM, McAllister TW, Arciniegas DB, editors. Textbook of traumatic brain injury. 3rd edition. Washington, DC: American Psychiatric Pub; 2019. p. 677–96.
3. Asken BM, Snyder AR, Clugston JR, et al. Concussion-like symptom reporting in non-concussed collegiate athletes. Arch Clin Neuropsychol 2017;32(8):963–71.
4. Zasler ND. Post-traumatic sensory disorders in TBI. In: Arciniegas D, Vanderploeg R, Zasler ND, et al, editors. Management of adults with traumatic brain injury. Washington, DC: American Psychiatric Publishing, Inc; 2013. p. 395–420.
5. Hammond FM, Masel T. Cranial nerve disorders. In: Zasler N, Katz D, Zafonte R, editors. Brain injury medicine: principles and practice. 2nd edition. New York: Demos Medical Publishing; 2012. p. 635–748.
6. Matuszak JM, McVige J, McPherson J, et al. A practical concussion physical examination toolbox evidence-based physical examination for concussion. Sports Health 2016;8(3):260–9.
7. Haider MN, Leddy JJ, Du W, et al. Practical management: brief physical examination for sport-related concussion in the outpatient setting. Clin J Sport Med 2018. Online ahead of print.
8. Ellis MJ, Leddy JJ, Willer B. Physiological, vestibulo-ocular and cervicogenic post-concussion disorders: an evidence-based classification system with directions for treatment. Brain Inj 2015;29(2):238–48.
9. Kontos AP, Jorgensen-Wagers K, Trbovich AM, et al. Association of time since injury to the first clinic visit with recovery following concussion. JAMA Neurol 2020;77(4):435–40.
10. Master CL, Scheiman M, Gallaway M, et al. Vision diagnoses are common after concussion in adolescents. Clin Pediatr 2016;55(3):260–7.
11. Alvarez TL, Kim EH, Vicci VR, et al. Concurrent vision dysfunctions in convergence insufficiency with traumatic brain injury. Optom Vis Sci 2012;89(12):1740–51.
12. Heitger MH, Jones RD, Macleod A, et al. Impaired eye movements in post-concussion syndrome indicate suboptimal brain function beyond the influence of depression, malingering or intellectual ability. Brain 2009;132(10):2850–70.
13. Heitger MH, Anderson TJ, Jones RD, et al. Eye movement and visuomotor arm movement deficits following mild closed head injury. Brain 2004;127(3):575–90.
14. Anzalone AJ, Blueitt D, Case T, et al. A positive Vestibular/Ocular Motor Screening (VOMS) is associated with increased recovery time after sports-related concussion in youth and adolescent athletes. Am J Sports Med 2017;45(2):474–9.

15. Von Noorden G, Campos E. Physiology of the ocular movements. Binocular vision and ocular motility: theory and management of strabismus. 6th edition. St Louis (MO): Mosby; 2002. p. 52–84.
16. Abraham NG, Srinivasan K, Thomas J. Normative data for near point of convergence, accommodation, and phoria. Oman J Ophthalmol 2015;8(1):14.
17. Zahid AB, Hubbard ME, Lockyer J, et al. Eye tracking as a biomarker for concussion in children. Clin J Sport Med 2018. Online ahead of print.
18. Howell DR, Brilliant AN, Master CL. Reliability of objective eye-tracking measures among healthy adolescent athletes. Clin J Sport Med 2018. Online ahead of print.
19. Lawrence JB, Haider MN, Leddy JJ, et al. The King-Devick test in an outpatient concussion clinic: assessing the diagnostic and prognostic value of a vision test in conjunction with exercise testing among acutely concussed adolescents. J Neurol Sci 2019;398:91–7.
20. Maruta J, Spielman LA, Rajashekar U, et al. Association of visual tracking metrics with post-concussion symptomatology. Front Neurol 2018;9:611.
21. Broglio SP, Collins MW, Williams RM, et al. Current and emerging rehabilitation for concussion: a review of the evidence. Clin Sports Med 2015;34(2):213–31.
22. Heick JD, Bay C, Dompier TP, et al. Relationships among common vision and vestibular tests in healthy recreational athletes. Int J Sports Phys Ther 2017; 12(4):581.
23. Kolev OI, Sergeeva M. Vestibular disorders following different types of head and neck trauma. Funct Neurol 2016;31(2):75.
24. Yorke AM, Smith L, Babcock M, et al. Validity and reliability of the vestibular/ ocular motor screening and associations with common concussion screening tools. Sports Health 2017;9(2):174–80.
25. Oliva M, Martín MG, Bartual J, et al. The head-thrust test (HTT): physiopathological considerations and its clinical use in daily practice. Acta Otorrinolaringol Esp 1998;49(4):275–9.
26. Morganroth J, Galetta S, Balcer L. Vision-based concussion testing in a youth ice hockey cohort: effects of age and visual crowding. Neurology 2014; 82(10):267.
27. Howell DR, Brilliant AN, Meehan WP III. Tandem gait test-retest reliability among healthy child and adolescent athletes. J Athl Train 2019;54(12):1254–9.
28. Howell DR, Oldham JR, DiFabio M, et al. Single-task and dual-task gait among collegiate athletes of different sport classifications: implications for concussion management. J Appl Biomech 2017;33(1):24–31.
29. Johnston W, Coughlan GF, Caulfield B. Challenging concussed athletes: the future of balance assessment in concussion. QJM 2017;110(12):779–83.
30. Bhattacharyya N, Gubbels SP, Schwartz SR, et al. Clinical practice guideline: benign paroxysmal positional vertigo (update). Otolaryngol Head Neck Surg 2017;156(3_suppl):S1–47.
31. Treleaven J. Sensorimotor disturbances in neck disorders affecting postural stability, head and eye movement control. Man Ther 2008;13(1):2–11.
32. Treleaven J, Jull G, Sterling M. Dizziness and unsteadiness following whiplash injury: characteristic features and relationship with cervical joint position error. J Rehabil Med 2003;35(1):36–43.
33. Zasler ND, Katz DI, Zafonte RD. Brain injury medicine: principles and practice. New York: Demos Medical Publishing; 2012.
34. Bogduk N. The anatomical basis for cervicogenic headache. J Manipulative Physiol Ther 1992;15(1):67–70.

35. Iwanaga J, Fisahn C, Alonso F, et al. Microsurgical anatomy of the hypoglossal and C1 nerves: description of a previously undescribed branch to the atlanto-occipital joint. World Neurosurg 2017;100:590–3.

36. Yin W, Willard F, Dixon T, et al. Ventral innervation of the lateral C1–C2 joint: an anatomical study. Pain Med 2008;9(8):1022–9.

37. Zhao Z, Cope DK. Nonsurgical interventional pain-relieving procedures. Handbook of pain and palliative care. New York: Springer; 2018. p. 507–45.

38. Travell JG, Simons DG. Myofascial pain and dysfunction: the trigger point manual. Philadelphia: Lippincott Williams & Wilkins; 1983.

39. Davidoff R. Trigger points and myofascial pain: toward understanding how they affect headaches. Cephalalgia 1998;18(7):436–48.

40. Shabat S, Leitner Y, David R, et al. The correlation between Spurling test and imaging studies in detecting cervical radiculopathy. J Neuroimaging 2012; 22(4):375–8.

41. Tong HC, Haig AJ, Yamakawa K. The Spurling test and cervical radiculopathy. Spine (Phila Pa 1976) 2002;27(2):156–9.

42. Glaser JA, Curé JK, Bailey KL, et al. Cervical spinal cord compression and the Hoffman sign. The Iowa orthopaedic journal 2001;21:49.

43. Chang C-W, Chang K-Y, Lin S-M. Quantification of the Trömner signs: a sensitive marker for cervical spondylotic myelopathy. Eur Spine J 2011;20(6):923–7.

44. Mitchell JA. Changes in vertebral artery blood flow following normal rotation of the cervical spine. J Manipulative Physiol Ther 2003;26(6):347–51.

45. Leddy JJ, Baker JG, Merchant A, et al. Brain or strain? Symptoms alone do not distinguish physiologic concussion from cervical/vestibular injury. Clin J Sport Med 2015;25(3):237–42.

46. Jackson R. Cervical trauma: not just another pain in the neck. Geriatrics 1982; 37(4):123–6.

47. Campbell DG, Parsons CM. Referred head pain and its concomitants: report of preliminary experimental investigation with implications for the post-traumatic "Head" syndrome. J Nerv Ment Dis 1944;99(5):544–51.

48. Kaneoka K, Ono L, Inami S, et al. Motion analysis of cervical vertebrae during whiplash loading. Spine (Phila Pa 1976) 1999;24(8):763–70.

49. Cole A, Farrel J, Stratton S. Functional rehabilitation of cervical spine athletic injuries. Functional rehabilitation of sports and musculoskeletal injuries. Gaithersburg (MD): Aspen Publishers; 1998. p. 127–48.

50. Mense S. Nociception from skeletal muscle in relation to clinical muscle pain. Pain 1993;54(3):241–89.

51. Morin M, Langevin P, Fait P. Cervical spine involvement in mild traumatic brain injury: a review. J Sports Med 2016;2016:1590161.

52. Bogduk N, Govind J. Cervicogenic headache: an assessment of the evidence on clinical diagnosis, invasive tests, and treatment. Lancet Neurol 2009;8(10): 959–68.

53. Barnsley L, Lord SM, Wallis BJ, et al. The prevalence of chronic cervical zygapophysial joint pain after whiplash. Spine (Phila Pa 1976) 1995;20:20–5. Philadelphia-Harper and Row Publishers then JB Lippincott Company.

54. Pearson AM, Ivancic PC, Ito S, et al. Facet joint kinematics and injury mechanisms during simulated whiplash. Spine 2004;29(4):390–7.

55. Crock H. A reappraisal of intervertebral disc lesions. Med J Aust 1970;1(20): 983–9.

56. Brinjikji W, Luetmer PH, Comstock B, et al. Systematic literature review of imaging features of spinal degeneration in asymptomatic populations. AJNR Am J Neuroradiol 2015;36(4):811–6.

57. Luedtke K, Boissonnault W, Caspersen N, et al. International consensus on the most useful physical examination tests used by physiotherapists for patients with headache: a Delphi study. Man Ther 2016;23:17–24.

58. Hall TM, Robinson KW, Fujinawa O, et al. Intertester reliability and diagnostic validity of the cervical flexion-rotation test. J Manipulative Physiol Ther 2008; 31(4):293–300.

59. Rubio-Ochoa J, Benítez-Martínez J, Lluch E, et al. Physical examination tests for screening and diagnosis of cervicogenic headache: a systematic review. Man Ther 2016;21:35–40.

60. Ogince M, Hall T, Robinson K, et al. The diagnostic validity of the cervical flexion–rotation test in C1/2-related cervicogenic headache. Man Ther 2007; 12(3):256–62.

61. Cheever K, Kawata K, Tierney R, et al. Cervical injury assessments for concussion evaluation: a review. J Athl Train 2016;51(12):1037–44.

62. Osmotherly PG, Rivett DA, Rowe LJ. Construct validity of clinical tests for alar ligament integrity: an evaluation using magnetic resonance imaging. Phys Ther 2012;92(5):718–25.

63. Hutting N, Scholten-Peeters GG, Vijverman V, et al. Diagnostic accuracy of upper cervical spine instability tests: a systematic review. Phys Ther 2013;93(12): 1686–95.

64. Uitvlugt G, Indenbaum S. Clinical assessment of atlantoaxial instability using the Sharp-Purser test. Arthritis Rheum 1988;31(7):918–22.

65. Clausen M, Pendergast DR, Wilier B, et al. Cerebral blood flow during treadmill exercise is a marker of physiological postconcussion syndrome in female athletes. J Head Trauma Rehabil 2016;31(3):215–24.

66. Fife TD, Giza C, editors. Posttraumatic vertigo and dizziness. Seminars in neurology. New York: Thieme Medical Publishers; 2013.

67. Leddy JJ, Kozlowski K, Fung M, et al. Regulatory and autoregulatory physiological dysfunction as a primary characteristic of post concussion syndrome: implications for treatment. NeuroRehabilitation 2007;22(3):199–205.

68. Orr R, Bogg T, Fyffe A, et al. Graded exercise testing predicts recovery trajectory of concussion in children and adolescents. Clin J Sport Med 2018. Publish Ahead of Print.

69. Dematteo C, Volterman KA, Breithaupt PG, et al. Exertion testing in youth with mild traumatic brain injury/concussion. Med Sci Sports Exerc 2015;47(11): 2283–90.

70. Leddy JJ, Hinds AL, Miecznikowski J, et al. Safety and prognostic utility of provocative exercise testing in acutely concussed adolescents: a randomized trial. Clin J Sport Med 2018;28(1):13–20.

71. Haider MN, Leddy JJ, Wilber CG, et al. The predictive capacity of the buffalo concussion treadmill test after sport-related concussion in adolescents. Front Neurol 2019;10:395.

72. Leddy JJ, Baker JG, Kozlowski K, et al. Reliability of a graded exercise test for assessing recovery from concussion. Clin J Sport Med 2011;21(2):89–94.

73. Haider MN, Johnson SL, Mannix R, et al. The buffalo concussion bike test for concussion assessment in adolescents. Sports Health 2019;11(6):492–7.

74. Gibbons RJ, Balady GJ, Bricker JT, et al. ACC/AHA 2002 guideline update for exercise testing: summary article: a report of the American College of

Cardiology/American Heart Association Task Force on Practice Guidelines (Committee to Update the 1997 Exercise Testing Guidelines). J Am Coll Cardiol 2002;40(8):1531–40.

75. Leddy JJ, Haider MN, Ellis M, et al. Exercise is medicine for concussion. Curr Sports Med Rep 2018;17(8):262–70.

76. Leddy J, Baker JG, Haider MN, et al. A physiological approach to prolonged recovery from sport-related concussion. J Athl Train 2017;52(3):299–308.

77. Collins MW, Kontos AP, Okonkwo DO, et al. Statements of agreement from the targeted evaluation and active management (TEAM) approaches to treating concussion meeting held in Pittsburgh, October 15-16, 2015. Neurosurgery 2016;79(6):912–29.

78. Grabowski P, Wilson J, Walker A, et al. Multimodal impairment-based physical therapy for the treatment of patients with post-concussion syndrome: a retrospective analysis on safety and feasibility. Phys Ther Sport 2017;23:22–30.

79. Carrick FR, Clark JF, Pagnacco G, et al. Head–eye vestibular motion therapy affects the mental and physical health of severe chronic Postconcussion Patients. Front Neurol 2017;8:414.

80. Leddy JJ, Haider MN, Ellis MJ, et al. Early subthreshold aerobic exercise for sport-related concussion: a randomized clinical trial. JAMA Pediatr 2019; 173(4):319–25.

81. Schneider KJ, Meeuwisse WH, Nettel-Aguirre A, et al. Cervicovestibular rehabilitation in sport-related concussion: a randomised controlled trial. Br J Sports Med 2014;48(17):1294–8.

82. Siddharth K, Thangarajan R, Theruvedhi N, et al. Android mobile applications in eye care. Oman J Ophthalmol 2019;12(2):73–7.

83. Schneider KJ, Meeuwisse WH, Nettel-Aguirre A, et al. Cervico-vestibular physiotherapy in the treatment of individuals with persistent symptoms following sport related concussion: a randomised controlled trial. Br J Sports Med 2014;48(17):1294–8.

84. Ellis MJ, Leddy J, Willer B. Multi-disciplinary management of athletes with post-concussion syndrome: an evolving pathophysiological approach. Front Neurol 2016;7:136.

85. Kristjansson E, Treleaven J. Sensorimotor function and dizziness in neck pain: implications for assessment and management. J Orthop Sports Phys Ther 2009;39(5):364–77.

86. Jull G, Trott P, Potter H, et al. A randomized controlled trial of exercise and manipulative therapy for cervicogenic headache. Spine 2002;27(17):1835–43.

87. Garcia JD, Arnold S, Tetley K, et al. Mobilization and manipulation of the cervical spine in patients with cervicogenic headache: any scientific evidence? Front Neurol 2016;7:40.

88. Hecht JS. Occipital nerve blocks in postconcussive headaches: a retrospective review and report of ten patients. J Head Trauma Rehabil 2004;19(1):58–71.

89. Maerlender A, Rieman W, Lichtenstein J, et al. Programmed physical exertion in recovery from sports-related concussion: a randomized pilot study. Dev Neuropsychol 2015;40(5):273–8.

90. Coupe M, Fortrat J, Larina I, et al. Cardiovascular deconditioning: from autonomic nervous system to microvascular dysfunctions. Respir Physiol Neurobiol 2009;169:S10–2.

91. Tan CO, Meehan WP 3rd, Iverson GL, et al. Cerebrovascular regulation, exercise, and mild traumatic brain injury. Neurology 2014;83(18):1665–72.

92. Leddy JJ, Wilber CG, Willer BS. Active recovery from concussion. Curr Opin Neurol 2018;31(6):681–6.

93. Kostyun RO, Milewski MD, Hafeez I. Sleep disturbance and neurocognitive function during the recovery from a sport-related concussion in adolescents. Am J Sports Med 2015;43(3):633–40.

94. Ahlskog JE, Geda YE, Graff-Radford NR, et al. Physical exercise as a preventive or disease-modifying treatment of dementia and brain aging. Mayo Clin Proc 2011;86(9):876–84.

95. Leddy JJ, Haider MN, Hinds AL, et al. A preliminary study of the effect of early aerobic exercise treatment for sport-related concussion in males. Clin J Sport Med 2019;29(5):353–60.

96. Gauvin-Lepage J, Friedman D, Grilli L, et al. Effectiveness of an exercise-based active rehabilitation intervention for youth who are slow to recover after concussion. Clin J Sport Med 2018. Online ahead of print.

97. Micay R, Richards D, Hutchison MG. Feasibility of a postacute structured aerobic exercise intervention following sport concussion in symptomatic adolescents: a randomised controlled study. BMJ Open Sport Exerc Med 2018;4(1): e000404.

98. Lawrence DW, Richards D, Comper P, et al. Earlier time to aerobic exercise is associated with faster recovery following acute sport concussion. PLoS One 2018;13(4):e0196062.

99. Majerske CW, Mihalik JP, Ren D, et al. Concussion in sports: postconcussive activity levels, symptoms, and neurocognitive performance. J Athl Train 2008; 43(3):265–74.

100. Griesbach GS, Tio DL, Vincelli J, et al. Differential effects of voluntary and forced exercise on stress responses after traumatic brain injury. J Neurotrauma 2012; 29(7):1426–33.

101. Peres G, Vandewalle H, Havette P. Heart rate, maximal heart rate and pedal rate. J Sports Med Phys fitness 1987;27(2):205.

102. Zasler N, Haider MN, Grzibowski NR, et al. Physician medical assessment in a multidisciplinary concussion clinic. J Head Trauma Rehabil 2019;34(6):409–18.

103. Ellenbogen RG, Batjer H, Cardenas J, et al. National football league head, neck and spine committee's concussion diagnosis and management protocol: 2017-18 season. Br J Sports Med 2018;52(14):894–902.

Neuroimaging in Sports-Related Concussion

Gaurav Jindal, MD[a],*, Rajan R. Gadhia, MD[b], Prachi Dubey, MD, MPH[c]

KEYWORDS

- Concussion • Traumatic brain injury • Diffusion tensor imaging
- Volumetric morphometry • Spectroscopy • Susceptibility-weighted imaging
- Perfusion imaging • Functional MRI

KEY POINTS

- Conventional neuroimaging techniques like head computed tomography and traditional magnetic resonance imaging (MRI) anatomic sequences are relatively insensitive to microstructural or functional abnormalities that are associated with mild traumatic brain injuries (mTBIs).
- Several advanced neuroimaging techniques, specifically MRI related, are being developed to gain insight into microstructural, functional, and metabolic changes secondary to brain trauma and have become pivotal in understanding mTBI pathophysiology.
- None of the current available techniques can yet be implemented in individual patients seen in a clinical setting.

INTRODUCTION

Sports-related concussions (SRCs) affect millions of athletes worldwide each year. In the United States, approximately 3.8 million concussions are diagnosed per year, which is thought to be a gross underestimation because a large number of SRCs go unreported.[1,2]

SRCs also have attracted considerable attention in the public health domain due to possible risk of long-term neurologic sequelae from repetitive head injuries.[3–5] Although concussions are a subset of mild traumatic brain injury (mTBI), the terms often are used interchangeably; for the purpose of this article as well, mTBI and SRC are used interchangeably.[4]

Noncontrast head CT is the imaging test of choice in evaluating and triaging patients with acute head trauma. The primary role of imaging in the acute setting is detection of

[a] Warren Alpert School of Medicine at Brown University, Rhode Island Hospital, 593 Eddy Street, Providence, RI 02903, USA; [b] Stanley H. Appel Department of Neurology, Houston Methodist Hospital, 6560 Fannin Street, Suite 802, Houston, TX 77030, USA; [c] Neuroradiology, Houston Methodist Hospital, 6560 Fannin Street, Houston, TX 77030, USA
* Corresponding author.
E-mail address: GAURAV.JINDAL@LIFESPAN.ORG

Clin Sports Med 40 (2021) 111–121
https://doi.org/10.1016/j.csm.2020.08.004
0278-5919/21/© 2020 Elsevier Inc. All rights reserved.
sportsmed.theclinics.com

intracranial hemorrhage and fractures. Brain contusions often may remain occult in the hyperacute stage; however, they can be seen on noncontrast computed tomography (CT) in the acute to subacute state, underscoring the need for close follow-up in the acute setting.[6]

Magnetic resonance imaging (MRI) anatomic sequences can depict contusions and gross hemorrhage in traumatic brain injury (TBI); however, traditional sequences are relatively insensitive to microstructural or functional abnormalities that are associated with mTBI. These abnormalities could serve as a key prognostic biomarker to predict long-term functional neurologic and cognitive status. As a result, the American college of Radiology, American Academy of Neurology, and the American Medical Society for Sports Medicine do not recommend any routine imaging in patients with mTBI.[7]

The goal of advanced neuroimaging techniques, specifically MRI, is to try to gain insight into microstructural, functional, and metabolic changes secondary to brain trauma and establish potential objective imaging biomarkers that could help predict outcomes.

Structural MRI techniques have focused on studying both macrostructural changes using quantitative morphometry to analyze posttraumatic changes in brain volumes and microstructural white matter changes using diffusion tensor imaging (DTI). Susceptibility-weighted imaging (SWI) is used to detect posttraumatic microhemorrhages. Functional cortical mapping is performed via blood oxygenation level–dependent (BOLD) MRI techniques that use certain imaging sequences sensitive to blood oxygenation levels and are able to evaluate changes in brain connectivity at rest as well as while performing tasks. Proton magnetic resonance spectroscopy (MRS) has been studied to evaluate metabolic changes in the brain after injury. Lastly, studies also have examined changes in cerebral blood flow (CBF) using magnetic resonance (MR) perfusion imaging techniques. These techniques are described in further detail.

DIFFUSION TENSOR IMAGING

Among the advanced imaging modalities currently being studied in evaluating patients with mTBI, DTI has been studied most extensively.[8]

DTI of the brain relies on evaluation of brownian motion of water molecules. This diffusion may be isotropic—that is, similar in all directions, such as unrestricted motion in cerebrospinal fluid—or anisotropic—that is, preferentially in 1 direction. Diffusion in intact white matter tracts is anisotropic preferentially along the direction of tracts. Apparent diffusion coefficient (ADC), mean diffusivity, and fractional anisotropy (FA) are commonly used estimates that can be computed to quantitatively assess the diffusion properties in the brain, acting as a surrogate for structural organization. The FA estimate gives an estimate of degree of anisotropic diffusion along the interrogated tissue volume[9,10] (Fig. 1).

DTI can aid assessment of white matter injury resulting from shearing strain seen in the setting of rapid acceleration and deceleration, often without leading to gross disruption in anatomic connections. These changes often are occult on conventional anatomic MRIs.

Imaging analysis in DTI is multifaceted, including evaluation of scalar multiparametric maps for whole-brain FA, MD, and ADC as well as assessment of vector or directionality information available on the color codes maps. This multipronged approach can assist not only in detecting the burden of abnormality but also in characterizing the anatomic location more precisely to assess for clinical functional impact of the injury. Although qualitative assessment of the DTI-based multiparametric maps can

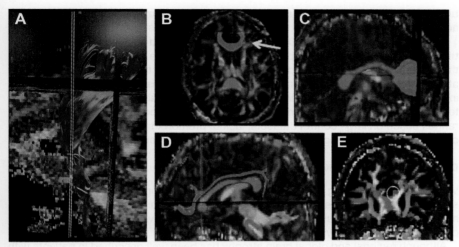

Fig. 1. DTI-based 3-D reconstructions of some of the fiber pathways that previously have been implicated in mTBI, Coricospinal/bulbar tracts (*A*), corpus callosum (frontal lobe connection through genu are depicted) (*B, C*), and cingulum bundle (*D, E*).

be used in individual clinical settings, they often yield greatest information in quantitative evaluation of in grouped comparisons. This can be based on anatomic region of interest–based assessment; deterministic, probabilistic 3-dimensional (3-D) tractographic approach; or global analysis using tract-based spatial statistics.[11]

In a review by Hulkower and colleagues,[12] examining more than 100 studies assessing the role of DTI in TBI, an overwhelming majority of studies demonstrated reduced FA values in TBI regardless of injury severity or time of injury. Brain anatomic areas implicated most commonly in TBI-related DTI studies include the corpus callosum, frontal lobes, internal capsule, and cingulum. Although it is likely that these structures are inherently more susceptible to abnormalities in TBI due to susceptibility to sheer stress–related injuries, it also is possible that being one of the highest FA tracts of the brain, these are more likely to yield statistically significant detectable abnormalities. The abnormalities in these structures also were noted in 7 of 8 studies specifically evaluating DTI in SRC.

Having an adequate control population is also one of the limitations for accurately understanding the DTI changes, because there is inherent variability in normal brain structural organization. In a recently published study by Niogi and colleagues[13] evaluating DTI in active professional football players, the investigators ascertained that comparing athletes' postconcussion scans to their own premorbid baseline scans might be superior to comparing the study population to healthy age-matched controls.

Changes in DTI parameters are not limited to athletes with clinically diagnosed concussion. Bahrami and colleagues[14] examined the effects of subconcussive impacts resulting from a single season of youth football on changes in specific white matter tracts detected with DTI and found statistically significant changes in FA values in the inferior fronto-occipital fasciculus and the superior longitudinal fasciculus, even in absence of clinically diagnosed concussion.

One of the major limitations of DTI is the lack of ability to resolve multiple fiber orientations within a single voxel. Newer methodologies being investigated to improve the resolution of crossing fibers include high angular resolution diffusion imaging, diffusion spectrum imaging, neurite orientation dispersion and density imaging model, and Q-ball imaging.[15,16]

Despite multiple advances, DTI still remains primarily a research tool. Challenges that have precluded wider adoption of DTI for clinical use are due mainly to the fact that the abnormalities seen are predominantly quantitative in nature; they are detected at a group level, and these findings cannot be reliably translated to individual patients in a standardized fashion. Additionally, there remain inconsistencies and differences in techniques between the reported studies, lack of technically rigorous normative ranges based on large control datasets, lack of premorbid baseline data, and unclear correlation between imaging abnormalities and long-term clinical outcome.[17]

QUANTITATIVE BRAIN MORPHOMETRY

Volumetric brain imaging is performed using high-resolution 3-D T1-weighted imaging sequences, which can be obtained on most MR scanners in routine clinical use. Automated software can be used to segment gray matter and white matter structures and perform volumetric analysis.[18,19]

Although regional and global brain atrophy has been well described in patients with moderate and severe TBI, it has not been well studied in mTBI.[20]

Zhou and colleagues[21] evaluated longitudinal changes in brain volume after mTBI over a 1-year period and described decrease in global brain volume as well as volume loss in anterior cingulate white matter, cingulate gyrus isthmus, and precuneus gray matter in concussed patients compared with age-matched controls. Furthermore, the investigators also reported correlation of volumetric changes with postconcussion symptoms.

Burrowes and colleagues[22] studied 51 mTBI patients with and without history of posttraumatic headache by obtaining MRI scans at 4 time points, within 10 days of injury and then at 1 month, 6 months, and 18 months postinjury. The investigators found decreased gray matter volume in mTBI patients compared with healthy controls and also reported regional decrease in gray matter volumes in patients with posttraumatic headache versus asymptomatic mTBI patients. This suggests that symptomatic mTBI patients may have an exaggerated long-term clinical course compared with asymptomatic mTBI, particularly as it relates to cognitive sequela, which have been shown to be associated with volumetric estimates.

In another recently study, Patel and colleagues[23] studied 70 military personnel with mTBI were found to have reduced mean volume in different regions of the frontal, parietal, and temporal lobes compared with controls. Limitations of morphometric studies include intersubject variations in brain morphology, lack of comparison to patient's preinjury scans, and relatively small cohort of patients studied. Further larger longitudinal studies may help in establishing a clinical role of morphometric studies in the management of patients with mTBI.

PROTON MAGNETIC RESONANCE SPECTROSCOPY

Proton MRS like DTI has been studied extensively in patients with mTBI.

Proton MRS, thought to hold promise as a noninvasive tool that can be utilized in individual patients, also known as virtual biopsy, relies on exploiting small changes in the precessing frequency of protons based on their chemical environment, yielding estimates of metabolite peaks (at specific parts per million) with quantifiable concentrations.[24]

When a single voxel is sampled, the interpretation relies on the concentrations as depicted by metabolite ratios or absolute concentrations. When whole-brain multivoxel sampling is performed, however, a metabolite map or MRS imaging can be performed, yielding both quantitative and qualitative information.[25]

Commonly detected metabolites in normal brain include N-acetyl-aspartate (NAA), which is considered a neuronal marker; choline (Cho), which is a measure of cell membrane turnover; creatine (Cr), which is a marker of energy metabolism (and commonly used as an internal reference); myoinositol (ML), which is marker for glial cells; and glutamate and glutamine (combined peak, referred to as Glx) an excitatory neurotransmitter.[25,26]

MRS can be performed using single-voxel or multivoxel techniques. Single-voxel technique has a higher signal-to-noise ratio but it interrogates only a small volume of brain tissue at a time, therefore making placement/selection of the volume of interest crucial. Multivoxel technique on the other hand interrogates a much larger volume of tissue at the expense of lower signal-to-noise ratio and longer acquisition time.[27]

Several studies have evaluated the role of MRS in patients with concussion. NAA, Cho, and Cr are studied most commonly studied. The most consistent finding in most studies is reduced NAA levels in gray matter and white matter and elevated Cho levels. The magnitude of these changes increases with increase in injury severity.[17]

Decreased NAA levels seen in the acute phase after injury may return to normal or remain depressed in the subacute phase, which does not necessarily correlate with neuropsychological recovery.[28]

Elevated Cho levels are believed to be related to cell membrane breakdown in the acute stage and likely secondary to glial proliferation in the chronic stage. Although some studies have shown elevated Cho levels in mTBI, others have demonstrated no statistically significant difference in Cho levels on spectroscopy.[17]

MRS study of symptomatic former National Football League (NFL) players revealed decreased parietal white matter Cr and NAA levels compared with controls. Reduced Cr levels were associated with higher cumulative head impact index. The study also revealed positive correlation between levels of Glx and ML in anterior cingulate gyrus with presence of behavioral or mood symptoms.[17,29]

Overall, the diagnostic utility of proton MRS as a biomarker for mTBI is highly debatable. It is fair to say that it remains to be studied in larger longitudinal studies to evaluate sensitivity and specificity of MRS in mTBI before it can be applied reliably to individual patients.

MAGNETIC RESONANCE SUSCEPTIBILITY–WEIGHTED IMAGING

SWI is the most sensitive MR imaging sequence to detect intracranial hemorrhage, including microhemorrhage that can remain occult on conventional anatomic imaging. Presence of unpaired electrons in deoxyhemoglobin in the acute stage and methemoglobin in subacute stage of hemorrhage result in abnormal magnetic susceptibility detected as areas of signal loss on the SWI image[27] (**Fig. 2**).

Another advantage of SWI is its ability to distinguish between small foci of calcification from hemorrhage utilizing the phase maps.[19]

SWI preferably is performed on a 3T magnet to obtain better sensitivity and higher signal-to-noise ratio; however, higher field strength also is associated with greater magnetic field inhomogeneity; thus, resulting artifacts, particularly around the air/bone interface, which are commonly sites prone to abnormality in the acceleration/deceleration pattern of injury and around areas of gross hemorrhage, such as seen with gross contusions. Research studies have shown even further improvement in detection of microbleeds at 7T.[30] However, 7T remains susceptible to these pitfalls

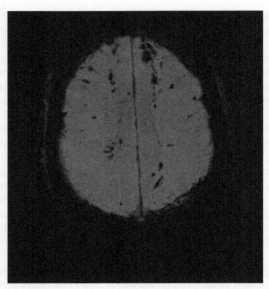

Fig. 2. SWI in a 46-year-old man with severe TBI shows multiple round and linear foci of signal loss in bilateral subcortical and deep white matter consistent with traumatic microhemorrhages.

to an even greater extent, indicating a need for technique optimization before widespread utilization in mTBI patients.

Although traumatic microbleeds are commonly described in moderate and severe head injury,[31] Griffin and colleagues[32] in their study of more than 400 patients recently reported presence of microbleeds in approximately 30% patients with mTBI. Patients with microbleeds also were noted to be twice as likely to be symptomatic at 30-day or 90-day follow-up. The investigators also suggested vascular injury as a possible underlying etiology of traumatic microbleeds. In a study of 30 mTBI patients, Studerus-Germann and colleagues[33] reported worse cognitive outcomes in mTBI patients with microbleeds detected on SWI.

One of the limitations of SWI is inability to establish mTBI as a definitive cause of microbleed in the absence of prior imaging studies. There remains a high prevalence of subclinical vasculopathies, including that which may be related to vascular risk factors, such as hypertension and amyloid angiopathy.[27]

BLOOD OXYGENATION LEVEL–DEPENDENT FUNCTIONAL MAGNETIC RESONANCE IMAGING

BOLD is an MR technique developed to identify functionally active areas of the brain at rest and while the patient is performing specific tasks. Currently, the main clinical application of BOLD functional MRI (fMRI) is preoperative planning for cortical mapping using task-based signal alteration to detect functionally active cortices especially the eloquent cortices.[34,35]

Oxyhemoglobin, which has 4 paired electrons, is diamagnetic whereas deoxyhemoglobin, with 4 unpaired electrons, is strongly paramagnetic. The paramagnetic properties of deoxyhemoglobin results in dephasing on T2*-weighted sequence used for fMRI. The interaction between neuronal activation, CBF, and changes in deoxyhemoglobin concentration–related dephasing, yields a measurable signal, forming the basis of neurovascular coupling, the fundamental principle underlying BOLD imaging.[36]

Task-based fMRI detects changes in BOLD signal while performing a task compared with baseline. BOLD signal fluctuations also are seen, however, in certain brain areas at rest. These changes are evaluated using resting state (RS)-fMRI techniques. Both task-based and RS-fMRI have been studied in patients with TBI.

In a meta-analysis of task-related fMRI studies in acute mTBI and subacute mTBI, the investigators reported decreased activation in the prefrontal region (middle frontal gyrus) in patients with cognitive impairment as the most consistent finding across multiple published studies.[37] Whether this is as result of neuronal injury in the cortex or a function of aberrations in underlying structural connectivity as established on prior DTI studies remains unclear.

On the other hand, there also are studies showing increased local functional connectivity in RS and task-based evaluation. A longitudinal study evaluating RS-fMRI in 92 concussed athletes and 82 controls[38] imaged patients at multiple time points, including acutely (within 24–48 hours) after concussion, after clearance to return to play (RTP), and 7 days after unrestricted RTP. The investigators reported elevated local connectivity in the right middle and superior frontal gyri, which returned to normal at the asymptomatic/RTP visit. In another longitudinal study, Churchill and colleagues[39] scanned 28 athletes within 1 week after concussion, at RTP, and 1 year after RTP. The investigators reported elevated connectivity in the frontal, temporal, and parietal regions and posterior cingulate early after concussion and at RTP with normalization of findings at 1 year.

fMRI studies have also been used to evaluate retired athletes with history of multiple prior concussions. Guell and colleagues[40] reported abnormal functional connectivity in cerebellar lobule V on RS-fMRI on 32 retired rugby players, suggesting a possible link between repetitive brain injury and cerebellar dysfunction. This suggests there potentially may be a temporal influence with a more widespread cumulative effect of repetitive injuries over time.

In another task-based fMRI study of 13 retired NFL players, the investigators reported increased activation in the dorsolateral prefrontal cortex and reduced connectivity in the dorsal frontoparietal network while performing tasks to assess executive function. This suggests that both increased and decreased connectivity/activation prefrontal cortical patterns can be seen with task-based methods.[41]

This multitude of abnormalities suggests lack of a specific signature for mTBI using BOLD fMRI methodology. This likely is a result of complex interplay of acute and chronic injury characteristics (extent, duration, magnitude, topology of injury itself, and personal factors, such as age, race, comorbidities, and so forth), underlying impact on structural network (as seen with DTI and morphometry), and vascular factors (vascular injury/perfusion abnormalities). Until this complex interplay is fully understood, the interpretation of BOLD changes in mTBI will remain challenging.

PERFUSION-WEIGHTED IMAGING

Perfusion-weighted imaging (PWI) can be performed readily using CT and MRI as well as nuclear medicine studies, such as PET and single-photon emission CT. MR perfusion studies can be performed both without and with intravenous contrast.

Arterial spin labeling is an MRI technique that enables obtaining quantitative perfusion data without injecting intravenous contrast. The technique thus is entirely noninvasive and involves no radiation exposure. Arterial spin labeling techniques, however, allow only information-related CBF into a tissue volume, whereas the contrast-enhanced techniques allow a multiparametric assessment, such as CBF, cerebral blood volume, mean transit time, and time to peak.[42]

Similar to BOLD, the results with PWI also are mixed and likely a complex interplay of structural and neurophysiologic aberrations as a function of injury pattern. Some studies report elevated CBF after injury and others report reductions in blood flow after concussion.

In a study evaluating 15 concussed teenage athletes at 2 weeks and 6 weeks after concussion, Stephens and colleagues[43] reported significantly elevated relative CBF in left dorsal anterior cingulate cortex and insula compared with controls. Whether this is a short-term direct response to an injury or an adaptive/redirectional response to a regional injury is unclear.

Churchill and colleagues[39] performed a multimodal longitudinal MRI study scanning 24 athletes with concussion at different time points after injury. The investigators reported significantly elevated CBF in the early symptomatic phase after injury in the superior frontal gyri. Perfusion imaging at 1 year after RTP, however, revealed reduced CBF in the middle frontal and temporal regions.

Based on these studies, it is tempting to expect increase in regional CBF in acute settings as the common theme; however, there are other studies that show the reverse pattern within a comparable time frame. For example, in a recently published study, Wang and colleagues[44] evaluated changes in CBF in 24 athletes with acute SRC and compared those with age-matched controls. The investigators reported a significant decrease in CBF in multiple brain regions in concussed athletes compared with controls. The same group also described statistically significant reduction in CBF in 18 concussed football players at 8 days compared with what was seen within 24 hours posttrauma.[45]

There is significant heterogeneity in the published literature regarding the changes in PWI; similar to BOLD imaging, PWI also is susceptible to complex interplay between injury/injured characteristics and structural underpinnings, thus making its diagnostic or prognostic utility as an isolated metric questionable.

SUMMARY

There is significant morbidity, albeit usually transient, due to SRC-associated mTBI. Conventional anatomic neuroimaging is relatively insensitive, however, to mTBI abnormalities. Advanced neuroimaging, therefore, has become pivotal in understanding mTBI pathophysiology.

Several DTI studies indicate white matter microstructural deficits, particularly in corpus callosum, internal capsule, frontal white matter, and cingulum bundle. There are additional gross volumetric abnormalities seen on morphometric studies. This likely is related to sheer stress structural injuries as can be expected in mTBI. SWI studies show a higher prevalence of microbleeds in mTBI, indicating associated axonal/vascular injury.

On the other hand, abnormalities on BOLD, PWI and proton MRS do not have a specific signature and are relatively challenging to interpret in isolation. They reflect a complex interplay of many factors, including injury/injured characteristics and underlying structural and functional substrates. It is unclear as to where precisely these changes fall along the spectrum of adaptive healing response to long-term irreversible damage.

Most importantly, none of the current available techniques can yet be implemented in individual patients seen in a clinical setting. Current imaging techniques lack reliable diagnostic or prognostic markers in acute or chronic mTBI.

Multimodal large-scale longitudinal imaging techniques are required to establish objective biomarkers that may correlate with SRC associated pathophysiologic changes and can be implemented in individual patients to detect changes early. The hope is that imaging biomarkers may be found to help determine a timeline for safe RTP and additionally predict long-term neurocognitive outcomes.

DISCLOSURE

The authors have nothing to disclose.

REFERENCES

1. Harmon KG, Drezner J, Gammons M, et al. American Medical Society for Sports Medicine position statement: concussion in sport. Clin J Sport Med 2013; 23(1):1–18.
2. Taylor CA, Bell JM, Breiding MJ, et al. Traumatic brain injury-related emergency department visits, hospitalizations, and deaths - United States, 2007 and 2013. MMWR Surveill Summ 2017;66(9):1–16.
3. Biagianti B, Stocchetti N, Brambilla P, et al. Brain dysfunction underlying pro-longed post-concussive syndrome: a systematic review. J Affect Disord 2020; 262:71–6.
·4. McKeithan L, Hibshman N, Yengo-Kahn AM, et al. Sport-related concussion: evaluation, treatment, and future directions. Med Sci (Basel) 2019;7(3):44.
5. McAllister TW, Ford JC, Flashman LA, et al. Effect of head impacts on diffusivity measures in a cohort of collegiate contact sport athletes. Neurology 2014; 82(1):63–9.
6. Guenette JP, Shenton ME, Koerte IK. Imaging of Concussion in young athletes. Neuroimaging Clin N Am 2018;28(1):43–53.
7. Giza CC, Kutcher JS, Ashwal S, et al. Summary of evidence-based guideline update: evaluation and management of concussion in sports: report of the guideline development subcommittee of the American academy of neurology. Neurology 2013;80(24):2250–7.
8. Hellewell SC, Nguyen VPB, Jayasena RN, et al. Characteristic patterns of white matter tract injury in sport-related concussion: an image based meta-analysis. Neuroimage Clin 2020;26:102253.
9. Mukherjee P, Berman JI, Chung SW, et al. Diffusion tensor MR imaging and fiber tractography: theoretic underpinnings. AJNR Am J Neuroradiol 2008;29(4): 632–41.
10. Mukherjee P, Chung SW, Berman JI, et al. Diffusion tensor MR Imaging and fiber tractography: technical considerations. Am J Neuroradiol 2008;29(5):843–52.
11. Smith SM, Jenkinson M, Johansen-Berg H, et al. Tract-based spatial statistics: voxelwise analysis of multi-subject diffusion data. Neuroimage 2006;31(4): 1487–505.
12. Hulkower MB, Poliak DB, Rosenbaum SB, et al. A decade of DTI in traumatic brain injury: 10 years and 100 articles later. AJNR Am J Neuroradiol 2013; 34(11):2064–74.
13. Niogi SN, Luther N, Kutner K, et al. Increased sensitivity to traumatic axonal injury on postconcussion diffusion tensor imaging scans in national football league

players by using premorbid baseline scans. J Neurosurg 2019;1–9. https://doi.org/10.3171/2019.3.JNS181864.

14. Bahrami N, Sharma D, Rosenthal S, et al. Subconcussive head impact exposure and white matter tract changes over a single season of youth football. Radiology 2016;281(3):919–26.

15. Mohammadian M, Roine T, Hirvonen J, et al. High angular resolution diffusion-weighted imaging in mild traumatic brain injury. Neuroimage Clin 2017;13:174–80.

16. Wu Y-C, Mustafi SM, Harezlak J, et al. Hybrid diffusion imaging in mild traumatic brain injury. J Neurotrauma 2018;35(20):2377–90.

17. Wintermark M, Sanelli PC, Anzai Y, et al, American College of Radiology Head Injury Institute. Imaging evidence and recommendations for traumatic brain injury: advanced neuro- and neurovascular imaging techniques. AJNR Am J Neuroradiol 2015;36(2):E1–11.

18. Hellstrøm T, Westlye LT, Sigurdardottir S, et al. Longitudinal changes in brain morphology from 4 weeks to 12 months after mild traumatic brain injury: associations with cognitive functions and clinical variables. Brain Inj 2017;31(5):674–85.

19. Adams LC, Bressem K, Böker SM, et al. Diagnostic performance of susceptibility-weighted magnetic resonance imaging for the detection of calcifications: a systematic review and meta-analysis. Sci Rep 2017;7(1):15506.

20. Ding K, Marquez de la Plata C, Wang JY, et al. Cerebral atrophy after traumatic white matter injury: correlation with acute neuroimaging and outcome. J Neurotrauma 2008;25(12):1433–40.

21. Zhou Y, Kierans A, Kenul D, et al. Mild traumatic brain injury: longitudinal regional brain volume changes. Radiology 2013;267(3):880–90.

22. Burrowes SAB, Rhodes CS, Meeker TJ, et al. Decreased grey matter volume in mTBI patients with post-traumatic headache compared to headache-free mTBI patients and healthy controls: a longitudinal MRI study. Brain Imaging Behav 2019. https://doi.org/10.1007/s11682-019-00095-7.

23. Patel JB, Wilson SH, Oakes TR, et al. Structural and volumetric brain MRI findings in mild traumatic brain injury. AJNR Am J Neuroradiol 2020;41(1):92–9.

24. Oz G, Alger JR, Barker PB, et al. Clinical proton MR spectroscopy in central nervous system disorders. Radiology 2014;270(3):658–79.

25. de Graaf RA. In vivo NMR spectroscopy: principles and techniques. New York: John Wiley & Sons; 1998.

26. Di Costanzo A, Trojsi F, Tosetti M, et al. Proton MR spectroscopy of the brain at 3 T: an update. Eur Radiol 2007;17(7):1651–62.

27. Kirov II, Whitlow CT, Zamora C. Susceptibility-weighted imaging and magnetic resonance spectroscopy in concussion. Neuroimaging Clin N Am 2018;28(1):91–105.

28. Koerte I, Hufschmidt J, Muehlmann M, Lin A, Shenton M. Advanced neuroimaging of mild traumatic brain injury. Translational Research in Traumatic Brain Injury 2015;277–98. https://doi.org/10.1201/b18959-14.

29. Alosco ML, Tripodis Y, Rowland B, et al. A magnetic resonance spectroscopy investigation in symptomatic former NFL players. Brain Imaging Behav 2019. https://doi.org/10.1007/s11682-019-00060-4.

30. Moenninghoff C, Kraff O, Maderwald S, et al. Diffuse axonal injury at ultra-high field MRI. PLoS One 2015;10(3):e0122329.

31. Riedy G, Senseney JS, Liu W, et al. Findings from structural MR imaging in military traumatic brain injury. Radiology 2016;279(1):207–15.

32. Griffin AD, Turtzo LC, Parikh GY, et al. Traumatic microbleeds suggest vascular injury and predict disability in traumatic brain injury. Brain 2019;142(11):3550–64.
33. Studerus-Germann AM, Gautschi OP, Bontempi P, et al. Central nervous system microbleeds in the acute phase are associated with structural integrity by DTI one year after mild traumatic brain injury: a longitudinal study. Neurol Neurochir Pol 2018;52(6):710–9.
34. Stippich C. Clinical functional MRI: presurgical functional neuroimaging. Springer Science & Business Media; 2007.
35. Stippich C. Presurgical functional MRI and diffusion tensor imaging. Clinical Functional MRI 2015;1–12. https://doi.org/10.1007/978-3-662-45123-6_1.
36. Barkhof F, Haller S, Rombouts SARB. Resting-state functional MR imaging: a new window to the brain. Radiology 2014;272(1):29–49.
37. Cook MJ, Gardner AJ, Wojtowicz M, et al. Task-related functional magnetic resonance imaging activations in patients with acute and subacute mild traumatic brain injury: a coordinate-based meta-analysis. Neuroimage Clin 2020;25:102129.
38. Meier TB, Giraldo-Chica M, España LY, et al. Resting-State fMRI metrics in acute sport-related concussion and their association with clinical recovery: a study from the NCAA-DOD CARE consortium. J Neurotrauma 2020;37(1):152–62.
39. Churchill NW, Hutchison MG, Graham SJ, et al. Mapping brain recovery after concussion: from acute injury to 1 year after medical clearance. Neurology 2019;93(21):e1980–92.
40. Guell X, Arnold Anteraper S, Gardner AJ, et al. Functional connectivity changes in retired rugby league players: a data-driven, functional magnetic resonance imaging study. J Neurotrauma 2020. https://doi.org/10.1089/neu.2019.6782.
41. Hampshire A, MacDonald A, Owen AM. Hypoconnectivity and hyperfrontality in retired American football players. Sci Rep 2013;3:2972.
42. Haller S, Zaharchuk G, Thomas DL, et al. Arterial spin labeling perfusion of the brain: emerging clinical applications. Radiology 2016;281(2):337–56.
43. Stephens JA, Liu P, Lu H, et al. Cerebral blood flow after mild traumatic brain injury: associations between symptoms and post-injury perfusion. J Neurotrauma 2018;35(2):241–8.
44. Wang Y, Nencka AS, Meier TB, et al. Cerebral blood flow in acute concussion: preliminary ASL findings from the NCAA-DoD CARE consortium. Brain Imaging Behav 2019;13(5):1375–85.
45. Wang Y, Nelson LD, LaRoche AA, et al. Cerebral blood flow alterations in acute sport-related concussion. J Neurotrauma 2016;33(13):1227–36.

Medical Therapies for Concussion

Jacob C. Jones, MD[a,b,]*, Michael J. O'Brien, MD[c,d,e,f]

KEYWORDS

- Concussion • Medication • Supplements • Postconcussive headache
- Postconcussion syndrome • Sports

KEY POINTS

- Medications and supplements are used primarily to treat concussion symptoms during prolonged recovery beyond the expected typical course.
- No medications or supplements are currently recommended to speed up recovery from concussion, and there are no US Food and Drug Administration–approved medications with specific indications for concussion.
- There are recent and ongoing clinical trials of supplements including docosahexaenoic acid regarding their role in concussion recovery.
- Providers should be aware of possible medications to treat prolonged concussion symptoms, including potential side effects.

INTRODUCTION

In a world where medications are commonly requested by patients, concussion is one diagnosis where they are not commonly prescribed. Although clinicians hope to speed the process of recovery, to this date there is no medicine or supplement clinically proved to reliably improve concussion recovery times. However, there are recent and ongoing clinical trials of certain supplements that may provide an opportunity to minimize symptoms during recovery. Note that there are no medications that are US Food and Drug Administration approved specifically for the treatment of concussion, and any medications prescribed would be considered off-label use.

Over-the-counter supplements are typically readily available, have a favorable risk/benefit profile, and may be useful as an adjunctive treatment, particularly early in the concussion recovery course. Prescription medications more commonly carry the risk

[a] Department of Sports Medicine, Texas Scottish Rite Hospital for Children, Dallas, TX, USA;
[b] Department of Orthopaedic Surgery and Pediatrics, University of Texas Southwestern, Dallas, TX, USA; [c] The Micheli Center for Sports Injury Prevention, Waltham, MA, USA; [d] Division of Sports Medicine, Department of Orthopedics, Boston Children's Hospital, Boston, MA, USA; [e] Department of Orthopaedic Surgery, Harvard Medical School, Boston, MA, USA; [f] Boston Children's Sports Medicine, 319 Longwood Avenue, Boston, MA 02115, USA
* Corresponding author. Sports Medicine, Scottish Rite for Children, 5700 Dallas Parkway, Frisco, TX 75034.
E-mail address: Jacob.jones@tsrh.org

Clin Sports Med 40 (2021) 123–131
https://doi.org/10.1016/j.csm.2020.08.005
0278-5919/21/© 2020 Elsevier Inc. All rights reserved.

for more significant side effects and are instituted only when certain criteria are met, most commonly in the cases of prolonged recovery or heavy symptom burden without improvement with standard care.

Posttraumatic headaches are a common sequela of concussion, and headache is the most common symptom reported with concussion.[1–5] Headaches may be persistent and episodically exacerbated by triggers commonly found in a student-athletes' lives, including stress (cognitive or physical), light (including digital devices), noise, movement, and peripheral movement (eg, crowded cafeterias or being a passenger in a motor vehicle).

Most patients recover from concussion within a period of days to weeks,[1,4,6–8] but some patients (perhaps up to 15%[9]) still have symptoms beyond a 3-month period.[9,10]

Prescription medications are typically considered only if the duration of symptoms exceeds the typical expected recovery period, symptom burden is significantly affecting quality of life (eg, activities of daily living, such as school attendance and participation, sleep quality, or basic light noncontact exercise), and the potential benefits of the medication outweigh the risks.[1] Medication therapy is not intended to return athletes to the playing field more quickly. If medication is initiated, the athlete should have successful resolution of all symptoms (as well as normalization of cognitive function and balance testing) during treatment and for a sustained amount of time after the withdrawal of the medication to be considered for potential return to contact sports. Of course, the prescribing clinician must be knowledgeable about the medication's dosing schedule, side effect profile, interactions with other medications, and pretreatment testing that may be necessary for any prescription.

Clinicians have tended to group the most common symptoms of concussion into domains or symptom clusters. Most commonly, the symptoms are categorized as somatic (most commonly headache), sleep disturbances, emotional symptoms, and cognitive symptoms.[1,11]

HEADACHES

Headache is a common symptom after concussion.[12] Interestingly, headaches are even more common after mild traumatic brain injury (TBI), such as concussion, compared with moderate and severe TBI.[1,2,13–15] Headaches may be described in several ways, including constant, episodic, band or tensionlike, or migrainous (eg, associated with light and noise sensitivity or nausea). They are often classified according to the International Headache Society classification system as a means to tailor treatment.[1] Even in the setting of postconcussion syndrome, clinicians should be aware of the many other common causes of headaches, including dehydration, poor nutrition, decreased visual acuity, stress, allergies, and menstrual cycle. The original injury may also have had concomitant cervical myofascial injury (whiplash), or triggered neuropathic scalp pain, so the evaluation of the patient should always include palpation of the occipital, cervical, and periscapular areas to look for areas of tenderness, trigger points, or allodynia. These examinations may be opportunities to alleviate nonconcussion contributors to headache with physical therapy, massage, acupuncture, or, in rare cases, occipital nerve blocks.

The characteristics of a headache can help guide potential treatment options. Of patients with postconcussive headaches, a study showed that about half of the patients have migrainelike features, whereas 32% to 37% have characteristics of tension-type headache.[16] Cervicogenic headache was third at around 4% and unclassified averaged around 11%.[16] Many, including the American Medical Society of Sports Medicine (AMSSM),[17] recommend that headaches be treated based on the characteristics and type of headache.[13]

Most people with concussion self-treat their headaches with over-the-counter medications, including nonsteroidal antiinflammatory drugs (NSAIDs) and/or acetaminophen, regardless of the type of headache.[16] However prolonged daily use of NSAIDs carries the potential risk of rebound headaches, which may complicate recovery.[1,2,15,18]

NSAIDs and acetaminophen are used principally as an abortive treatment, but, for patients with daily disruptive headaches, a preventive medication may be warranted. For prevention of migrainelike postconcussive headaches, tricyclic antidepressants (TCAs) and antiepileptics are commonly used.[1,19,20]

For many years, amitriptyline (a TCA) has been a common option.[21–24] Although the data are not universal, some retrospective studies have shown that up to 90% of patients achieve excellent or good recovery when treated with amitriptyline for posttraumatic headaches.[23] It has been found to be helpful for migrainous and tension-type headaches.[1,3,15,25] TCAs are typically prescribed at much lower doses compared with the levels needed for antidepressant treatment. This fact may be used as a clarification point for patients and families who may be shocked at the suggestion that an antidepressant may be prescribed for their child. It is also wise to obtain an electrocardiograph to confirm that the patient does not have prolonged-QT syndrome because TCAs can drive this condition into an arrhythmia.[25] Among the most common side effects of amitriptyline and other TCAs is drowsiness, especially on initiation of treatment. For this reason, a TCA is typically dosed before bedtime, and it may have a particular advantage in those patients with both headache and insomnia. If daytime somnolence is particularly disruptive, nortriptyline could be considered as a potentially less sedating alternative to amitriptyline. Although less common than fatigue, all TCAs still carry the risk of increased emotionality, palpitations, or orthostasis. In our practice, we aim for the lowest effective dose between 10 mg and 50 mg, commonly starting at a low dose of 10 mg and, over several weeks, reassessing clinically to evaluate for tolerance and effectiveness.

Other classes of medications that have commonly been used include antiepileptics. Valproic acid seems to be an additional, relatively safe option for treatment of persistent headaches after trauma.[26]

Topiramate is another viable option for postconcussive headache.[27] As with all medications, providers should be aware of the side effect profile and be comfortable with prescribing these and titrating them to effect. Gabapentin has also been used frequently for prolonged headaches, particularly if there is clinical evidence of neuropathic scalp pain or allodynia, despite the fact that it lacks good evidence for its efficacy in treating migraines.[28] Especially on initiation, this medicine can cause fatigue. Similar to some of the other medications, prescribers can use this to advantage by starting the medication at nighttime while the patient builds a tolerance to the side effects. Gabapentin has a large therapeutic window so it can be titrated to effect as long as the patient tolerates it. Also remember that, when it is time to stop this medication, a gradual tapering will help reduce potential withdrawal symptoms.[29]

β-Blockers, most commonly propranolol, are another class of medications that are commonly used in migraine prophylaxis and may be considered in posttraumatic headache treatment when it is migraine type.[1,3,15,18,22,26] As with the other medications, clinicians must be aware of the side effects of this drug. Avoid prescribing this medication in patients with asthma and low blood pressure, among other conditions, because of unfavorable beta-blockade side effects. In some patients, β-blockers can have an anxiolytic effect; however, they may also potentially exacerbate the symptoms of depression, which is a common comorbidity in patients with prolonged headache and postconcussion syndrome after minor TBI (mTBI).[30,31]

SLEEP

Sleep patterns are commonly affected following concussion[32] and disruptions in quality sleep can exacerbate symptoms of anxiety and mood.[33] Sleep disruption itself can create most of the symptoms seen on the Postconcussion Symptom Scale, including fatigue, irritability, difficulty concentrating, difficulty remembering, not feeling right, and so forth. Ideally, restoring sleep patterns should be attempted without medication when possible.[17] The first thing to address is sleep hygiene, which includes eliminating screen time in the evening before bedtime; sleeping in a dark, cool room; avoiding caffeine and alcohol consumption; minimizing daytime napping; reducing noise; and performing daily exercise.[34] Sleep hygiene is key when working with postconcussive patients.

Melatonin levels, which naturally regulate the sleep/wake cycle in the brain, decrease in the setting of bright lights.[35] Therefore, in postconcussive patients, suggestions include avoiding digital screens and dimming lights at least an hour before bedtime. TBI may alter melatonin levels, and late-night screen time may further exacerbate this phenomenon.[33,36,37] Naps are also common during the concussion recovery, especially when patients are particularly somnolent in the initial phase, or when they are out of their normal pattern of school attendance and sports or exercise during prolonged recovery. Care must be taken to avoid deconditioning and to maintain the circadian rhythm. Daytime naps should be brief and should be avoided if nighttime sleep has become interrupted. Allowing for some daily daytime sun exposure; light activity, including walking; and avoidance of daytime naps may help mitigate some of the nighttime insomnia that can come with circadian dysregulation.

After addressing sleep hygiene, nightly melatonin supplements are a common, safe recommendation to help reregulate the circadian rhythm. Melatonin is safe, available over the counter, and low cost. Interestingly, melatonin has not only been shown to improve sleep in patients with TBI but has improved cognition in animal TBI models.[38] However, the application of melatonin as a cognitive therapy is far from being considered well established.

Some medications used for insomnia, such as benzodiazepines and atypical GABA (gamma-aminobutyric acid) agonists may have negative effects on cognition and judgment; therefore, they should be avoided in the setting of concussion recovery.[17,39] Cognitive behavior therapy has been beneficial in general cases of insomnia, with some small studies showing that it helps anxiety and depression in postconcussion patients.[33]

OTHER SYMPTOMS

Following head injury, depression and other anxiety are potential comorbidities.[30,31] Unlike the paradoxic pattern with headaches, where headaches are often more disruptive in mTBI than in more severe trauma, these psychological conditions tend to be more common in severe injuries.[40–42] The AMSSM recommends consideration of medications for mood disturbance only after 6 to 12 weeks of continued symptoms. It also endorses the role of cognitive-based therapy, in place of or in conjunction with medications.[17] Furthermore, the AMSSM recommendations state that stimulants should not be used for acute attention problems acquired from a concussion, which are expected to be temporary.[17] However, if a patient had a previously diagnosed attention disorder and was on a stimulant medication preinjury, we withhold these medications only during the acute phase (24–48 hours) while also recommending brief cognitive and exercise restrictions during that time. Withholding this medication for a prolonged period of time may make it difficult to identify the cause of any ongoing attention difficulties. At present, there seems to be no evidence-based reason for prolonged withholding of stimulant medications in the setting of concussion recovery.

There have been proposed medical treatments, including memantine, β-blockers, betahistine, and oxcarbazepine, for oculomotor and vestibular disorders that may occur after concussion.[43] These medications are not routinely prescribed by providers managing concussions, but they may be considered by otolaryngology specialists, ocular specialists, or others with appropriate subspecialty experience.

Other over-the-Counter Supplements

Magnesium has often been used in headache prevention and may be applied as a safe, over-the-counter option for posttraumatic headaches. In patients with migraine headaches, studies have discovered that free magnesium levels are often low.[44–46] Other studies have shown that magnesium can be a good option in reducing the severity and frequency of migraine headaches.[47]

Magnesium glycinate and magnesium citrate are best absorbed by the body, whereas magnesium oxide, which is cheaper but poorly absorbed, may result in more of a tendency toward loose stools or diarrhea. Riboflavin, commonly known as vitamin B_2, is also used as a migraine prophylaxis.[48,49] This water-soluble vitamin is another safe option for posttraumatic headache with migraine characteristics. For migraine prophylaxis, magnesium dosages range from 360 to 600 mg daily in adults (most commonly, 400 mg daily).[50–53] Riboflavin is typically dosed at 400 mg daily in adults.[54–56] Younger children can even benefit from and tolerate daily doses of 200 mg of riboflavin.[57] There are proprietary blends of magnesium with riboflavin combinations, often with additional supplements such as feverfew, which have been effective for migraine prophylaxis for some patients. Other supplements often mentioned as remedies for migraine prevention include coenzyme q10, alpha-lipoic acid, and butterbur.[58,59]

OMEGA-3 FATTY ACIDS

Although there are no recommended medical treatments to prevent concussion or speed recovery from concussion, one supplement that seems to have the most promise may be omega-3 fatty acids. One particular omega-3 fatty acid, docosahexaenoic acid (DHA), has been a focus of research because it is the predominant omega-3 fatty acid found in the phospholipid membranes of neurons.[60,61] Following TBI, phospholipid membranes break down and DHA levels are altered.[61,62] In addition, DHA plays a role in the cellular signaling cascade helping to protect against cell death,[61,63,64] regulates neurotransmitter levels,[65] and possesses antiinflammatory properties.[65] Perhaps more importantly, there are several animal studies that investigated the benefit of omega-3 fatty acid supplementation in both preventing and treating concussion.[61,65–68] In humans, there are reports that DHA could improve cognition in patients with TBI,[65,66] and may even benefit others with attention-deficit/hyperactivity disorder or depression.[61] The interest in using DHA in human patients with concussion has grown and this has led to a recent, small feasibility clinical trial that showed that 2000 mg of daily DHA may hasten recovery in the concussed pediatric population.[67] Because of the promising results, a larger, multicenter clinical trial of DHA in concussions could lead to future recommendations in concussion recovery. Considered relatively safe,[67] common side effects of taking DHA, or other fish oils, are generally benign and include fishlike breath, belches, looser stools, reflux, and nausea.[68] Concerns raised about omega-3 fatty acids increasing bleeding risks were not supported in studies, including with patients already taking other antithrombotic medications.[69]

SUMMARY

The medications that are used in postconcussion syndrome are typically used to help manage or minimize disruptive symptoms while recovery proceeds. These medications are not routinely used in most patients with concussion, who recover within days to weeks. However, it is beneficial to be aware of medication options that may be used in athletes with prolonged concussion symptoms or for those that have symptom burdens that preclude entry into basic concussion protocols, such as school reentry and light noncontact exercise. Clinicians who manage concussions frequently should become familiar with the options that are being used and investigated. Medications and supplements remain a small part of the concussion treatment plan, which may include temporary academic adjustments, physical therapy, vestibular and ocular therapy, psychological support, and graded noncontact exercise.

DISCLOSURE

The authors have no financial relationships relevant to this study to disclose. Dr J.C. Jones has no relevant affiliations or financial involvement with any organization or entity with a financial interest in or financial conflict with the subject matter or materials discussed in this article, including employment, consultancies, honoraria, stock ownership or options, expert testimony, grants or patents received or pending, or royalties. Peer reviewers on this article have no relevant financial relationships to disclose. Dr M.J. O'Brien is reimbursed by Wolters Kluwer Publishing for authorship and ongoing editing of 2 concussion-related sections for *UptoDate* online clinical resource. He has no conflicts of interest to disclose.

REFERENCES

1. Meehan WP. Medical therapies for concussion. Clin Sports Med 2011;30(1): 115–24, ix.
2. Packard RC. Epidemiology and pathogenesis of posttraumatic headache. J Head Trauma Rehabil 1999;14(1):9–21.
3. Weiss HD, Stern BJ, Goldberg J. Post-traumatic migraine: chronic migraine precipitated by minor head or neck trauma. Headache 1991;31(7):451–6.
4. Guskiewicz KM, McCrea M, Marshall SW, et al. Cumulative effects associated with recurrent concussion in collegiate football players: the NCAA Concussion Study. JAMA 2003;290(19):2549–55.
5. Guskiewicz KM, Weaver NL, Padua DA, et al. Epidemiology of concussion in collegiate and high school football players. Am J Sports Med 2000;28(5):643–50.
6. McCrory P, Meeuwisse W, Dvořák J, et al. Consensus statement on concussion in sport-the 5th international conference on concussion in sport held in Berlin, October 2016. Br J Sports Med 2017;51(11):838–47.
7. Iverson GL, Brooks BL, Collins MW, et al. Tracking neuropsychological recovery following concussion in sport. Brain Inj 2006;20(3):245–52.
8. Guskiewicz KM, Ross SE, Marshall SW. Postural stability and neuropsychological deficits after concussion in collegiate athletes. J Athl Train 2001;36(3):263–73.
9. Kuczynski A, Crawford S, Bodell L, et al. Characteristics of post-traumatic headaches in children following mild traumatic brain injury and their response to treatment: a prospective cohort. Dev Med Child Neurol 2013;55(7):636–41.
10. Gavett BE, Stern RA, McKee AC. Chronic traumatic encephalopathy: a potential late effect of sport-related concussive and subconcussive head trauma. Clin Sports Med 2011;30(1):179–88, xi.

11. Reddy CC. A treatment paradigm for sports concussion. Brain Injury Professional 2004;4:24–5.
12. McConnell B, Duffield T, Hall T, et al. Post-traumatic headache after pediatric traumatic brain injury: prevalence, risk factors, and association with neurocognitive outcomes. J Child Neurol 2020;35(1):63–70.
13. Lucas S. Characterization and management of headache after mild traumatic brain injury. In: Kobeissy FH, editor. Brain neurotrauma: molecular, neuropsychological, and rehabilitation aspects. Frontiers in neuroengineering. Boca Raton (FL): CRC Press/Taylor & Francis; 2015. Available at: http://www.ncbi.nlm.nih.gov/books/NBK299177/. Accessed January 18, 2020.
14. Couch JR, Bearss C. Chronic daily headache in the posttrauma syndrome: relation to extent of head injury. Headache 2001;41(6):559–64.
15. Lenaerts ME, Couch JR, Couch JR. Posttraumatic Headache. Curr Treat Options Neurol 2004;6(6):507–17.
16. DiTommaso C, Hoffman JM, Lucas S, et al. Medication usage patterns for headache treatment after mild traumatic brain injury. Headache 2014;54(3):511–9.
17. Harmon KG, Drezner JA, Gammons M, et al. American Medical Society for Sports Medicine position statement: concussion in sport. Br J Sports Med 2013;47(1): 15–26.
18. Lane JC, Arciniegas DB. Post-traumatic Headache. Curr Treat Options Neurol 2002;4(1):89–104.
19. Langdon R, Taraman S. Posttraumatic Headache. Pediatr Ann 2018;47(2):e61–8.
20. Mittenberg W, Canyock EM, Condit D, et al. Treatment of post-concussion syndrome following mild head injury. J Clin Exp Neuropsychol 2001;23(6):829–36.
21. Comper P, Bisschop SM, Carnide N, et al. A systematic review of treatments for mild traumatic brain injury. Brain Inj 2005;19(11):863–80.
22. Lew HL, Lin P-H, Fuh J-L, et al. Characteristics and treatment of headache after traumatic brain injury: a focused review. Am J Phys Med Rehabil 2006;85(7): 619–27.
23. Tyler GS, McNeely HE, Dick ML. Treatment of post-traumatic headache with amitriptyline. Headache 1980;20(4):213–6.
24. Label L. Treatment of post-traumatic headaches: maprotiline or amitriptyline? Neurology 1991;41(Suppl 1):247.
25. Alvarez PA, Pahissa J. QT alterations in psychopharmacology: proven candidates and suspects. Curr Drug Saf 2010;5(1):97–104.
26. Packard RC. Treatment of chronic daily posttraumatic headache with divalproex sodium. Headache 2000;40(9):736–9.
27. Erickson JC. Treatment outcomes of chronic post-traumatic headaches after mild head trauma in US soldiers: an observational study. Headache 2011;51(6): 932–44.
28. Ha H, Gonzalez A. Migraine Headache Prophylaxis. Am Fam Physician 2019; 99(1):17–24.
29. Norton JW. Gabapentin withdrawal syndrome. Clin Neuropharmacol 2001;24(4): 245–6.
30. Wei C-B, Jia J-P, Wang F, et al. Overlap between headache, depression, and anxiety in general neurological clinics: a cross-sectional study. Chin Med J 2016; 129(12):1394–9.
31. Cole WR, Arrieux JP, Dennison EM, et al. The impact of administration order in studies of computerized neurocognitive assessment tools (NCATs). J Clin Exp Neuropsychol 2017;39(1):35–45.

32. Schreiber S, Barkai G, Gur-Hartman T, et al. Long-lasting sleep patterns of adult patients with minor traumatic brain injury (mTBI) and non-mTBI subjects. Sleep Med 2008;9(5):481–7.
33. Sandsmark DK, Elliott JE, Lim MM. Sleep-wake disturbances after traumatic brain injury: synthesis of human and animal studies. Sleep 2017;40(5). https://doi.org/10.1093/sleep/zsx044.
34. Irish LA, Kline CE, Gunn HE, et al. The role of sleep hygiene in promoting public health: A review of empirical evidence. Sleep Med Rev 2015;22:23–36.
35. Lewy AJ, Wehr TA, Goodwin FK, et al. Light suppresses melatonin secretion in humans. Science 1980;210(4475):1267–9.
36. Figueiro MG, Wood B, Plitnick B, et al. The impact of light from computer monitors on melatonin levels in college students. Neuro Endocrinol Lett 2011;32(2):158–63.
37. Shekleton JA, Parcell DL, Redman JR, et al. Sleep disturbance and melatonin levels following traumatic brain injury. Neurology 2010;74(21):1732–8.
38. Barlow KM, Esser MJ, Veidt M, et al. Melatonin as a treatment after traumatic brain injury: a systematic review and meta-analysis of the pre-clinical and clinical literature. J Neurotrauma 2019;36(4):523–37.
39. Larson EB, Zollman FS. The effect of sleep medications on cognitive recovery from traumatic brain injury. J Head Trauma Rehabil 2010;25(1):61–7.
40. Dikmen SS, Bombardier CH, Machamer JE, et al. Natural history of depression in traumatic brain injury. Arch Phys Med Rehabil 2004;85(9):1457–64.
41. O'Donnell ML, Creamer M, Pattison P, et al. Psychiatric morbidity following injury. Am J Psychiatry 2004;161(3):507–14.
42. Deb S, Lyons I, Koutzoukis C, et al. Rate of psychiatric illness 1 year after traumatic brain injury. Am J Psychiatry 1999;156(3):374–8.
43. Strupp M, Thurtell MJ, Shaikh AG, et al. Pharmacotherapy of vestibular and ocular motor disorders, including nystagmus. J Neurol 2011;258(7):1207–22.
44. Lodi R, Montagna P, Soriani S, et al. Deficit of brain and skeletal muscle bioenergetics and low brain magnesium in juvenile migraine: an in vivo 31P magnetic resonance spectroscopy interictal study. Pediatr Res 1997;42(6):866–71.
45. Lodi R, Iotti S, Cortelli P, et al. Deficient energy metabolism is associated with low free magnesium in the brains of patients with migraine and cluster headache. Brain Res Bull 2001;54(4):437–41.
46. Ramadan NM, Halvorson H, Vande-Linde A, et al. Low brain magnesium in migraine. Headache 1989;29(7):416–9.
47. Chiu H-Y, Yeh T-H, Huang Y-C, et al. Effects of intravenous and oral magnesium on reducing migraine: a meta-analysis of randomized controlled trials. Pain Physician 2016;19(1):E97–112.
48. Thompson DF, Saluja HS. Prophylaxis of migraine headaches with riboflavin: A systematic review. J Clin Pharm Ther 2017;42(4):394–403.
49. Namazi N, Heshmati J, Tarighat-Esfanjani A. Supplementation with riboflavin (vitamin b2) for migraine prophylaxis in adults and children: a review. Int J Vitam Nutr Res 2015;85(1–2):79–87.
50. Peikert A, Wilimzig C, Köhne-Volland R. Prophylaxis of migraine with oral magnesium: results from a prospective, multi-center, placebo-controlled and double-blind randomized study. Cephalalgia 1996;16(4):257–63.
51. Facchinetti F, Sances G, Borella P, et al. Magnesium prophylaxis of menstrual migraine: effects on intracellular magnesium. Headache 1991;31(5):298–301.
52. Schuck P, Böhmer K, Resch KL. [Migraine and prevention of migraine: the value of magnesium]. Schweiz Med Wochenschr 1999;129(3):63–70.

53. Yablon LA, Mauskop A. Magnesium in headache. In: Vink R, Nechifor M, editors. Magnesium in the central nervous system. Adelaide (AU): University of Adelaide Press; 2011. p. 129–31. Available at: http://www.ncbi.nlm.nih.gov/books/NBK507271/. Accessed January 18, 2020.

54. Boehnke C, Reuter U, Flach U, et al. High-dose riboflavin treatment is efficacious in migraine prophylaxis: an open study in a tertiary care centre. Eur J Neurol 2004;11(7):475–7.

55. Maizels M, Blumenfeld A, Burchette R. A combination of riboflavin, magnesium, and feverfew for migraine prophylaxis: a randomized trial. Headache 2004; 44(9):885–90.

56. Schoenen J, Jacquy J, Lenaerts M. Effectiveness of high-dose riboflavin in migraine prophylaxis. A randomized controlled trial. Neurology 1998;50(2): 466–70.

57. Talebian A, Soltani B, Banafshe HR, et al. Prophylactic effect of riboflavin on pediatric migraine: a randomized, double-blind, placebo-controlled trial. Electron Physician 2018;10(2):6279–85.

58. D'Onofrio F, Raimo S, Spitaleri D, et al. Usefulness of nutraceuticals in migraine prophylaxis. Neurol Sci 2017;38(Suppl 1):117–20.

59. Guilbot A, Bangratz M, Ait Abdellah S, et al. A combination of coenzyme Q10, feverfew and magnesium for migraine prophylaxis: a prospective observational study. BMC Complement Altern Med 2017;17(1):433.

60. Bazan NG. Neuroprotectin D1 (NPD1): a DHA-derived mediator that protects brain and retina against cell injury-induced oxidative stress. Brain Pathol 2005; 15(2):159–66.

61. Bailes JE, Patel V. The potential for DHA to mitigate mild traumatic brain injury. Mil Med 2014;179(11 Suppl):112–6.

62. Homayoun P, Rodriguez de Turco EB, Parkins NE, et al. Delayed phospholipid degradation in rat brain after traumatic brain injury. J Neurochem 1997;69(1): 199–205.

63. Huang WL, King VR, Curran OE, et al. A combination of intravenous and dietary docosahexaenoic acid significantly improves outcome after spinal cord injury. Brain 2007;130(Pt 11):3004–19.

64. Pan H-C, Kao T-K, Ou Y-C, et al. Protective effect of docosahexaenoic acid against brain injury in ischemic rats. J Nutr Biochem 2009;20(9):715–25.

65. Barrett EC, McBurney MI, Ciappio ED. ω-3 fatty acid supplementation as a potential therapeutic aid for the recovery from mild traumatic brain injury/concussion. Adv Nutr 2014;5(3):268–77.

66. Lewis M, Ghassemi P, Hibbeln J. Therapeutic use of omega-3 fatty acids in severe head trauma. Am J Emerg Med 2013;31(1):273.e5–8.

67. Miller SM, Zynda AJ, Sabatino MJ, et al. Docosahexaenoic acid (dha) for the treatment of pediatric sport-related concussion: results of a feasibility trial. Orthop J Sports Med 2019;7(3_suppl). 2325967119S0000.

68. Trojian TH, Jackson E. Ω-3 polyunsaturated fatty acids and concussions: treatment or not? Curr Sports Med Rep 2011;10(4):180–5.

69. Bays HE. Safety considerations with omega-3 fatty acid therapy. Am J Cardiol 2007;99(6A):35C–43C.

Female Athlete and Sports-Related Concussions

Katherine H. Rizzone, MD, MPH[a],*, Kathryn E. Ackerman, MD, MPH[b]

KEYWORDS

- Concussion • Female athlete • Injury epidemiology • Gender disparity

KEY POINTS

- In matched sports (eg, soccer and basketball), female athletes experience higher rates of sports-related concussion compared with their male counterparts.
- Female athletes have longer recovery times compared with male athletes after a sports-related concussion.
- There are anatomic, biomechanical, and biochemical differences between the sexes that may contribute to the epidemiologic disparity of incidence and recovery between the sexes.

INTRODUCTION

Female athletes are participating in athletics at all levels (scholastic, collegiate, and professional) at higher rates than previously.[1] Although male athletes still comprise the majority of participants in sports like football, many collision and contact sports, such as soccer, basketball, lacrosse, hockey, and wrestling, have seen increased female participation in recent years.[2] Female athletes also compete in sports, such as gymnastics,[3] cheerleading,[4] and competitive dance, in greater numbers than their male counterparts. Although these sports often are not considered collision or contact sports in the traditional sense, several athletes experience sports-related concussions (SRCs) while participating, because they are using their bodies as projectiles.[5–7] Post-concussion, women report greater symptomatology,[8] score more poorly on neuro-cognitive testing,[9] and are noted to have higher mortality rates compared with their male equivalents.[10] This article discusses the epidemiology of concussions in girls and women; what is known about female risk factors for concussions; suggestions for concussion treatment and prevention; and future directions to improve knowledge and care of female athletes susceptible to concussion.

[a] Orthopaedics and Pediatrics, University of Rochester Medical Center, 601 Elmwood Avenue Box 665, Rochester, NY 14642, USA; [b] Medicine, Harvard Medical School, Boston Children's Hospital, Massachusetts General Hospital, Sports Medicine, 319 Longwood Avenue 6th Floor, Boston, MA 02115, USA
* Corresponding author.
E-mail address: katherine_rizzone@urmc.rochester.edu

Clin Sports Med 40 (2021) 133–145
https://doi.org/10.1016/j.csm.2020.08.006
0278-5919/21/© 2020 Elsevier Inc. All rights reserved.

EPIDEMIOLOGY

Female athletes experience concussions in similar sports as their male counterparts (eg, soccer, basketball, lacrosse, and softball) but also have unique activities in which they participate in greater numbers than male athletes (eg, cheerleading, gymnastics, and field hockey), which are associated with high concussion rates.[11] Although male athletes experience a greater number of overall concussions, female athletes have a greater incidence of SRCs compared with male athletes.[11–13] Of the youth sports with the highest rates of concussion, women's soccer is second only to football with concussion injury burden[11,14] and more recent data have highlighted that high school female soccer players actually may have a greater incidence of concussions compared with high school football players.[15] In sex-comparable sports (basketball, ice hockey, soccer, and baseball/softball), high school female athletes had 1.4-times greater concussion incidence than male athletes.[16] In soccer and basketball, collegiate female athletes had a higher duration of time loss from sports after concussion compared with their male counterparts.[14]

Ice hockey and lacrosse are some of the fastest growing sports in the United States.[17] Play is different in the respective genders, because the rules are designed to encourage less contact in the female versions of these sports (eg, no body checking).[18,19] Researchers tracking concussions during international hockey tournaments found that adult female hockey players had lower rates of concussion than adult male hockey players (1.0/1000 player-games for women and 1.4/1000 player-games for men). At the under-18 level of participation, however, female players and male players had similar concussion rates (1.4/1000 player-games for both girl and boy hockey players).[20] Youth-level coaches (28% of whom were women) of female hockey players had similar levels of concussion knowledge as coaches of male youth hockey players.[21]

Men's lacrosse is a collision sport, whereas women's lacrosse has been considered a contact sport. Injuries have been decreasing in men's lacrosse but have been noted to be increasing in women's lacrosse.[22] Recent rule changes may be leading to more contact in women's lacrosse (eg, subbing on the fly and establishment of the shot clock). Over the past 2 decades, women's lacrosse has added protective eyewear and in some regions also has added protective helmets.[23] As women's sports continue to evolve to involve more contact, injury rates will likely go up, as they have in women's lacrosse, despite equipment modifications. Early research examining the effect of soft headgear on injury rates in women's lacrosse found no significant reduction in linear or rotational impacts from high-velocity ball impacts or lateral impact response for stick impact. The soft headgear, however, did lead to a small decrease in frontal impacts of stick impact to the head.[24] More research is needed to better ascertain risk reduction from head equipment.

Baseball and softball are similar sports but with important differences. The distance from the pitcher's mound to the batter is shorter in softball compared with baseball, as is the difference between the bases. A systematic review examined traumatic brain injuries (TBIs) in baseball and softball. Female softball players were more than twice as likely to experience a concussion compared with male baseball players.[25] In high school players, a majority of concussions were experienced by the catcher in softball (29.7%), but by the batter in baseball (50.6%). At the collegiate level, a majority of TBIs occurred to the batter in softball and to the middle infielder in baseball.[25]

Female athletes participate in gymnastics, competitive dance, and cheerleading at higher rates than athletes.[3,4,26,27] There is a lack of understanding of the full epidemiologic concussion burden in these activities, but the few published studies demonstrate that there is concussion injury burden in these sports.[14,28,29] Uncertainty of SRC rates in competitive dance and cheer has been compounded by evolving definitions of what is considered a sport. Competitive cheerleading only recently has been classified a sport, which contributes to the paucity of injury data. Additionally, there is a deficit of specific tracking information for competitive dance in sports injury epidemiology.[30]

ANATOMY/PHYSIOLOGY/CHEMICAL DIFFERENCES

Concussion symptoms are thought to result from an alteration and dysregulation of cerebral blood flow.[31] Thus, research has focused on monitoring brain perfusion during the recovery process. Studies have shown a baseline sex difference in healthy, noninjured young adults, with female athletes having a higher global cerebral blood flow compared with male athletes on PET scan.[32] In a study of 9 concussed female athletes and 13 nonconcussed, healthy athlete controls, cerebral blood flow was monitored via transcranial Doppler (TCD). Concussed athletes demonstrated significantly lower minute ventilation and CO_2 sensitivity but greater cerebral blood flow at similar exercise workloads in association with symptom onset and premature exercise cessation. These findings were thought to be due to increased perfusion needs from injury. The minute ventilation, CO_2 sensitivity, and cerebral blood flow changes of the concussed athletes improved after subsymptom threshold aerobic exercise treadmill therapy.[33] In contrast, a TCD study of 58 postconcussive adolescent athletes ages 14 years old to 19 years old demonstrated that female athletes had no changes on TCD even when still reporting symptoms subjectively; this was not observed in the male participants.[34] This suggests that there are subclinical changes that differ by sex that need to be considered both in clinical evaluation and within research studies examining cerebral perfusion changes.

In both in vitro rat and human stem cell axonal cultures, female axons were consistently smaller than male axons and displayed greater damage with dynamic stretch-injury mechanics compared with male axons. This led to greater swelling and loss of normal calcium signaling in female tissues compared with male tissues.[35] These axonal level findings could help explain symptomology differences between the sexes but need to be evaluated with greater depth in further human studies.

Chronic traumatic encephalopathy (CTE) is caused by repetitive TBI and defined by neuropathology showing degenerative changes in brain tissue on autopsy: hyperphosphorylated tau in gray matter, myelin loss, axonal injury, and white matter microstructural changes.[36] Much of the anatomic research involving long-term effects of concussion, in particular those of CTE, have focused on the brains of male athletes, whereas data are lacking in female athletes.[37–39] In 1 small study of female athletes, 8 young adult, nonconcussed female soccer and hockey players were compared with 10 soccer, hockey, and water polo female players who were 6 months postconcussion. There were no differences on diffusion tensor imaging in the corticospinal tract between the 2 groups, but, within the corpus callosum, the concussed group had lower diffusivity in the area that leads to the prefrontal cortex (whose responsibilities include planning and high-level thinking).[40] Because the function of the corpus collosum is to synthesize motor, sensory, and cognitive functions of the 2 hemispheres of the brain, such a finding suggests considerable neurocognitive deficiencies that should be explored further in athletes of both sexes.

Autonomic responses to postural changes were examined in a study that compared 65 concussed adolescent athletes (60% female) to a control group of 54 nonconcussed athletes (46% female). Heart rate variability, heart rate, and blood pressure were monitored during 6 weekly clinic visits. Less heart rate variability was found in concussed versus nonconcussed female athletes, with no significant difference noted between the male athlete groups. In the overall cohort, the postconcussive participants had greater baseline seated blood pressures and heart rates compared with the controls. These parameters resolved by the end of the study, but the heart rate variability decrease did not resolve in the female participants, suggesting a possible autonomic dysregulation sex disparity, potentially contributing to longer duration of symptomatology.[41] Because vestibular coordination is known to be a factor in symptomatology and is related to postural motions, understanding this difference in the body's autonomic response to injury may help explain the prolonged recovery repeatedly observed in female athletes postinjury.

An area of concussion research that is expanding rapidly and leading to new areas of focus in diagnosis, management, and time to recovery is the field of concussive biomarkers. In a cohort of 415 healthy, nonconcussed collegiate athletes (39% female), β-amyloid 42, total tau, S100 calcium binding protein B (S100B), ubiquitin carboxy-terminal hydrolyzing enzyme L1 (UCH-L1), glial fibrillary acidic protein, microtubule-associated protein 2, and 2′,3′-cyclic-nucelotide 3′-phosphodiesterase (CNPase) serum concentrations were measured. There were baseline biomarker differences between female athletes and male athletes; notably, female athletes had higher CNPase and lower UCH-L1 and S100 B compared with male athletes.[42] In the same cohort, there were no differences found between the sexes in terms of previous concussions, even though male athletes had a statistically significant higher number of years of cumulative exposure to collision sports (10.2 years ± 5.2 years in male athletes compared with 8.5 years ± 6.1 years in female athletes). Biomarkers were examined in the context of reported number of prior concussions and no differences were found specific to sex.[43] Although athletes and clinicians are eager to find the ideal concussion-related biomarker for diagnosis and recovery tracking, there is no conclusive evidence that any specific serum or blood biomarker is useful to date.

Additionally, physiologic differences from hormonal regulation have also been suggested.[44] In women with typical menstrual cycles, estrogen is low in the early follicular phase (menses), slowly rises and peaks right before ovulation, abruptly drops, slowly increases to a lower mid–luteal phase peak, and then declines into its nadir again during menses (early follicular phase). Progesterone is low throughout the follicular phase, increases after ovulation, gradually peaks mid–luteal phase, and drops with its nadir again during the follicular phase. The average menstrual cycle is 29 days, with a normal range of 24 days to 35 days, because there is large interindividual and intraindividual variability.[45] As with other sports injuries, it has been postulated that female athletes may be more susceptible to concussion during a particular phase of their menstrual cycles. In a preliminary report of 18 eumenorrheic female athletes who experienced an SRC, two-thirds experienced SRC during the late luteal phase or during the first 2 days of menstruation (a 9-day span), suggesting increased SRC risk when estrogen and progesterone are low.[46] Wunderle and colleagues[47] studied 144 premenopausal female patients (16–60 years old) who presented to the emergency department within 4 hours of a mild TBI (mTBI), assessed phase of menstrual cycle via interview and laboratory testing, and assessed recovery 1 month postinjury. Women who sustained a mTBI during the luteal phase (n = 37) had a significantly lower quality of life and were in worse health 1 month after mTBI than those who were injured during the follicular phase (n = 72) or were on hormonal contraceptives (HCs) (n = 35).[47] The investigators proposed a "withdrawal hypothesis," suggesting that women may fare worse if they sustained a TBI when progesterone levels were high and then decreasing or if the concussion led to an abrupt drop in progesterone, but hormone levels were not assessed to verify if there were changes in progesterone over time.[47]

In a study of 68 adolescent and young adult female athletes post-SRC versus 61 female athletes post–other sports-related orthopedic injuries, 23.5% of the SRC group experienced 2 or more abnormal menstrual cycles during the study follow-up period (120 days) versus only 5% of the nonhead orthopedic injury group. All participants previously had been eumenorrheic, suggesting at least transient disruption of the hypothalamic-pituitary-ovarian axis in some female athletes postconcussion.[48] This is consistent with findings in adults with TBI. In a prospective study of 46 consecutive patients with TBI (33% female), 76% had early laboratory testing consistent with hypogonadism or hypothyroidism, with long-term hypopituitarism frequent only in severe TBI.[49]

In a study of collegiate athletes, 24 female athletes using HCs and 25 not using hormonal birth control when concussed were compared. Non-HC users had higher symptom severity than HC users but no significant difference in length of recovery.[44] Because it was small study, with little description of type or timing of HC (1 was using NuvaRing), it makes it difficult to draw conclusions about the potential benefits of HC and various hormone levels.

In an early rodent model (1993), male rats given estrogen prior to induced brain trauma had improved concussion outcomes (eg, higher brain-free magnesium concentration, greater brain cytosolic phosphorylation potential, and better 1-week posttrauma motor function) whereas female rats post–brain trauma had higher mortality than the male rats in general, and those with estrogen treatment had even lower cytosolic phosphorylation potential postinjury.[50] This suggests that estrogen was neuroprotective in male rats and exacerbated brain injury in female rats. In contrast, in another series of experiments, acute survival post-TBI was much greater in female rats versus male rats and female rats had a less dramatic drop in and better recovery of cortical blood flow than male rats. When rats were given 2 weeks of daily 17β-estradiol injections prior to injury, postinjury cortical blood flow was higher in both female rats and male rats compared with those given sham injections.[51] Estrogen is known to have antioxidant effects and enhance endothelial nitric oxide synthase, improving vasodilation; thus, a microvascular benefit from estrogen is plausible. Progesterone also has potential neuroprotective properties and may enhance repair of damaged nerve cells via neurotrophic, anti-inflammatory, antiexcitotoxicity, anti–lipid peroxidase, and antiapoptotic mechanisms.[52] Rubin and Lipton[53] reviewed 50 publications of TBI in animal models that included male models and female models (rats, mice, and piglets). There was substantial variability in study design and results were somewhat model-dependent, but overall female models seemed to have better behavioral outcomes and less pathology after TBI compared with male models. Progesterone, in particular, was associated most commonly with beneficial effects.[53] In the few human studies using estrogen or progesterone as a treatment post-TBI, neither hormone has shown a consistent decrease in mortality or clear clinical benefit.[54]

More human studies are needed to determine if consistent hormone levels throughout injury and recovery are beneficial and if hormonal testing post-SRC and possible hormonal supplementation are warranted. At a minimum, it will expand knowledge in this field for medical providers managing SRC in women to ask about phases of the menstrual cycle at time of injury and to track menstrual cycle patterns more closely during recovery.

Psychosocial factors could an additional explanation to the observed sex and gender difference in concussion rates, becaus it has been suggested female athletes may be more likely to report symptoms postinjury.[55] A study of 435 Irish adolescent athletes found no significant differences in concussion reporting behaviors between the sexes.[56] But a large study of more than 30,000 Maine high school athletes found that nonconcussed female athletes reported concussion-like symptoms at baseline in greater numbers than male athletes.[57] A systematic review and meta-analysis of 21 studies of 12 year olds to 26 year olds reported that female athletes consistently reported more symptoms at baseline and postconcussion on the Post-Concussion scale and the Sport Concussion Assessment Tool (SCAT) (2nd version), than male athletes, but that the difference was not clinically significant.[58] It is unclear why symptom reporting varies between the sexes and it is likely a multifactorial reason that should be investigated further in order to better diagnosis and symptomatically managed post-concussive athletes of both genders.

BIOMECHANICAL FACTORS

Recent literature has proposed that decreased neck strength and lower control in head motion may be a risk factor for concussion. Females' overall smaller head circumferences, thinner skull cortices, and differences in spinal musculature all have been proposed sex-specific anatomic findings that may contribute to the sex disparity in concussion incidence.[59,60]

Youth female soccer players were found to have higher peak linear and rotational accelerations during a study monitoring forces during controlled soccer headers, exposing them to an increased risk of injury.[61] In a small study of college soccer players who wore accelerometers while heading the ball, female players had lower cervical/neck strength and neck girth and greater head velocities during impact compared with male players.[62] In youth soccer players ages 11 to 14, male athletes had more head impacts than female athletes but female athletes experienced head impacts of greater magnitude than male athletes.[63] A small study of collegiate female hockey players showed that players had lower peak linear accelerations during head impacts compared with linear accelerations previously reported in male players, but peak rotational accelerations were similar.[64]

An innovative, exploratory study reviewed pictures of soccer players on Google and found that there were significantly more pictures of female soccer players than male soccer players heading the ball with their eyes closed. These big data methods clearly have limitations but should prompt more investigation into the effects visual cues may contribute to increased risk of concussion in female athletes.[65]

Additional, unexplored potential risk contributors include environmental factors, such as different coaching styles in women's sports, game conditions, and even athletes' hair length. Coaches may play starting athletes at rates different from male athletes, increasing exposure and leading to increased risk for starting players. Games and matches may be held in less optimal spaces (eg, poor field conditions with less upkeep), leading to an increased risk of injury. Consideration of the barriers to girls and women in sports regarding funding and accessibility to optimal playing conditions should be incorporated in future risk assessment work.

A hot topic for concussion clinicians has been whether protective headgear decreases the risk of concussive injury. The theory behind this equipment utility is that the headgear may decrease the force to the head during heading. A large randomized controlled trial of adolescent soccer players examined the effectiveness of headgear in reducing concussion. There was no protective effect of headgear for male athletes or female athletes.[66] This may be because the most common mechanism for concussion in soccer players is from contact from other players, not because of trauma from headers.[67]

Further research should continue to examine possible preventive biomechanical mechanisms for concussion and these interventions should be tested on both male athletes and female athletes to ensure that findings are potentially pertinent to both sexes.

CONCUSSION TESTING DIFFERENCES

Neurocognitive testing frequently is utilized for concussion diagnosis, postconcussion symptom monitoring, and clearance for return to play. In 1 study, approximately 300 high school and collegiate athletes' baseline and postconcussion ImPACT and Post-Concussion Symptom Scale scores were analyzed. Female athletes had significantly lower visual memory scores compared with male athletes on ImPACT testing and also reported more concussive symptoms.[68] In a study of 79 collegiate athletes (48% female) who took ImPACT tests prior to injury and then postconcussion, there were no differences in baseline scores between the sexes. In a large study of high school athletes, there were significant differences in baseline ImPACT testing scores, with female athletes reporting more symptoms and slower reaction times on the computer-based test.[69] Postconcussion, female athletes demonstrated lower visual memory scores.[70] In a study of 188 collegiate athletes with a previous history of concussion (47% female), female athletes with 2 prior concussions and those with 3 or more concussions had higher visual memory scores compared with male athletes with the same concussion burden history. Additionally, male athletes scored lower on processing speed and reaction time compared with female athletes with the same concussion history.[71]

The SCAT was developed to allow for sideline assessment of concussion in athletes. Scores range from 0 to 100 with lower scores indicating more difficulty with cognitive and physical function. More than 1000 high school athletes were given the SCAT (2nd version) prior to concussion. Female athletes had higher overall scores compared with male athletes.[72] Examining SCAT (3rd version) in more than 2000 high school and collegiate athletes demonstrated that female athletes had higher baseline symptom scores on the testing but better Balance Error Scoring System scores compared with male athletes.[73]

MANAGEMENT OF SYMPTOMS

In a study of 277 high school athletes (47.5% female), adolescent girls and boys had similar SRC knowledge, but the female athletes were more likely to report their symptoms to an adult.[74] Comparing approximately 300 female atheletes and male athletes after concussion, female athletes reported more physical and somatic symptoms than their male counterparts.[75] In those experiencing their first lifetime concussion, female athletes reported a greater number of symptomatic days compared with male athletes regardless of age.[76] In a robust study of more than 300 concussed adolescents who were evaluated within 10 days of injury, gender was not a predictive factor in symptom resolution (an abnormal Romberg test was the largest predictor in a multivariate analysis), but female athletes had an odds ratio of 1.37 for longer symptom duration compared with male athletes.[77]

Female athletes have been shown to have prolonged symptoms in specific domains, including vestibular oculomotor motion screening (VOMS) and vestibular ocular reflex (VOR) scores. A small study of concussed young athletes showed that female gender explained 45% of the variance in the horizontal VOR scores postconcussion but there were no differences between sexes in the other VOMS scores.[78] Comparing gait tasks postconcussion in adolescent male athletes and female athletes (49% female), female athletes had a greater change in cadence. Both genders had shorter stride lengths compared with controls but there was no difference in reported symptom scales between male athletes and female athletes.[79]

Recently, more literature is highlighting that early aerobic exercise may quicken recovery from concussion. The research group that pioneered the Buffalo Concussion Treadmill Test has examined the impact of gender on this interaction. Relative rest and a stretching program were less effective than subsymptomatic threshold aerobic exercise in both male athletes and female athletes. There was a trend for female athletes to have more symptoms when prescribed rest.[80]

RETURN TO SPORT

This area of concussion has become a recent focus as more athletes and their families are looking for guidance postinjury. A large Canadian study that followed patients (ages 5–18 years) postconcussion found that most children ages 5 years to 7 years of age recovered within the initial 2 weeks after injury. For children ages 8 years old to 18 years old, recovery was closer to 4 weeks. Adolescent girls had significantly longer recovery time compared with adolescent boys, showing that most female athletes had not recovered by week 12.[81] This group currently is conducting a randomized controlled trial to compare full physical rest until completely asymptomatic versus returning to sport within 72 hours postinjury, regardless of symptoms.

A cohort of 726 adolescent athletes were followed over a 7-step return to play protocol that included an initial return to school prior to initiation of light exercise. Female athletes took almost a full week longer to reach step 3 and step 6 compared with their male counterparts.[82] A prospective cohort study of 355 children (ages 8–17 years) who had an active rehabilitation intervention postconcussion found that female athletes had greater symptom levels but recovered from their symptoms faster than male athletes.[83]

A recent retrospective chart review of 579 middle school, high school, and collegiate athletes who experienced a concussion showed that female athletes took 6 days longer than their age-matched male counterparts to begin a return-to-play protocol.[84] In a study of 170 SRCs, female hockey players took longer to return to sport compared with concussed male hockey players, but male basketball players took longer to recover than their female counterparts.[85]

Long-term recovery from concussion also appears to have some gender-related differences. A group of approximately 200 athletes was studied more than 6 months after their concussion for cognitive and executive functions. Female athletes responded more slowly than male athletes on dual-task testing. No other sex-differences were seen in cognitive testing.[86]

Other studies, however, have found no difference in time to resolution of concussive symptoms. These include the important high school reporting information online data that involved 100 high schools and 812 concussions, which showed no difference in return to play between the genders.[8] A study of 215 moderate to severe SRCs also showed no difference in recovery times between female athletes and male athletes 18 years and younger.[87] In a study of adolescent and young adult athletes in primary care sports clinic prolonged return to play in 100 SRCs, there was no difference between sexes but the study consisted primarily of male athletes (90%).[88] Additionally, a study of 468 college athletes (57% female), found that female athletes suffered higher rates of ankle or knee injury after experiencing a concussion compared with their male counterparts postconcussion.[89] Such work suggests the need for further research to examine potential modifiable factors to minimize injury risk during the immediate phase of return to play for athletes.

SUMMARY

As female athlete participation continues to increase, greater awareness of prevention and management of SRC in female athletes should be emphasized because of the gender disparities detailed in this article. Women have greater risk for SRC versus male athletes participating in comparable sports and also have risks in sports in which they participate in higher numbers than male athletes (ie, cheerleading). Because SRC has been identified as an important concern for female athletes, the science must be advanced to truly understand the interplay among rules of play, equipment, biomechanics, and hormonal contribution to SRC susceptibility and recovery, because there is a paucity of published research on the topic. Large prospective studies, including female athletes from a variety of sports and with close monitoring of menstrual cycle patterns and hormonal testing, are warranted. Small studies with female athletes as a minority of subjects will not clarify the magnitude women's physiology may play in SRC susceptibility and treatment response. With further work, it may be found that women's physiology can be used to an advantage to prevent SRCs and improve the care of female athletes.

DISCLOSURE

The author, K.H. Rizzone, do not have any commercial or financial conflicts of interest. I have a grant funded by the American Medical Society of Sports Medicine. The author, K.E. Ackerman, do not have any commercial or financial conflicts of interest. I have received grant funding from the National Institutes of Health, the Department of Defense, the American Medical Society of Sports Medicine, the American College of Sports Medicine, and the International Olympic Committee.

REFERENCES

1. Senne J. Examination of gender equity and female participation in sport. Sport J 2016;21.
2. Associations, N.F.o.S.H.S., High School Sports Participation Increases for 29th Consecutive Year. 2018.
3. Statista. Number of participants in US high school gymnastics from 2009/10 to 2018/19. 2019. Available at: https://www.statista.com/statistics/511355/participation-in-us-high-school-gymnastics/.
4. Statista, Number of participants in US high school competitive spirit squads from 2009/10 to 2018/19. 2019.
5. O'Kane J, et al. Survey of injuries in seattle area levels 4 to 10 female club gymnasts. Clin J Sports Med 2011;21(6):486–92.
6. Currie D, et al. Cheerleading injuries in United States High Schools. Pediatrics 2016;137(1).
7. Stein C, et al. Dance-related concussion: a case series. J Dance Med Sci 2014; 18(2):53–61.
8. Frommer L, et al. Sex differences in concussive symptoms of high school athletes. J Athl Train 2011;46:76–84.
9. Covassin T, et al. Are there differences in neurocognitive function and symptoms between male and female soccer players after concussions? Am J Sports Med 2013;41:2890–5.

10. Farace E, Alves W. Do women fare worse? A meta-analysis of gender differences in outcome after traumatic brain injury. J Neurosurg 2000;93:539–45.

11. Marar M, et al. Epidemiology of concussions among United States high school athletes in 20 sports. Am J Sports Med 2012;40(4):747–55.

12. Lincoln A, et al. Trends in concussion incidence in high school sports: a propsective 11-year study. Am J Sports Med 2011;39(5):958–63.

13. Zuckerman S, et al. Epidemiology of sports-related concussion in NCAA Athletes From 2009-2010 to 2013-2014: incidence, recurrence and mechanisms. Am J Sports Med 2015;43(11):2654–62.

14. Covassin T, Moran R, Elbin R. Sex differences in reported concussion injury rate and time loss from participation: an update of the National Collegiate Athletic Association injury surveillance program from 2004-2005 through 2008-2009. J Athl Train 2016;51(3):189–94.

15. Schallmo M, Weiner J, Hsu W. Sport anad sex-specific reporting trends in the epidemiology of concussions sustained by high school athletes. J Bone Joint Surg 2017;99(15):1314–20.

16. Meehan WP, et al. Assessment and management of sport-related concussions in the united states high schools. Am J Sports Med 2011;39(11):2304–10.

17. Fuse Explores the surge in sports participation: why teens play and why they don't. Available at: https://www.businesswire.com/news/home/20180712005864/en/Fuse-Explores-Surge-Sports-Participation-Teens-Play.

18. Putukian M, Lincoln A, Crisco J. Sports-specific issues in men's and women's lacrosse. Curr Sports Med Rep 2014;13(5):334–40.

19. Men's vs. Women's Hockey-What are the main differences. Available at: https://busyplayinghockey.com/mens-vs-womens/.

20. Touminen M, et al. Injuries in women's international ice hockey: an 8-year study of the World Championship tournaments and Olympic Winter Games. Br J Sports Med 2016;50(22):1406–12.

21. Guo D, Verweel L, Reed N. Exploring gaps in concussion knowledge and knowledge in translation among coaches of youth female hockey players. Clin J Sports Med 2017;1–8.

22. Cooley C, et al. A comparison of head injuries in male and female lacrosse participants seen in US emergency departments from 2005 to 2016. Am J Emerg Med 2019;37(2):199–203.

23. Free movement among rule changes for high school girls in 2020. 2019. Available at: https://www.uslacrosse.org/blog/free-movement-among-rule-changes-for-high-school-girls-in-2020.

24. Rodowicz K, Olberding J, Rau A. Head injury potential and the effectiveness of headgear in women's lacrosse. Ann Biomed Eng 2015;43(4):949–57.

25. Cusimano M, Zhu A. Systematic review of traumatic brain injuries in baseball and softball: a framework for prevention. Front Neurol 2017;8:492.

26. Vassallo A, et al. Epidemiology of dance-realted injuries presenting to emergency departments in the United States 2000-2013. Med Probl Perform Art 2017;32(3):170–5.

27. Cain K, et al. Physical activity in youth dance classes. Pediatrics 2015;135(6):1066–73.

28. Shields B, Fernandez S, Smith G. Epidemiology of cheerleading stunt-related injuries in the United States. J Athl Train 2009;44(6):586–94.

29. McIntyre L, Lierderback M. Concussion knowledge and behaviors in a sample of the dance community. J Dance Med Sci 2016;20(2):79–88.

30. Green L. Impact of competitive cheer laws, regulations on Title IX compliance. National Federation of State High School Associations; 2019.
31. Len T, Neary J. Cerebrovascular pathophysiology following mild traumatic brain injury. Clin Physiol Funct Imaging 2010;31(2):85–93.
32. Esposito G, et al. Gender differences in cerebral blood flow as a function of cognitive state with PET. J Nucl Med 1996;37:559–64.
33. Clausen M, et al. Cerebral blood flow during treadmill exercises is a marker of physiological postconcussion syndrome in female athletes. J Head Trauma Rehabil 2016;31(3):215–24.
34. Thibeault C, et al. Sex-based differences in transcranial doppler ultraouns and self-reported symptoms after mild traumatic brain injury. Front Neurol 2019; 10:590.
35. Dolle J, et al. Newfound sex differences in axonal structure underlie differential outcomes from in vitro traumatic axonal injury. Exp Neurol 2018;300:121–34.
36. Holleran L, et al. Axonal disruption in white matter underling cortical sulcus tau pathology in chronci traumatic encephalopathy. Acta Neuropathol 2017;133(3): 367–80.
37. Meehan W III, et al. Chronic traumatic encephalopathy and athletes. Neurology 2015;85(17):1504–11.
38. Eme R, Gilbertson K, Oehler S. Persistent cognitive impairment in a multiply concussed femael athlete: is it chronic traumatic encephalopathy? a case study. The Practitioner Scholar: Journal of Counseling and Professional Psychology 2013;2: 43–51.
39. Bieniek KF, Blessing MM, Heckman MG, et al. Association between contact sports participation and chronic traumatic encephalopathy: a retrospective cohort study. Brain Pathol 2020;30(1):63–74.
40. Charmard E, et al. Long-term abnormalities in the corpus callosum of female concussed athletes. J Neurotrauma 2016;33(13):1220–6.
41. Balestrini C, et al. Autonomic dysregulation in adolescent concussion is sex-and posture-dependent. Clin J Sports Med 2019. https://doi.org/10.1097/JSM. 0000000000000734.
42. Asken B, et al. Concussion biomarkers assessed in collegiate student-athletes (BASICS) I: normative study. Neurology 2018;91(23):e2109–22.
43. Asken B, et al. Concussion BASICS II: baseline serum biomarkers, head impact exposure, and clinical measures. Neurology 2018;91(23):e2123–32.
44. Gallagher V, et al. The effects of sex differences and hormonal contraception on outcomes after collegiate sports-related concussion. J Neurotrauma 2018;35(11): 1242–7.
45. Bull JR, et al. Real-world menstrual cycle characteristics of more than 600,000 menstrual cycles. NPJ Digit Med 2019;2:83.
46. La Fountaine MF, et al. Preliminary evidence for a window of increased vulnerability to sustain a concussion in females: a brief report. Front Neurol 2019;10:691.
47. Wunderle K, et al. Menstrual phase as predictor of outcome after mild traumatic brain injury in women. J Head Trauma Rehabil 2014;29(5):E1–8.
48. Snook ML, et al. Association of concussion with abnormal menstrual patterns in adolescent and young women. JAMA Pediatr 2017;171(9):879–86.
49. Klose M, et al. Acute and long-term pituitary insufficiency in traumatic brain injury: a prospective single-centre study. Clin Endocrinol (Oxf) 2007;67(4):598–606.
50. Emerson CS, Headrick JP, Vink R. Estrogen improves biochemical and neurologic outcome following traumatic brain injury in male rats, but not in females. Brain Res 1993;608(1):95–100.

51. Roof RL, Hall ED. Estrogen-related gender difference in survival rate and cortical blood flow after impact-acceleration head injury in rats. J Neurotrauma 2000; 17(12):1155–69.

52. Wei J, Xiao GM. The neuroprotective effects of progesterone on traumatic brain injury: current status and future prospects. Acta Pharmacol Sin 2013;34(12): 1485–90.

53. Rubin TG, Lipton ML. Sex differences in animal models of traumatic brain injury. J Exp Neurosci 2019;13. 1179069519844020.

54. Brotfain E, et al. Neuroprotection by estrogen and progesterone in traumatic brain injury and spinal cord injury. Curr Neuropharmacol 2016;14(6):641–53.

55. Halstead M, Walter K. Council on sports medicine and fitness, Clinical report: sport-related concussion in children and adolescents. Pediatrics 2010;126: 597–615.

56. Sullivan L, Molcho M. Gender differences in concussion-related knowledge, attitudes and reporting-behaviours among high school student-athletes. Int J Adolesc Med Health 2018. https://doi.org/10.1515/ijamh-2018-0031.

57. Iverson G, et al. Factors associated with concussion-like symptom reporting in high school athletes. JAMA Pediatr 2015;169(12):1132–40.

58. Brown D, et al. Differences in symptom reporting between males and females at baseline and after a sports-related concussion: a systematic review and meta-analysis. Sports Med 2015;45:1027–40.

59. Tierney R, et al. Gender differences in head-neck segment dynamic stabilization during head acceleration. Med Sci Sports Exerc 2005;37:272–9.

60. Collins C, et al. Neck strength: a protective factor reducing risk for concussion in high school sports. J Prim Prev 2014;35:309–19.

61. Caccese J, et al. Sex and age differences in head acceleration during purposeful soccer heading. Res Sports Med 2018;26(1):64–74.

62. Bretzin A, et al. Sex differences in anthropometrics and heading kinematics among division I soccer athletes. Sports Health 2017;9(2):168–73.

63. Chrisman S, et al. Head impact exposure in youth soccer and variation by age and sex. Clin J Sports Med 2019;29(1):3–10.

64. Wilcox B, et al. Biomechanics of head impacts associated with diagnosed concussion in female collegiate ice hockey players. J Biomech 2015;48(10): 2201–4.

65. Clark J, et al. Lack of eye discipline during headers in high school girls soccer: a possible mechanism for increased concussion rates. Med Hypotheses 2017; 100:10–4.

66. McGuine T, et al. Does soccer headgear reduce the incidence of sport-related concussion? A cluster, randomised controlled trial of adolescent athletes. Br J Sports Med 2019;54(7):408–13.

67. Rhea C, et al. Neuromotor and neurocognitive performance in female American football players. Athl Train Sports Health Care 2019;11(5):224–33.

68. Covassin T, et al. The role of age and sex in symptoms, neurocognitive performance, and postural stability in athletes after concussion. Am J Sports Med 2012;40(6):1303–12.

69. Mormile M, Langdon J, Hunt T. The role of gender in neuropsychological assessment in healthy adolescents. J Sports Rehabil 2018;27(1):16–21.

70. Covassin T, Schatz P, Swanik C. Sex differences in neuropsychological function and post-concussion symptoms of concussed collegiate athletes. Neurosurgery 2007;61(2):345–51.

71. Covassin T, et al. Investigating baseline neurocognitive performance between male and female athletes with a history of multiple concussions. Neurol Neurosurg Psychiatry 2010;81(6).
72. McLeod TV, et al. Representative baseline values on the sport concussion assessment tool 2 (SCAT2) in adolescent athletes vary by gender, grade, and concussion history. Am J Sports Med 2012;40(4):927–33.
73. Chin E, et al. Reliability and validity of the sport concussion assessment tool-3 (SCAT3) in high school and collegiate athletes. Am J Sports Med 2016;44(9): 2276–85.
74. Wallace J, Covassin T, Beidler E. Sex differences in high school athletes' knowledge of sport-related concussion symptoms and reporting behaviors. J Athl Train 2017;52(7):682–8.
75. Clair R, et al. Gender differences in quality of life and symptom expression during recovery from concussion. Appl Neuropsychol 2020;9(3):206–14.
76. Neidecker J, et al. First-time sports-related concussion recovery: the role of sex, age and sport. J Am Osteopath Assoc 2017;117(10):635–42.
77. Howell D, et al. Clinical predictors of symptom resolution for chilren and adolescents with sport-related concussion. J Neurosurg Pediatr 2019;1–8.
78. Sufrinko A, et al. Sex differences in vestibular/pcular and neurocognitive outcomes after sport-related concussion. Clin J Sports Med 2017;27(2):133–8.
79. Howell D, et al. Dual-task gait differences in female and male adolescents following sport-related concussion. Gait Posture 2017;54:284–9.
80. Willer B, et al. Comparison of rest to aerobic exercise and placebo-like treatment of acute sport-related concussion in male and female adolescents. Arch Phys Med Rehabil 2019;100(12):2267–75.
81. Ledoux A, et al. Natural progression of symptom change and recovery from concussion in a pediatric population. JAMA Pediatr 2019;173(1):e183820.
82. Tamura K, et al. Concussion recovery timeline of high school athletes using a stepwise return-to-play protocol: age and sex effects. J Athl Train 2020; 55(1):6–10.
83. Gauvin-Lepage J, et al. Effect of sex on recovery from persistent postconcussion symptoms in children and adolescents participating in an active rehabilitation intervention. J Head Trauma Rehabil 2019;34(2):96–102.
84. Stone S, et al. Sex differences in time to return to play progression after sport-related concussion. Sports Health 2017;9(1):41–4.
85. Bloom G, et al. The prevalence and recovery of concussed male and female collegiate athletes. Eur J Sports Soc 2008;8:295–303.
86. Sicard V, Moore R, Ellemberg D. Long-term cognitive outcomes in male and female athletes following sport-related concussions. Int J Psychophysiol 2018; 132:3–8.
87. Cantu R, Guskiewicz K, Register-Mihalik J. A retrospective clinical analysis of moderate to severe athletic concussions. Phys Med Rehabil 2010;2:1088–93.
88. Asplund C, McKeag D, Olsen C. Sport-related concussion: factors associated with prolonged reutn to play. Clin J Sports Med 2004;14:339–43.
89. Houston M, et al. Sex and number of concussions influence the association between concussion and musculoskeletal injury history in collegiate athletes. Brain Inj 2018;32(11):1353–8.

Sports-Related Concussions and the Pediatric Patient

Stessie Dort Zimmerman, MD[a], Brian T. Vernau, MD, CAQSM[b],
William P. Meehan III, MD[c], Christina L. Master, MD, CAQSM[d],*

KEYWORDS

- Pediatric concussions • Adolescent concussions • Head injury • Return to learn
- Return to sport

KEY POINTS

- Most pediatric patients will recover from their concussion within 4 weeks; however, 10% to 33% will have persistent postconcussive symptoms beyond 4 weeks.
- Guiding the patient and family through the return to full academic demands is an essential part of concussion management in the pediatric population.
- "Cocoon therapy" following concussion is no longer recommended as standard of care. After 24 to 48 hours, graduated supervised exercise can be safe in the adolescent patient.
- Learning disabilities, attention-deficit/hyperactivity disorder, mood, and sleep disorders can result in higher symptom severity scores and require focused attention for successful concussion management.
- Little is known about concussions in young children; however, age-appropriate screening tools should be used when available.

INTRODUCTION

Concussion diagnoses are on the increase in the pediatric population owing, in part, to increased sports participation, as well as increased recognition and awareness. By the age of 16, one in 5 pediatric patients will experience a traumatic brain injury (TBI).[1] Most pediatric patients will recover from their concussion within 4 weeks. However, about 10% to 33% of pediatric patients will suffer persistent postconcussive symptoms (PPCS) beyond 4 weeks.[2] Although they present with similar symptoms to their

[a] Urgent Care, Seattle Children's Hospital, 4800 Sand Point Way Northeast, M/S MB.7.520, Seattle, WA 98105, USA; [b] Pediatric and Adolescent Sports Medicine, Division of Pediatric Orthopedics, The Children's Hospital of Philadelphia, 34th and Civic Center Boulevard, Philadelphia, PA 19104, USA; [c] Division of Sports Medicine, The Micheli Center for Sports Injury Prevention, Boston Children's Hospital, Harvard Medical School, 9 Hope Avenue–Suite 100, Waltham, MA 02453, USA; [d] Minds Matter Concussion Program, Pediatric and Adolescent Sports Medicine, Division of Pediatric Orthopedics, Perelman School of Medicine at the University of Pennsylvania, The Children's Hospital of Philadelphia, 34th and Civic Center Boulevard, Philadelphia, PA 19104, USA
* Corresponding author.
E-mail address: masterc@email.chop.edu

Clin Sports Med 40 (2021) 147–158
https://doi.org/10.1016/j.csm.2020.08.010
0278-5919/21/© 2020 Elsevier Inc. All rights reserved.

adult counterparts, pediatric patients have unique life circumstances and developmental needs that require consideration to ensure excellent clinical care. Many concussions sustained during childhood and adolescence are sport related; however, accidents and free play account for many concussions sustained by patients less than 18 years of age. Furthermore, primary care providers, particularly pediatricians, are often the first point of clinical contact for concussion management.[3] By developing expertise in the management of concussions, including the return to learn and return to play processes, pediatricians are able to guide most patients to complete recovery, but will ideally have the support of sports medicine physicians for those patients who are not recovering within the first few weeks.

BODY
Return to Learn

Most pediatric patients need to return to the high cognitive demand and workload of school. Guiding the patient and family through this return to full academic demands is an essential part of concussion management in the pediatric population. The timing of cognitive rest may impact the duration of symptoms. A retrospective study in elementary, high-school, and collegiate students showed that nearly 45% returned to the learning environment prematurely, resulting in the recurrence and worsening of concussion symptoms.[4] One study found that pediatric patients starting cognitive rest immediately after concussion recovered more quickly than those who delayed cognitive rest for several days after injury.[5] On the other hand, prescribing strict rest beyond a couple of days has been shown to increase emotional symptoms in adolescents with acute concussion.[6] Current consensus guidelines suggest an initial rest period 24 to 48 hours after injury as symptoms abate, followed by a gradual return to cognitive activity while monitoring for symptom exacerbation is appropriate for pediatric patients.[7] The primary role of the physician is to guide patients after concussion through a gradual return to academic activity while minimizing symptoms, stress, missed tests, makeup work, and unnecessary grade repetition or retention.

There is little evidence to guide recommendations for return to learn, but several reviews and guidelines have outlined common school accommodations to ease the transition.[8,9] School accommodations should be patient centered and account for the physical examination findings and symptoms the patient is reporting with examples provided in **Box 1**.[8] Visiovestibular symptoms are seen in up to 69% of adolescents[10] and may provoke headaches and dizziness, cause blurry vision, and make it difficult to read or take notes. Autonomic symptoms, such as lightheadedness, can be seen with position changes throughout the school day. Cognitive, sleep, and mood-related symptoms make it difficult to focus on schoolwork. All these difficulties exacerbate PPCS and impair functioning in school. A graded return to learn progression can help guide the injured student to reengage in cognitive activity in the days following a concussion (**Table 1**).[8] Preexisting conditions and postinjury clinical findings may further complicate the school reentry process and thus are important to note when obtaining the pediatric patient's medical history (**Box 2**).[8,11] Many of these diagnoses have symptoms that overlap with concussion symptoms and can augment symptom scores, complicating school reentry. Any symptoms present before concussion may worsen during the concussion.

In addition to the psychological stress surrounding return to cognitive work, prolonged time out of school can have detrimental effects on the patient's social life. Adolescents are highly connected to social media through their mobile devices. In addition, they often require electronic devices to communicate regarding schoolwork.

Box 1
Recommendations for school accommodations for pediatric patients with concussions

Frequent breaks as needed in quiet areas to rest during class (may need to be scheduled in younger patients).

Limit the number of classes in a day.

Initially limit test taking. Once they return to test taking, limit the number of tests per day. Permit breaks during tests.

Temporary use of sunglasses, dimmed screens, and/or paper printouts.

Temporary use of earplugs/headphones in loud busy places.

Delayed return to gym class or outdoor recess.

Permit initially school reentry to include a listening day without note taking or reading.

Vertical saccades deficits: limit note taking and provide preprinted notes.

Horizontal saccade deficits: Provide larger text font, double-spaced lines, audio books, recorded lectures, movies, and so forth.

Convergence deficits: larger font (size 18), preprinted teachers notes, recorded lectures.

Data from Grady MF, Master CL. Return to School and Learning after Concussion: Tips for Pediatricians. Pediatric Annals; Thorofare. 2017;46(3):e93-98.

There is no evidence to date to suggest that symptom-limited screen time has detrimental effects on recovery. Therefore, prolonged strict avoidance of all electronic devices is discouraged. Beyond working collaboratively with a multidisciplinary team, physicians should determine each child's social support and resilience. Physicians should continue to teach the important role these social networks play in the recovery period to school professionals and families.[12,13]

Overall, clear communication with pediatric patients and their caregivers is critical to achieve successful school reentry without significant setbacks. Effective coordination with elementary, middle, and high schools is essential for patients and physicians to implement proposed temporary accommodations. Schools face many barriers to implementing state concussion laws because of lack of resources, and physicians play a key role in educating all stakeholders in the latest understanding of concussion management.[14]

Return to Activity and Sport

The phase of metabolic mismatch following concussion in pediatric patients supports the hypothesis that some initial rest is important for patients in the early stages of physiologic recovery in order to minimize the exacerbation of symptoms.[15] However, the optimal length of rest, including the timing of reintroduction of exercise, is still being explored. There is increasing evidence suggesting that supervised exercise is safe during the acute stages of concussion among adolescent patients.[16–18] Specifically recommended exercises that are safe include jogging or riding a stationary bicycle in a symptom-limited approach, exercising to the point of new symptom onset or worsening of existing symptoms, but not beyond. "Cocoon therapy," which is sustained avoidance of all activities following concussion, is no longer recommended as standard of care, because there are data that strict rest for multiple days can increase symptoms and does not improve cognitive performance.[6]

There are also emerging data that exercise not only is safe but also may be beneficial for concussion recovery. One trial of 103 adolescents with acute concussion

Table 1
Graduated return to school approach

Stage		Activity	Goal of Stage
1	Physical and cognitive rest	Home and leisure activities during the day that do not increase symptoms (eg, reading, texting, screen time). Minimal physical activity	Gradual return to daily activities
2	Prepare for school reentry	Subsymptom cognitive activity (eg, light schoolwork at home over shorter stretches of time compared with usual). Social encounters with 1 or 2 friends	Increase tolerance of cognitive work
3	Back to school	Increase cognitive activity in a school environment with accommodations. Start with 1 h, half days, or every other day school attendance, as needed. Begin with listening-only days, attend less stressful classes, temporarily avoiding music or gym class, or preferential seating as needed. Extra time to complete homework/classwork as needed	Increase academic activities
4	Normal routine with some restrictions	Back to full days of school (but can be <5 d a week, if needed). Completing as much homework in longer stretches of time as tolerated. Resume tests and quizzes as tolerated, with extended time if needed. Allow students to catch up on missed tests or work gradually while working to keep up with learning new material	Return to full academic activities and catch up on missed work
5	Full reintegration	This should include regular attendance, regular homework, regular tests, extracurricular activities	

Adapted from Grady MF, Master CL. Return to School and Learning after Concussion: Tips for Pediatricians. Pediatric Annals; Thorofare. 2017;46(3):e93-98; with permission.

Box 2
Preinjury and postinjury influencing factors in concussion recovery

Preinjury predictors or effect modifiers of slower clinical recovery from concussion
  Female sex
  High-school age
  Personal or family history of migraine
  Personal or family history of mental health problems

Postinjury clinical risk factors for persistent concussion symptoms greater than 1 month
  Initial severity of cognitive deficits
  Development of subacute headaches
  Development of subacute depression

Data from Iverson GL, Gardner AJ, Terry DP, et al. Predictors of clinical recovery from concussion: a systematic review. *Br J Sports Med*. 2017;51(12):941-948.

---

randomized participants to either exercise or placebo-like stretching protocol. The exercise group recovered faster and did not demonstrate an increased rate of prolonged recovery.[19] Assessment of exercise capacity may be beneficial in concussion prognosis as well, as demonstrated in a randomized controlled trial by Leddy and colleagues,[16] whereby adolescents with a lower heart rate at time of symptom exacerbation during the Buffalo treadmill test were more likely to have PPCS greater than 4 weeks. Thus, using treadmill or bicycle tests may prove to be useful in the initial evaluation of concussion to help guide treatment and offer anticipatory guidance.[16,17]

There is well-established evidence for exercise in patients who have PPCS for greater than 4 weeks in the adult literature, making exercise one of the cornerstones for managing chronic concussion symptoms.[20] Kurowski and colleagues[21] demonstrated in a randomized trial of 30 adolescents that symptom scores improved in the aerobic exercise group compared with a placebo stretching group, although adherence rates for the exercise group were low. A larger retrospective study of adolescents with PPCS showed an exponential reduction in symptoms following initiation of a subsymptom threshold exercise program.[22] One cohort in a tertiary care pediatric concussion program found 59% of patients with PPCS had a normal tolerance for heavy aerobic activity.[23] In these pediatric patients, daily subsymptom aerobic exercise working up to 30 minutes per day, including running, elliptical, exercise bike, and sport-related training and drills, should be encouraged. Patients should be specifically instructed to avoid contact drills, scrimmages, games, and other activities that increase the risk of trauma to the head until they have made a full recovery.

Pediatric patients are often motivated to make a full return to sport as soon as possible. However, coordinating sport reentry with the return to school process is important, because students may sometimes be less motivated to return to academic activities. Return to sport after concussion recovery should be navigated in a staged process similar to the return to learn process (**Table 2**).[7,24] The goal of this staged return to sports progression is to prevent worsening of symptoms as the athlete returns slowly back to full physical activity. Working closely with an interdisciplinary team can assist in timely and safe sport reentry. Athletic trainers are increasingly available to athletes in high schools in the United States. They are skilled in assessing patients and facilitating the transition from stage to stage in the return to activity process. This type of exercise progression can also be used to guide the intensity of exercise for those with PPCS just starting out on their exercise plan.

Table 2
Graduated return to activity approach

Stage	Aim	Activity	Goal of Stage
1	Symptom-limited activity	Day-to-day activities that do not provoke symptoms	Gradual reintroduction of school activities
2	Light aerobic exercise	Walking or stationary biking at slow to medium pace. No resistance training	Increase heart rate
3	Sport-specific exercise	Running or skating drills. No head-impact activities	Add movement
4	Noncontact practice	More difficult training drills (eg, passing drills, rapid starts and stops). May start progressive resistance training	Increased cognition, exercise, and coordination
5	Full contact practice	Following medical clearance, normal training activities	Restore confidence and assess functional skill
6	Return to sport	Regular game play	

NOTE: Athletes should be at each stage for at least 24 h or longer. If symptoms worsen during physical activity, the athlete should go back to the previous step. Resistance training should not be added until stage 3 at the earliest. If symptoms are persistent for greater than 1 mo, the athlete should be referred to a health care professional who is an expert in managing concussions.

Adapted from Consensus statement on concussion in sport—the 5th international conference on concussion in sport held in Berlin, October 2016 | British Journal of Sports Medicine. https://bjsm.bmj.com/content/51/11/838.long. Accessed January 29, 2020; with permission.

Pediatric Concussions, Learning Disabilities, and Attention-Deficit/Hyperactivity Disorder

Comorbidities, such as learning disabilities and attention-deficit/hyperactivity disorder (ADHD), are important risk factors for a complicated return to school and recovery from a concussion.[25] One of the most common neurodevelopmental disorders in children is ADHD, affecting nearly 10% of the pediatric population according to 2016 surveillance studies.[26] This disease is characterized by periods of inattentiveness, hyperactivity, and compulsive behaviors. These individuals are at increased risk for accidents and injuries. A cross-sectional study from data gathered from the National Survey of Children with Special Health Care Needs adds that the severity of ADHD is an independent risk factor for mild traumatic brain injury (mTBI).[27] A systematic review demonstrated that there is a higher incidence of having a previous history of ADHD for children with a history of mTBI than those who have not had an mTBI.[28] It is hypothesized that this is due to the increased impulsivity, which may impede self-protective mechanisms during sports and play.

It is likely that physicians who provide postconcussion management will see patients with ADHD. Not surprisingly, pediatric patients with ADHD preinjury will report more concussion-like symptoms and have worse balance than controls without ADHD.[29] The presence of co-morbid ADHD may complicate the assessment following concussion, particularly when attempting to determine recovery to preinjury status. Goal-centered discussions with the patient, caregivers and a multidisciplinary team represent the optimal approach to managing these challenging patients. Physicians may need to advocate for updates to the individualized education plan for these patients to ensure ongoing support in the academic setting. Moreover, these data highlight the importance of remembering that concussion is still a clinical diagnosis. Although various tools exist to augment a physician's capacity to diagnose and manage concussions, these should not be used in isolation or in lieu of clinical judgment.

Impact of Concussions on Sleep in Pediatrics

It is well established that sleep plays a significant role in overall human function. Effective sleep is important for optimal physical, mental, and cognitive health of young athletes.[30] Sleep symptoms following concussion can include sleeping too much, sleeping too little, increased sleep latency, and feeling drowsy and fatigued.[31] In adolescents with sport-related concussions, disturbances in sleep are correlated with higher concussion symptom severity and poorer neurocognitive function.[31] In a retrospective review of pediatric patients who suffered sport-related concussions, those who reported poor sleep following the injury took 2 weeks longer to recover than those who reported good sleep quality.[32] In contrast, a study in the collegiate population did not demonstrate a difference in time to recovery based on initial sleep quality,[33] suggesting that age may influence the role of sleep in concussion recovery, and close attention should be given to sleep disturbances immediately following concussion in pediatric patients. Educating patients and family about good sleep hygiene may be needed. In addition, cognitive behavioral therapy should be considered to address insomnia because this can improve sleep and PPCS.[34]

Concussions and Mental Health in Adolescents

Many symptoms of concussion are nonspecific and may also be associated with anxiety, depression, and other mood disorders, which can confuse the clinical picture, making it difficult to distinguish the symptoms of concussion from those of preexisting mood disorders.[35,36] Furthermore, falling behind in school, cognitive difficulties, social isolation, and other factors that accompany concussions may exacerbate preexisting depression and anxiety, further complicating the clinical presentation. Thus, patients with a history of depression or anxiety should be encouraged to reconnect with their therapist during concussion recovery to mitigate further mood decline.[36] For most patients, mood symptoms resolve within 14 days of the injury, faster than cognitive disturbances.[37] Thus, once the patient's safety has been ensured, physicians should assess whether mood symptoms are affecting the patient's recovery process. If so, a psychologist familiar with concussions should participate in care.

In addition to anxiety and depression, somatization can also confound the care of pediatric patients following mTBIs. Somatic symptom disorder is the reporting of symptoms that are not fully described by any known physical disease. This disorder results in excessive use of costly, and sometimes invasive, medical resources. In addition, it significantly impairs one's social and academic function. Adolescent girls have a higher incidence of somatization disorders than boys. In addition, female adolescents with high somatization scores have a higher risk for prolonged concussion recovery (>4 weeks) even when controlling for anxiety, depression, loss of consciousness, history of prior concussions, history of migraines, and age.[38] Thus, if an athlete is not recovering as expected after a concussion, somatization should be considered in the differential diagnosis and treated when appropriate.

Special Considerations for Younger Children

Although there is little evidence guiding the management of concussions sustained by younger children, there are plenty of considerations that may be helpful in managing this population. In school-age children, concussion is recognized and diagnosed similarly to adolescents. However, there are modifications in some concussion screening tools that physicians should note. For example, the Child Sport Concussion Assessment Tool, 5th edition (child SCAT5), which is modified from the SCAT5 used in adolescents and adults, should be considered for athletes between the ages of 5 and 12 years of age.[39] Although concussion management data in this age group are limited, it is known that there are different academic, athletic, and social considerations for the 5- to 7-year-old patient compared with the 8- to 12-year-old patient. From a practical standpoint, dividing patients into developmentally appropriate subgroups can help with postconcussion management. For these younger patients, symptom scores with parent reporting can be helpful with the postconcussion symptom inventory (PCSI) and health and behavior inventory (HBI) being the most studied in this age group.[40,41] PCSI is a 26-item, 7-point Likert scale, with developmentally appropriate questions for the different age groups, including 5 to 7, 8 to 12, and 13+ years of age. PCSI also offers a teacher-reported symptom scale to help monitor school-related symptoms. The HBI is a 50-question inventory with a 4-point scale with both patient-reported and parent-reported symptoms, originally developed to be used with all severities of TBI. Vestibular-oculomotor and balance testing can be used to track recovery in this age group, keeping in mind the developmental stage. For example, patients in the 5- to 7-year-old age group who have short attention spans may require more interactive "games" when evaluating for oculomotor symptoms and fatigue. Foot-related errors may be seen frequently during tandem-gait testing in young patients, because tandem gait is normally expected by 6 years of age.[42] When assessing tandem gait, sway at the level of the trunk and shoulders would be considered abnormal.

Developmentally speaking, young children may be more likely to display changes in behavior rather than verbalize specific symptoms. Patients in this age group may manifest their concussion symptoms by having tantrums, napping more than usual, being inattentive, or being hyperactive. As such, these patients may have difficulty with the gradual return to cognitive and physical activity, because they are still learning how to regulate their activity and behavior in response to their symptoms. Parental guidance and school accommodations should reflect these limitations in the young patient and advocate for scheduled breaks before these signs become evident. In most settings, these young children should have accommodations that include breaks with the school nurse or in a quiet place to help manage their symptoms.

In young patients, restraint should also be exercised during return to organized sport, because it can be difficult to tell if they are completely symptom free during physical activity; however, return to low-risk, free play should be encouraged as soon as is tolerated. Some data suggest younger children improve more quickly than their adolescent counterparts,[43] and this may be related to the increased academic demands and social stressors facing the adolescent population. Children in the younger age groups do experience PPCS, although it is much more common in adolescents. Rehabilitation in younger children can involve vestibular therapy, vision therapy, and subsymptom threshold aerobic activity, as with the older patients.[44,45] This area continues to be an important area for future study.

SUMMARY

Pediatric patients with concussions have different needs throughout the recovery process than adults. Adolescents, in particular, may take longer to recover from concussion than adults. Initially, relative rest from academic and physical activities is recommended for 24 to 48 hours to allow symptoms to abate. After this time period, physicians should guide the return to activity and return to school process in a staged fashion using published guidelines. Special attention should be given to the return to school process because academic demands from school is "work" for the pediatric patient. Comorbidities can increase the time to recovery in the pediatric patient. These comorbidities include learning disabilities, ADHD, depression, anxiety, somatic symptom disorders, and sleep disorders. In addition, recognizing the type of reported symptoms (cognitive, autonomic, mood, visual, and vestibular symptoms) is important for directing the rehabilitation process for patient recovery. Further concussion research in pediatric patients, particularly those younger than high-school age, is needed to advance the management of this special population.

CLINICS CARE POINTS

- Following a concussion, current consensus guidelines recommend relative cognitive and physical rest for 24 to 48 hours to allow symptoms to abate in the pediatric patient.
- Delaying the start of cognitive rest following a concussion may lead to an increase in symptom severity score and prolong the time to recovery.
- Symptom-limited exercise is a safe treatment in both acute and prolonged concussion management.
- There is no evidence to date to suggest that symptom-limited screen time has detrimental effects on concussion recovery in the pediatric patient.
- In adolescents with sport-related concussions, disturbances in sleep are correlated with higher concussion symptom severity and poorer neurocognitive function.
- Pediatric patients with ADHD preinjury report more concussion-like symptoms and have worse balance than controls without ADHD.
- Patients with a history of depression or anxiety should be encouraged to reconnect with their therapist during concussion recovery to mitigate further mood decline.

DISCLOSURE

S.D. Zimmerman: The author has nothing to disclose. B.T. Vernau: The author has nothing to disclose. W.P. Meehan III: Dr W.P. Meehan receives royalties from (1) ABC-Clio publishing for the sale of his books, *Kids, Sports, and Concussion: A Guide for Coaches and Parents*, and *Concussions*; (2) Springer International for the book *Head and Neck Injuries in Young Athletes*; and (3) Wolters Kluwer for working as an author for *UpToDate*. His research is funded, in part, by philanthropic support from the National Hockey League Alumni Association through the Corey C. Griffin Pro-Am Tournament and a grant from the National Football League. C.L. Master: Dr C.L. Master does not have any conflicts of interest directly related to this article, but her research is funded by the National Institutes of Health–National Institute of Neurological Disorders and Stroke, National Eye Institute, and National Institute of Nursing Research, as well as the National Collegiate Athletic Association and Department of Defense, Pennsylvania Department of Health, and the Children's Hospital of Philadelphia Frontier Program.

REFERENCES

1. McKinlay A, Grace RC, Horwood LJ, et al. Prevalence of traumatic brain injury among children, adolescents and young adults: prospective evidence from a birth cohort. Brain Inj 2008;22(2):175–81.
2. Purcell L, Harvey J, Seabrook JA. Patterns of recovery following sport-related concussion in children and adolescents. Clin Pediatr 2016;55(5):452–8.
3. Arbogast KB, Curry AE, Pfeiffer MR, et al. Point of health care entry for youth with concussion within a large pediatric care network. JAMA Pediatr 2016;170(7): e160294.
4. Carson JD, Lawrence DW, Kraft SA, et al. Premature return to play and return to learn after a sport-related concussion: physician's chart review. Can Fam Physician 2014;60(6):e310–5.
5. Taubman B, Rosen F, McHugh J, et al. The timing of cognitive and physical rest and recovery in concussion. J Child Neurol 2016;31(14):1555–60.
6. Thomas DG, Apps JN, Hoffmann RG, et al. Benefits of strict rest after acute concussion: a randomized controlled trial. Pediatrics 2015;135(2):213–23.
7. McCrory P, Meeuwisse W, Dvorak J, et al. Consensus statement on concussion in sport - the 5th International Conference on Concussion in Sport held in Berlin, October 2016. Br J Sports Med 2018;51:838–47.
8. Grady MF, Master CL. Return to school and learning after concussion: tips for pediatricians. Pediatr Ann 2017;46(3):e93–8.
9. Halstead ME, McAvoy K, Devore CD, et al. Returning to learning following concussion. Pediatrics 2013;132(5):948–57.
10. Master CL, Scheiman M, Gallaway M, et al. Vision diagnoses are common after concussion in adolescents. Clin Pediatr 2016;55(3):260–7.
11. Iverson GL, Gardner AJ, Terry DP, et al. Predictors of clinical recovery from concussion: a systematic review. Br J Sports Med 2017;51(12):941–8.
12. Stalnacke BM. Community integration, social support and life satisfaction in relation to symptoms 3 years after mild traumatic brain injury. Brain Inj 2007;21: 933–42.
13. Sarmiento K, Waltzman D, Lumba-Brown A, et al. CDC Guideline on Mild Traumatic Brain Injury in Children: important practice takeaways for sports medicine providers. Clin J Sport Med 2018. https://doi.org/10.1097/JSM. 0000000000000704.
14. Coxe KA, Sullivan L, Newton A, et al. Barriers to the implementation of state concussion laws within high schools. J Adolesc Health 2019. https://doi.org/10. 1016/j.jadohealth.2019.08.01.
15. Giza CC, Hovda DA. The new neurometabolic cascade of concussion. Neurosurgery 2014;75:S24–33.
16. Leddy JJ, Hinds AL, Miecznikowski J, et al. Safety and prognostic utility of provocative exercise testing in acutely concussed adolescents: a randomized trial. Clin J Sport Med 2018;28(1):13–20.
17. Haider MN, Johnson SL, Mannix R, et al. The Buffalo Concussion Bike Test for concussion assessment in adolescents. Sports Health 2019;11(6):492–7.
18. Howell DR, Mannix RC, Quinn B, et al. Physical activity level and symptom duration are not associated after concussion. Am J Sports Med 2016;44(4):1040–6.
19. Leddy JJ, Haider MN, Ellis MJ, et al. Early subthreshold aerobic exercise for sport-related concussion: a randomized clinical trial. JAMA Pediatr 2019; 173(4):319–25.

20. Leddy JJ, Haider MN, Ellis M, et al. Exercise is medicine for concussion. Curr Sports Med Rep 2018;17(8):262–70.
21. Kurowski BG, Hugentobler J, Quatman-Yates C, et al. Aerobic exercise for adolescents with prolonged symptoms after mild traumatic brain injury: an exploratory randomized clinical trial. J Head Trauma Rehabil 2017;32(2):79–89.
22. Chrisman SPD, Whitlock KB, Somers E, et al. Pilot study of the Sub-Symptom Threshold Exercise Program (SSTEP) for persistent concussion symptoms in youth. NeuroRehabilitation 2017;40(4):493–9.
23. Johnson W, Wiebe S, Nixon-Cave D, et al. Exercise Tolerance in Pediatric Patients with Post-concussion syndrome (abstract). Poster Presented at American Medical Society for Sports Medicine 2015 Annual Meeting; Hollywood, FL, April 16, 2015.
24. DeMatteo C, Randall S, Falla K, et al. Concussion management for children has changed: new pediatric protocols using the latest evidence. Clin Pediatr 2020; 59(1):5–20.
25. Bernard CO, Ponsford JA, McKinlay A, et al. Predictors of post-concussive symptoms in young children: injury versus non-injury related factors. J Int Neuropsychol Soc 2016;22(8):793–803.
26. Danielson ML, Bitsko RH, Ghandour RM, et al. Prevalence of parent-reported ADHD diagnosis and associated treatment among U.S. Children and Adolescents, 2016. J Clin Child Adolesc Psychol 2018;47(2):199–212.
27. Karic S, DesRosiers M, Mizrahi B, et al. The association between attention deficit hyperactivity disorder severity and risk of mild traumatic brain injury in children with attention deficit hyperactivity disorder in the United States of America: a cross-sectional study of data from the national survey of children with special health care needs. Child Care Health Dev 2019;45(5):688–93.
28. Adeyemo BO, Biederman J, Zafonte R, et al. Mild traumatic brain injury and ADHD: a systematic review of the literature and meta-analysis. J Atten Disord 2014;18(7):576–84.
29. Cook NE, Kelshaw PM, Caswell SV, et al. Children with attention-deficit/hyperactivity disorder perform differently on pediatric concussion assessment. J Pediatr 2019;214:168–74.e1.
30. Copenhaver EA, Diamond AB. The value of sleep on athletic performance, injury, and recovery in the young athlete. Pediatr Ann 2017;46(3):e106–11.
31. Kostyun RO, Milewski MD, Hafeez I. Sleep disturbance and neurocognitive function during the recovery from a sport-related concussion in adolescents. Am J Sports Med 2015;43(3):633–40.
32. Chung JS, Zynda AJ, Didehbani N, et al. Association between sleep quality and recovery following sport-related concussion in pediatrics. J Child Neurol 2019; 34(11):639–45.
33. Hoffman NL, Weber ML, Broglio SP, et al. Influence of postconcussion sleep duration on concussion recovery in collegiate athletes. Clin J Sport Med 2017. https://doi.org/10.1097/JSM.0000000000000538.
34. Tomfohr-Madsen L, Madsen JW, Bonneville D, et al. A pilot randomized controlled trial of cognitive-behavioral therapy for insomnia in adolescents with persistent postconcussion symptoms. J Head Trauma Rehabil 2019. https://doi.org/10.1097/HTR.0000000000000504.
35. Iverson GL. Misdiagnosis of the persistent postconcussion syndrome in patients with depression. Arch Clin Neuropsychol 2006;21(4):303–10.

36. Kontos AP, Covassin T, Elbin RJ, et al. Depression and neurocognitive performance after concussion among male and female high school and collegiate athletes. Arch Phys Med Rehabil 2012;93(10):1751–6.
37. Mainwaring LM, Hutchison M, Bisschop SM, et al. Emotional response to sport concussion compared to ACL injury. Brain Inj 2010;24(4):589–97.
38. Root JM, Zuckerbraun NS, Wang L, et al. History of somatization is associated with prolonged recovery from concussion. J Pediatr 2016;174:39–44.e1.
39. Davis GA, Purcell L, Schneider KJ, et al. The Child Sport Concussion Assessment Tool 5th edition (Child SCAT5): background and rationale. Br J Sports Med 2017; 51(11):859–61.
40. Gioia GA, Schneider JC, Vaughan CG, et al. Which symptom assessments and approaches are uniquely appropriate for paediatric concussion? Br J Sports Med 2009;43(Suppl 1):i13–22.
41. Ayr LK, Yeates KO, Taylor HG, et al. Dimensions of postconcussive symptoms in children with mild traumatic brain injuries. J Int Neuropsychol Soc 2009;15(1): 19–30.
42. Scharf RJ, Scharf GJ, Stroustrup A. Developmental milestones. Pediatr Rev 2016; 37(1):25–38.
43. Ledoux A-A, Tang K, Yeates KO, et al. Natural progression of symptom change and recovery from concussion in a pediatric population. JAMA Pediatr 2019; 173(1):e183820.
44. Storey E, Wiebe D, D'Alonzo B, et al. Vestibular rehabilitation is associated with visuovestibular improvement in pediatric concussion. J Neurol Phys Ther 2018; 42(3):134–41.
45. Storey E, Master S, Lockyer J, et al. Near point of convergence after concussion in children. Optom Vis Sci 2017;94(1):96–100.

Prevention of Sport-Related Concussion

Peter K. Kriz, MD[a,b,]*, William O. Roberts, MD, MS[c]

KEYWORDS

- Concussion • Injury prevention • Protective equipment • Rule and policy change

KEY POINTS

- Few prospective, randomized controlled trials evaluating sport-related concussion (SRC) prevention strategies exist.
- Many initiatives and recommendations pertaining to elite adult athletes have been inappropriately extrapolated to groups of different ages and skill levels, including youth and adolescent athletes.
- Rule and policy changes remain promising tactics to reduce risk of SRC, but more research assessing their effectiveness in a variety of contact/collision sports and athlete age groups is needed, as is research pertaining to enforcement of these rule and policy changes.
- Educational institutions and sport organizations play an integral role in reducing SRC risk by ensuring recruitment practices in Division I collegiate athletics do not jeopardize the physical and mental health of prospective middle school and high school student athletes.

INTRODUCTION

Concussion remains a common injury among participants in youth, adolescent, and adult sports. An estimated 283,000 children seek care in US emergency departments each year for sport- or recreation-related traumatic brain injury (TBI); contact sports account for approximately 45% of these visits.[1] Although eliminating concussion in contact and collision sports is not a practical goal, implementing practices and strategies to reduce the risk of sport-related concussion (SRC) and their long-term sequalae should be a primary objective of sports organizations and their members. It is

[a] Division of Sports Medicine, Department of Orthopedics, Warren Alpert Medical School, Brown University, Rhode Island Hospital/Hasbro Children's Hospital, 1 Kettle Point Drive, Suite 300, East Providence, RI 02915, USA; [b] Department of Pediatrics, Warren Alpert Medical School, Brown University, Rhode Island Hospital/Hasbro Children's Hospital, 1 Kettle Point Drive, Suite 300, East Providence, RI 02915, USA; [c] Department of Family Medicine and Community Health, University of Minnesota, 516 Delaware Street Southeast, 6-240 Phillips-Wangensteen Building, Minneapolis, MN 5545, USA
* Corresponding author.
E-mail address: Peter_Kriz@brown.edu
Twitter: @DrPKrizBrownU (P.K.K.); @WilliamORoberts (W.O.R.)

Clin Sports Med 40 (2021) 159–171
https://doi.org/10.1016/j.csm.2020.08.007
0278-5919/21/© 2020 Elsevier Inc. All rights reserved.

essential for medical professionals involved in the care of these athletes to support concussion reduction strategies.

Initial prevention efforts primarily focused on protective equipment and rule changes. However, over the past few decades, initiatives involving educational programs, legislation, physiologic and behavior modifications, teaching proper body checking and tackling technique, and changing culture in sport have collectively shown promise in mitigating risk of concussion in contact and collision sports.

The effectiveness of concussion prevention strategies in reducing concussion risk in sport has recently been assessed by several working groups using systematic reviews.[2,3] Emery and colleagues[2] reviewed peer-reviewed full-text and abstracts of analytical study designs (including randomized controlled trials, quasi-experimental, cohort, case-control, cross-sectional, preexperimental, ecological) evaluating a concussion prevention intervention including human sport participants with concussions or head impacts. Schneider and colleagues[3] reviewed prospective study design full-text articles limited to sport and recreation examining the preventative effect of equipment, training modifications, or educational programs on the incidence of concussions in comparison to a control group.

Overall, there are few prospective, randomized controlled trials (RCTs) that evaluate concussion prevention strategies. Many initiatives and recommendations have focused on studies involving elite adult athletes, and their results have been extrapolated contentiously to youth and adolescent sports.[4,5]

The purpose of this article is to provide an update on the multifaceted approach to risk reduction of SRC in youth, adolescent, and adult sports. The focus will be on current evidence-based strategies and promising future directions that have yet to be rigorously studied.

PROTECTIVE EQUIPMENT
Helmets/Headgear

Significant morbidity and mortality in American football sparked the adoption of modern head protection. Mandatory helmet use was not instituted in American football until 1939 in the National Collegiate Athletic Association (NCAA) and 1943 in the National Football League. Even with required helmet use, serious head injuries including intracranial hemorrhages and skull fractures remained prevalent in American football throughout the mid-twentieth century. These troubling injuries prompted changes in the rules and coaching techniques. In 1969, the National Operating Committee on Standards for Athletic Equipment formed as a governing body to test and certify helmets and implemented the first football helmet safety standards in 1973.[6,7]

American football

Because the current sports concussion management guidelines were developed and refined through a rigorous consensus process,[8,9] few studies regarding the effectiveness of helmets in reducing head injury during American football play have been published. Studies conducted before the Prague/Zurich concussion consensus conferences tended to underreport concussive injuries, reported only the most severe concussive injuries, and relied on coach and certified athletic trainer for diagnosis.[6,10,11] Although newer helmet designs have the potential to reduce impact forces involving the crown of the helmet and the facemask, they are ineffective in mitigating the movement of the brain within the skull ("brain slosh"), resulting in suboptimal energy absorption for brain tissue protection.[3]

One of the most referenced prospective cohort studies involving American football helmet design was performed by Collins and colleagues during the 2002 to 2004 seasons comparing concussion rates and recovery times for 2141 high school football players. Nearly half the sample wore newer helmet technology (Riddell Revolution), and the remainder used reconditioned traditional helmet designs from various manufacturers. Over the course of the study, the concussion rate of the Revolution helmet group was 5.3% compared with 7.6% in the traditional helmet group (P<.03).[12] However, the impact exposure for the affected players was not tracked, which limited the comparison conclusions. In addition, the study was limited by lack of randomization of helmets among study participants, mean chronologic age discrepancies among study groups, and variability in helmet age, as the Revolution helmets were brand new, whereas traditional helmets were reconditioned.

McGuine and colleagues performed a prospective cohort study of 2081 high school football players during the 2012 and 2013 seasons to determine whether the type of protective equipment and player characteristics affect the incidence of SRC. There were 211 SRCs sustained by 206 players (9% of included athletes), for an incidence of 1.6 SRCs per 1000 athletic exposures (AEs). No difference in incidence of SRC for players wearing Riddell, Schutt, or Zenith helmets was identified. In addition, helmet age and recondition status did not affect the incidence of SRC.[13] Limitations of this study included lack of randomization of helmets among study participants and lack of impact exposure data to include in the analysis.

Rugby

Internationally, rugby is the most popular team collision sport. Headgear for rugby is made of soft polyethylene foam; current evidence is lacking regarding its effectiveness for reducing head impact forces or concussion incidence in rugby.[3,6] McIntosh and colleagues performed a 3-arm RCT involving 82 rugby union teams consisting of men younger than 13-, 15-, 18-, and 20-year age groups. There were 1493 participants in the control group (no headgear), 1128 participants who wore standard (10 mm thick) headgear, and 1474 participants who wore modified (16 mm thick) headgear. Participants were followed over 2 years. Compliance to random assignment was overall low, although in 46% of exposures, players wore standard headgear. No differences in the rates of head injury or concussion between controls and headgear arms was found following an intention-to-treat analysis.[14] However, poor compliance with control or intervention group assignment limits interpretation of the study's findings.

Ice hockey Similar to American football, ice hockey protective headgear has undergone technological advances, beginning with leather and felt construction in the 1950s and the introduction of plastic shells and foam liners in the 1970s, which could absorb energy and provide a comfortable fit. In 1979, the National Hockey League (NHL) adopted head protection 11 years following a fatal head injury during NHL play.[15] Despite the widespread use of helmets at both amateur and professional levels, brain injuries remain a serious concern.[16]

Soccer

Until recently, no RCT had been performed involving protective headgear for soccer players. Quality of evidence historically was low, limited to retrospective surveys and laboratory studies. In 2019, McGuine and colleagues published a randomized controlled trial involving high school male and female soccer players performed during the 2016/17 and 2017/18 seasons. Schools were randomly assigned to be in headgear and no headgear (control) groups based on stratified randomization by school enrollment size. Individuals were allowed to choose which headgear model to wear for the season. There were 2766 participants, and 130 participants (5.3% women, 2.2% men) sustained SRCs. Neither the incidence of SRC nor the days lost from SRC were different between the groups for either men or women.[17] Limitations of the study included potential selection bias, no video recording of concussion injury to document the head impacts or accelerometer data to record impact forces, and use of multiple headgear models in the headgear group.

Mouthguards

There are 3 main types of mouthguards: stock, boil-and-bite, and custom-fitted. Stock mouthguards are ready to wear, whereas boil-and-bite mouthguards must first be heated and then can be molded to the teeth while cooling. Custom mouthguards must be made by a dental professional and offer the best fit.[18] In theory, mouthguards reduce concussion risk by dissipating force absorbed by the mandible as the mandibular condyle approaches the mandibular fossa of the temporal bone, partially absorbing force that otherwise would reach the brain.[19]

There are no RCTs involving mouthguards and concussion prevention, given the questionable ethics of performing an RCT in collision sports where mouthguard use is mandated. Existing evidence is limited, and results have been inconclusive. Systematic reviews have cited small sample sizes, confounding factors including varying mouthguard thickness, inconsistent accounting for AEs, potential underreporting of injuries by athletic trainers, and self-report measurement bias.[2,3]

RULE AND POLICY CHANGES/ENFORCEMENT

Rule and policy changes in sport have the potential to reduce concussion risk and improve the health and safety of participants. In 2014, the Institute of Medicine's Committee on Sports-Related Concussions in Youth acknowledged that although some evidence from youth ice hockey and soccer demonstrates that rule modification and enforcement of player safety and Fair Play policies contribute to a reduction in sports-related injuries, including concussion, more research is necessary to measure the effectiveness of rules in reducing concussion.[18] In a 2017 systematic review of existing strategies to reduce the risk of concussion in sport, Emery and colleagues[2] concluded that the most compelling evidence involves body checking policies in youth ice hockey, where not allowing body checking demonstrates a significant protective effect in reducing concussion risk. A call for further research investigating rule changes in other sports and age groups has been brought forward by international committees.[9]

American Football

The kickoff return in American football, during which athletes run at high speeds toward each other over long distances, has historically been associated with a high concussion risk compared with other football plays. In 2016, the Ivy League introduced 2 key changes to its football kickoffs: (1) kickoffs were moved up from the 35-yard line to the 40, and (2) touchbacks were moved from the 20-yard line to the 25. The intent of these changes was to have more kickoffs land in the end zone, disincentivizing receivers from returning the kick and risking head injury from collisions with oncoming defenders. Wiebe and colleagues studied the effects of these rule changes on concussion rates in Ivy League football players during 5 seasons—3 preceding the rule change and 2 following the rule change (2013–15, 2016–17). The mean annual concussion rate per 1000 plays during kickoffs was 10.93 before and 2.04 after the rule change (difference, −8.88; 95% confidence interval [CI], −13.68 to −4.09).[20]

The successful 2016 Ivy League rule change inspired the National Collegiate Athletic Association (NCAA) to alter its kickoff procedures. In 2018, the NCAA (including the Ivy League) implemented a new rule allowing players to call for a fair catch on kickoffs that fall inside the 25-yard line—the equivalent of a touchback, where the ball is placed at the 25. As of this writing, no study has analyzed the effects of this rule change.

Baseball

Although the overall incidence of mild traumatic brain injuries (mTBIs) in professional baseball is low (0.42 mTBI per 1000 AEs) compared with professional American football (6.61 mTBI per 1000 AEs),[21] Green and colleagues[22] demonstrated that greater than 40% of mTBIs occurred among catchers while fielding, and 40% of these injuries were caused by home plate collisions. In response to these findings, both Major League Baseball (MLB) and Minor League Baseball (MiLB) adopted a rule in 2014 to regulate home plate collisions, prohibiting runners from purposefully initiating contact with the catcher or catchers from blocking the runner pathway if not in possession of the ball. Green and colleagues performed a retrospective review of data entered into professional baseball's electronic medical record system involving all active MLB and MiLB players from 2011 to 2017. Before the rule change (2011–13 seasons), a mean of 11 concussions attributed to home plate collisions occurred annually, compared with 2.3 per year following the rule change (2014–17 seasons) [$P = .0029$], with no MLB concussions due to home plate collisions following the rule change. The mean number of days per season missed due to concussion resulting from home plate collisions decreased from 276 before 2014 to 36 per season after 2014 ($P = .0001$).[23]

Ice Hockey

Body checking in ice hockey is a legal strategy for adolescent and adult male participants to separate a player from the puck. Given the increased risk of injury including concussion associated with body checking, its role in youth ice hockey has been deliberated in past decades. In 2010, Emery and colleagues compared concussion injury risk between Pee Wee (age 12 years and younger) youth ice hockey players in the Canadian provinces of Alberta, in which body checking was allowed, and Quebec, in which body checking was not allowed. The investigators found a greater than 3-fold increased risk of concussion and all game-related injury (including severe concussion with time loss >10 days and severe injury with time loss >7 days) in the Alberta league compared with the Quebec league.[24] Influenced by Emery's study findings, USA Hockey and Hockey Canada eliminated body checking at the 12-and-under level in 2011 and 2013, respectively.

Another rule change in ice hockey implemented to reduce head and cervical spine injury involves Fair Play (FP) rules. Considered a behavior modification program focused on eliminating intent-to-harm, head contact, and "targeting" behavior in collision sports, FP rule changes use team or individual player penalties to promote sportsmanship by positively reinforcing assertive play (eg, controlled play, no intent-to-injure behavior) and negatively reinforcing aggressive play (eg, hits to the head, checking from behind). Initiated in Nova Scotia and Quebec, FP has been used by Minnesota Hockey since 2004 and recently has been implemented in high school boys' hockey in Rhode Island.

Variations of FP rules and rule application exist in ice hockey. In the traditional model, points are rewarded to (or withheld from) teams that stay below (or exceed) a given number of penalty minutes allotted in a game. Team standings and tournament results are determined not only by wins and losses but also by team FP points. Roberts and colleagues have published results evaluating the effectiveness of FP rules reducing injury in ice hockey. During a 1994 Junior Gold Hockey (19-year-old and under and enrolled in high school) tournament in Minnesota, FP rules were used for 24 round-robin games, whereas regular rules (RR) were used for the tournament's championship round (7 games). The FP/RR injury ratio was 1:4.8, the average number of penalties per game was 7.1 in FP compared with 13 in RR, and the number of rough play/injury penalties was 4 times higher in RR games.[25]

In 2015, the Rhode Island Interscholastic League implemented an FP rule change in boy's high school ice hockey that suspended individual players who accumulated greater than or equal to 50 penalty minutes (PIM) for 2 league games. Players who accumulated an additional 20 PIM ($\geq$70 PIM) were suspended for the remainder of the season (including playoffs). Kriz and colleagues collected injury data from hospital systems and game/penalty data from the Rhode Island Hockey Coaches Association during 3 seasons before the rule change (2012/13–2014/15) and 3 seasons following the rule change (2015/16–2017/18). The PIM rule change was associated with a significant reduction in all injuries (odds ratio [OR], 0.55; 95% CI, 0.35–0.86), concussion/closed head injury (OR, 0.44; 95% CI, 0.23–0.85), and combined subgroups of concussion/closed head injury and upper body injury (OR, 0.50; 95% CI, 0.31–0.80).[26]

Other strategies that reduce ice hockey collision may have the potential to reduce concussion risk. Larger rink size tends to spread out game play and separate players. In a study looking at injury data from the Ontario Junior A Hockey League (ages 16–20 years old), game injury rates were inversely related to ice surface size ($P<.01$). Neurotraumas per game and aggressive penalty data did not show any difference related to ice rink size.[27] The World Junior Championships were played on different size rinks in 3 successive years (2002–2004). Wennberg used game video to assess player collisions and head impacts. The larger ice sheet had less collision and less head injury compared with intermediate and smaller size rinks.[28]

Decreasing the number of players on the ice may also reduce injury by spreading out the players. A historical precedent occurred when the team size, Silver Sevens (7 on a side), was reduced to 6 on a side, dropping the "deep center" position. On small rinks, 4 skaters plus the goalie on each side would functionally "enlarge" the skating surface.

Another strategy aimed at reducing flagrant penalties and modifying player behavior is to institute injury suspensions for illegal activities that lead to injury, where the injuring player would be prohibited from playing in the league until the injured player returned to the roster at full capacity plus an additional game restriction (ie, flagrant injury penalty = injury time off for the injured player + 3 games). Soccer and basketball rules require players who accumulate more than 2 to 4 penalties per game, respectively, to leave the game, and a similar strategy might be effective in ice hockey. These strategies require that officials call games uniformly and strictly enforce the rules.

Soccer

In soccer, yellow and red cards are used to discipline players for illegal play during game play. Yellow card accumulation policies (YCPs), which suspend players and/or coaches for illegal play or misconduct, have been used by soccer federations internationally[29] as well as at the state level in the United States, to discourage foul play and disqualify individual players and teams from playoff participation if yellow card foul thresholds are exceeded. Despite YCPs being used in high school boys' and girls' soccer for more than 25 years in the United States, the effectiveness of YCPs as an injury prevention strategy had not been formally evaluated until recently. Kriz and colleagues studied National Federation of State High School Associations YCPs and high school soccer competition injuries during seasons 2005/06 through 2017/18, with injury and AE data collected from High School RIO. There was no significant difference in injury rates between schools in states with and without YCPs. Among states with YCPs, injury rates were not significantly different between pre- and post-YCP implementation. Although a significantly lower proportion of injuries that resulted in greater than 3 weeks' time loss occurred in states with YCPs, no significant differences were observed in proportions of concussions, fractures, anterior cruciate ligament injuries, or injuries, resulting in surgery between states with/without YCPs. The investigators concluded that contrary to their intended impact, YCPs were not effective in lowering high school soccer competition–related athlete-athlete contact injury rates and that implementation of YCPs alone, without proper enforcement, may not be a sufficient injury prevention strategy (Kriz PK, Yang J, Arakkal A, et al. Fair play as an injury prevention intervention: do yellow card accumulation policies reduce high school soccer injuries? 2020. Submitted for publication).

EDUCATIONAL PROGRAMS

Sport governing bodies and medical organizations such as the Center for Disease Control and Prevention have recently stepped up their educational campaigns aimed at collision and body contact in youth sports, developing multimedia educational messages and online training programs for coaches, players, and parents.[30,31] Critics of these educational efforts have raised concerns that educational campaigns are largely ineffective if knowledge transfer and action stages do not occur. Educational program outcomes have primarily been evaluated using surveys, questionnaires, and quizzes; qualitative methods rarely have been implemented. Although studies report short-term improvement in participants' knowledge and attitudes, long-term benefits of educational programs are less clear. Kroshus and colleagues surveyed 146 players on 6 Division I male ice hockey teams before and after the players had received NCAA-mandated concussion educational interventions. Five teams had received education in a handout/e-mail format, whereas one team viewed an educational video. The investigators found that no significant improvements in concussion knowledge occurred among players and only a very small decrease in intention to continue playing with concussion.[32] Kerr and colleagues evaluated the effectiveness of USA Football's Heads Up Football (HUF) coaching education program and practice contact restriction in 2108 youth American football players aged 5 to 15 years participating in leagues using HUF programs, leagues without HUF programs (NHUF), and leagues implementing Pop Warner (PW) practice contact restrictions over a single season. Concussion rates during practice were lower in leagues that used both HUF and PW contact restrictions (HUF + PW) compared with NHUF leagues. HUF leagues saw no change in injuries sustained during games unless they also used PW practice restrictions (HUF + PW).[33]

Cusimano and colleagues assessed concussion knowledge among 503 survey respondents before and after exposure to one or more of 19 SRC education resources introduced through a Canadian national initiative. Concussion knowledge scores (CKS) were calculated for pre- and postexposure. Respondents in the post-survey had higher CKS than those in presurvey. Two out of 19 resources and 4 out of 6 modes of concussion education delivery (Web pages, written guidelines, phone apps, in-person resources, but not quizzes or videos) were successful in improving concussion knowledge, with Web page educational resources being the most effective delivery mode. In addition, using 3 or more resources was predictive of a statistically significant increase in CKS compared with using a single resource.[34]

LEGISLATION

The Zackery Lystedt Law passed by the State of Washington in 2009 has been model legislation for sport concussion law.[35] Within 5 years of its passage, all 50 states and the District of Columbia have adopted youth sports concussion laws. The Lystedt Law has 3 basic tenets: (1) education of athletes, parents, and coaches, (2) removal from practice/play a suspected concussion at time of injury, (3) medically supervised return to play. However, significant variability regarding delivery of concussion education continues to exist among states. Although some states have explicitly mandated annual education of coaches, the Lystedt Law, as written does not directly mandate coach education. In addition, not all states require athlete, parent, and coach education.[36] Variability also exists among states regarding which licensed health care providers trained in concussion management can medically clear concussed athletes, as many states have rural and underserved areas necessitating nonphysician providers be directly involved in concussion evaluation and management. Sports medicine providers should be familiar with their respective state's concussion laws and interpretation, as well as their communities' emergency action plans before engaging in game and event coverage.

PHYSIOLOGIC STRATEGIES TO REDUCE CONCUSSION
Neck Strengthening

Neck strengthening exercises—historically an integral part of strength and conditioning among American football players and wrestlers—have recently received renewed attention as a prevention strategy for concussion among contact/collision sport athletes. Collins and colleagues recently assessed neck strength and neck circumference measurements in more than 6700 high school athletes over a 2-year period. Concussed athletes had (1) smaller neck circumferences compared with athletes who did not report concussion over the study period, (2) smaller neck circumferences and larger head circumferences compared with nonconcussed athletes, and (3) less neck strength compared with nonconcussed athletes. The investigators determined that for every pound increase in neck strength, odds of concussion decreased by 5% (OR = 0.95, 95% CI 0.92–0.98).[37]

In addition to neck strengthening, anticipating collision has been proposed as a prevention strategy to reduce risk of SRC. Eckner and colleagues performed a biomechanical study in 46 male and female contact sport athletes aged 8 to 30 years. Maximum isometric neck strength was measured in various anatomic planes, and a loading apparatus then applied impulsive forces to the athletes' heads during both baseline and anticipatory cervical muscle activation conditions. The investigators determined that greater isometric neck strength and anticipatory activation were independently associated with decreased head peak linear velocity and peak angular velocity after impulsive loading across all planes of motion. The study concluded that neck strength and impact anticipation are potentially modifiable risk factors for SRC and suggested that interventions aimed at increasing neck strength and that reducing unanticipated head and body impacts may reduce SRC incidence among contact/collision sport athletes.[38]

Vision Training

There is emerging evidence that vision training has potential as a concussion injury risk reduction tool. Clark and colleagues examined the effectiveness of a preseason vision training (VT) program (light board training, strobe glasses, and tracking drills) in a Division I American football team over 4 seasons. Concussion incidence was compared with the previous 4 consecutive seasons. A statistically significant lower concussion rate was noted in players who underwent VT compared with those who did not (1.4 concussions per 100 player seasons vs 9.2 concussions per 100 game exposures, $P \leq .001$).[39] Limitations include retrospective study design, lack of randomization, no control group, small sample size, and nonuniform denominator measures of AE.

Jugular Vein Compression

In recent years, attention has been directed to novel approaches that may protect an athlete's brain from within by decreasing brain "slosh" during impact. Academic and industry researchers alike are investigating biomechanical modifications to cerebral blood flow. Placing a collar around an athlete's neck applies mild bilateral jugular vein compression (or occlusion) that diverts blood flow to the vertebral veins, prompting cerebral engorgement. The venous cerebral engorgement theoretically reduces intracranial energy absorption associated with head impact exposures, preserving integrity of brain white matter, which is susceptible to structural alterations as a result of concussive or subconcussive impacts. Proponents, including developers of commercial collars, have likened this physiologic modification to the woodpecker's mechanism for protecting its brain.[40] However, critics have challenged this claim, stating that nowhere in the woodpecker literature is such an evolutionary adaptation actually described or hypothesized.[41]

Nonetheless, several recent studies pertaining to jugular compression have been published.[42–44] Meyer and colleagues performed a prospective longitudinal neuroimaging study involving 50 high school female soccer players divided into collar-wearing and noncollar groups; collars were worn during games and practices during their competitive season. All underwent pre- and postseason MRI and diffuse tensor imaging (DTI) evaluation. Head impacts were monitored using wearable patch accelerometers. DTI analyses showed significant preseason to postseason white matter changes in the noncollar group, which resolved partially at 3 months off-season follow-up. No significant white matter changes were detected in the collar group despite similar head impact exposure, suggesting a potential prophylactic effect of the collar in preventing microstructural changes associated with repetitive head impacts.[44] Limitations of the study included potential confounding of hormonal fluctuations (hormonal cycling on intracranial pressure/volume, potential neuroprotective effect of progesterone after a TBI) and lack of correlation between DTI changes and athletes' physical or cognitive function.

SPORT CULTURE CHANGE

Several disturbing trends regarding sport culture persist in athletic communities and potentially contribute to SRC risk. Single-sport specialization in youth and adolescent sports, in which athletes play on multiple teams and attend numerous showcases in pursuit of college scholarships, not only has contributed to the epidemic of overuse injuries but is also a likely factor in concussion risk/susceptibility, as windows of opportunity for brain recovery following head impacts have become narrower as most sports have become 3-season or year-round commitments.

Educational institutions and organizations are also responsible for cultural changes in sport. In recent years, several Division I universities have offered college scholarships to eighth-grade football players,[45] and verbal commitments by high school underclassmen to play Division I sports are commonplace.[46,47] Such early commitments consequently create a culture of increased AEs at a younger age, transferring a higher volume and intensity of participation to a less physically mature population—an unintended consequence that has not been acknowledged in the literature but is apparent to clinicians treating these athletes. The NCAA has recently adopted rules to address early recruitment practices in Division I athletics, creating a "phased-in" recruiting approach that allows coaches to build relationships with prospective student-athletes through phone/electronic communication before allowing for visits and off-campus contact. Although some of the impetus of the rule change is to prevent early recruitment, variability between individual sports' recruiting rules remains. Men's ice hockey, for example, continues to allow contact with prospective student-athletes during January of sophomore year.[48] With more athletes "reclassifying"—repeating grades in order to gain physical maturity and size/stature advantages over their peers—additional age, size, and physical maturity discrepancies have been created in contact/collision sports at the adolescent level. Collectively, these developments have inevitably resulted in more athletes and their families risking recurrent, cumulative injury including SRC, hoping for a payoff in the form of a college athletic scholarship. As a result, sports medicine providers are treating more adolescent athletes with multiple concussions who are in jeopardy of being retired from sport early in their high school careers.

As skill level and competition for Division I ice hockey scholarships has increased, so has a trend for high school players to hone their skills in elite junior programs in the United States in an effort to continue their hockey careers at a US university or college. Just as professional ice hockey leagues, junior leagues permit fighting, a known risk factor for SRC and related complications including cognitive impairment.[49] Some of these junior program players accumulate recurrent SRC, which jeopardizes both their athletic and academic futures.

SUMMARY

Preventive strategies to reduce concussion risk in sport continue to evolve. Over the past decade, scientific evaluation of concussion prevention strategies has become more rigorous providing higher-quality evidence to judge the efficacy of the interventions. Technological advancements in fields such as neuroimaging and wearable accelerometers allow researchers to collect and disseminate information involving the effects of sport-related head impacts to athletes, coaches, and sports organizations. Inevitably, future directions in reducing concussion risk in sport will include commonsense interventions such as rule changes, behavioral modifications, and cultural change, which will become easier to implement as research critically evaluates their impact on sport concussion reduction. Educational programs will continue to play an integral role in reducing concussion risk, and transferring concussion knowledge into action that effectively reduces concussion will continue to be a high priority.

In the future, athletes, parents, coaches, and sport governing bodies will need to assess acceptable versus unacceptable injury to help set policy regarding higher risk activities within sport. It is clear that ice hockey is safest with no body checking or fighting; however, sport governing bodies have been slow to implement these simple interventions. Player attitude is also critical to safety, and as long as "bad behavior" is tolerated, the players who do follow the rules will be at risk from others who do not comply. Using "Fair Play" systems that reward teams abiding by the rules and punish individuals who break the rules is a simple strategy that has made a difference in some settings. Ultimately, a combination of rules compliance and strict enforcement works best for player safety and concussion reduction.

DISCLOSURE

The authors have nothing to disclose.

REFERENCES

1. Sarmiento K, Thomas KE, Daugherty J, et al. Emergency department visits for sports- and recreation-related traumatic brain injuries among children — United States, 2010–2016. Morb Mortal Wkly Rep 2019;68(10):237–42.
2. Emery CA, Black AM, Kolstad A, et al. What strategies can be used to effectively reduce the risk of concussion in sport? A systematic review. Br J Sports Med 2017;51(12):978–84.
3. Schneider DK, Grandhi RK, Bansal P, et al. Current state of concussion prevention strategies: a systematic review and meta-analysis of prospective, controlled studies. Br J Sports Med 2017;51(20):1473–82.
4. Emery CA. Injury prevention and future research. In: Caine D, Maffulli N, editors. Epidemiology of pediatric sports injuries: team sports. Basel (Switzerland): Karger Medical and Scientific Publishers; 2005. p. 170–91. https://doi.org/10.1159/000085396.
5. Emery C. Injury prevention and future research. In: Caine D, Maffulli N, editors. Epidemiology of pediatric sports injuries: individual sports. Basel (Switzerland): Karger Medical and Scientific Publishers; 2005. p. 179–200. https://doi.org/10.1159/000084289.
6. Daneshvar DH, Baugh CM, Nowinski CJ, et al. Helmets and mouth guards: the role of personal equipment in preventing sport-related concussions. Clin Sports Med 2011;30(1):145–63.
7. Bennett T. The NFL's official encyclopedic history of professional football. 2nd edition. New York: Macmillan; 1977.
8. McCrory P, Johnston K, Meeuwisse W, et al. Summary and agreement statement of the 2nd International Conference on Concussion in Sport, Prague 2004. Br J Sports Med 2005;39(4):196–204.
9. McCrory P, Meeuwisse W, Dvořák J, et al. Consensus statement on concussion in sport—the 5th international conference on concussion in sport held in Berlin, October 2016. Br J Sports Med 2017;51(11):838–47.
10. Covassin T, Elbin R, Stiller-Ostrowski JL. Current sport-related concussion teaching and clinical practices of sports medicine professionals. J Athl Train 2009; 44(4):400–4.
11. Notebaert AJ, Guskiewicz KM. Current trends in athletic training practice for concussion assessment and management. J Athl Train 2005;40(4):320–5.
12. Collins M, Lovell MR, Iverson GL, et al. Examining concussion rates and return to play in high school football players wearing newer helmet technology: a three-year prospective cohort study. Neurosurgery 2006;58(2):275–84.
13. McGuine TA, Hetzel S, McCrea M, et al. Protective equipment and player characteristics associated with the incidence of sport-related concussion in high school football players: a multifactorial prospective study. Am J Sports Med 2014;42(10): 2470–8.
14. McIntosh AS, McCrory P, Finch CF, et al. Does padded headgear prevent head injury in rugby union football? Med Sci Sports Exerc 2009;41(2):306–13.
15. Hoshizaki TB, Brien SE, Bailes JE, et al. The science and design of head protection in sport. Neurosurgery 2004;55(4):956–67.
16. Asplund C, Bettcher S, Borchers J. Facial protection and head injuries in ice hockey: a systematic review. Br J Sports Med 2009;43(13):993–9.

17. McGuine T, Post E, Pfaller AY, et al. Does soccer headgear reduce the incidence of sport-related concussion? A cluster, randomised controlled trial of adolescent athletes. Br J Sports Med 2019;1–6. https://doi.org/10.1136/bjsports-2018-100238.

18. Institute of Medicine and National Research Council. Sports-related concussions in youth: improving the science, changing the culture. Washington, DC: The National Academies Press; 2014.

19. Knapik JJ, Marshall SW, Lee RB, et al. Mouthguards in sport: activities history, physical properties and injury prevention effectiveness. Sports Med 2007;37(2):117–44.

20. Wiebe DJ, D'Alonzo BA, Harris R, et al. Association between the experimental kickoff rule and concussion rates in Ivy League football. JAMA 2018;320(19):2035–6.

21. Nathanson JT, Connolly JG, Yuk F, et al. Concussion incidence in professional football: position-specific analysis with use of a novel metric. Orthop J Sports Med 2016;4(1). https://doi.org/10.1177/2325967115622621.

22. Green GA, Pollack KM, D'Angelo J, et al. Mild traumatic brain injury in major and minor league baseball players. Am J Sports Med 2015;43(5):1118–26.

23. Green G, D'Angelo J, Coyles J, et al. Association between a rule change to reduce home plate collisions and mild traumatic brain injury and other injuries in professional baseball players. Am J Sports Med 2019;47(11):2704–8.

24. Emery CA, Kang J, Shrier I, et al. Risk of injury associated with body checking among youth ice hockey players. J Am Med Assoc 2010;303(22):2265–72.

25. Roberts WO, Brust JD, Leonard B, et al. Fair-play rules and injury reduction in ice hockey. Arch Pediatr Adolesc Med 1996;150:140–5.

26. Kriz PK, Staffa SJ, Zurakowski D, et al. Effect of penalty minute rule change on injuries and game disqualification penalties in high school ice hockey. Am J Sports Med 2019;47(2):438–43.

27. Watson RC, Nystrom MA, Buckolz E. Safety in Canadian junior ice hockey: the association between ice surface size and injuries and aggressive penalties in the Ontario Hockey League. Clin J Sport Med 1997;7(3):192–5. Available at: http://www.ncbi.nlm.nih.gov/pubmed/9262886. Accessed January 4, 2020.

28. Wennberg R. Effect of ice surface size on collision rates and head impacts at the World Junior Hockey Championships, 2002 to 2004. Clin J Sport Med 2005;15(2):67–72.

29. World Cup fair-play conduct points: what they are, why they matter - The Washington Post. Available at: https://www.washingtonpost.com/news/soccer-insider/wp/2018/06/28/everything-you-need-to-know-about-the-world-cups-fair-play-tiebreaker/. Accessed December 29, 2019.

30. HEADS UP to Youth Sports | HEADS UP | CDC Injury Center. Available at: https://www.cdc.gov/headsup/youthsports/index.html. Accessed December 29, 2019.

31. Concussion Awareness | US Lacrosse. Available at: https://www.uslacrosse.org/safety/concussion-awareness. Accessed December 29, 2019.

32. Kroshus E, Daneshvar DH, Baugh CM, et al. NCAA concussion education in ice hockey: an ineffective mandate. Br J Sports Med 2014;48(2):135–40.

33. Kerr ZY, Yeargin S, Valovich McLeod TC, et al. Comprehensive coach education and practice contact restriction guidelines result in lower injury rates in youth American football. Orthop J Sports Med 2015;3(7). https://doi.org/10.1177/2325967115594578.

34. Cusimano MD, Zhang S, Topolovec-Vranic J, et al. Pros and cons of 19 sport-related concussion educational resources in Canada: avenues for better care and prevention. Front Neurol 2018;9. https://doi.org/10.3389/fneur.2018.00872.

35. Ellenbogen RG. Concussion advocacy and legislation: a neurological surgeon's view from the epicenter. Neurosurgery 2014;75:S122–30.
36. Concannon LG. Effects of legislation on sports-related concussion. Phys Med Rehabil Clin N Am 2016;27(2):513–27.
37. Collins CL, Fletcher EN, Fields SK, et al. Neck strength: a protective factor reducing risk for concussion in high school sports. J Prim Prev 2014;35(5):309–19.
38. Eckner JT, Oh YK, Joshi MS, et al. Effect of neck muscle strength and anticipatory cervical muscle activation on the kinematic response of the head to impulsive loads. Am J Sports Med 2014;42(3):566–76.
39. Clark JF, Medicine R. An exploratory study of the potential effects of vision training on concussion incidence in football. Optom Vis Perform 2015;3(2):116–25.
40. Wang L, Cheung JT-M, Pu F, et al. Why do woodpeckers resist head impact injury: a biomechanical investigation. PLoS One 2011;6(10):e26490. Briffa M, ed.
41. Smoliga JM, Wang L. Woodpeckers don't play football: implications for novel brain protection devices using mild jugular compression. Br J Sports Med 2018;53(20). https://doi.org/10.1136/bjsports-2018-099594.
42. Yuan W, Barber Foss KD, Thomas S, et al. White matter alterations over the course of two consecutive high-school football seasons and the effect of a jugular compression collar: a preliminary longitudinal diffusion tensor imaging study. Hum Brain Mapp 2018;39(1):491–508.
43. Myer GD, Yuan W, Barber Foss KD, et al. Analysis of head impact exposure and brain microstructure response in a season-long application of a jugular vein compression collar: a prospective, neuroimaging investigation in American football. Br J Sports Med 2016;50(20):1276–85.
44. Myer GD, Barber Foss K, Thomas S, et al. Altered brain microstructure in association with repetitive subconcussive head impacts and the potential protective effect of jugular vein compression: a longitudinal study of female soccer athletes. Br J Sports Med 2018. https://doi.org/10.1136/bjsports-2018-099571.
45. Eighth grade football players racking up college-scholarship offers - schooled in sports - Education Week. Available at: http://blogs.edweek.org/edweek/schooled_in_sports/2013/06/eighth_grade_football_players_racking_up_college_scholarship_offers.html. Accessed December 29, 2019.
46. For boys lacrosse players, the recruiting process is starting earlier than ever - Baltimore Sun. Available at: https://www.baltimoresun.com/sports/bs-xpm-2012-03-16-bs-va-sp-spring-sports-preview-feature-2012-20120317-story.html. Accessed December 29, 2019.
47. Johns Hopkins gets two more commitments from freshmen - Baltimore Sun. Available at: https://www.baltimoresun.com/sports/bs-xpm-2013-12-27-bal-recruiting-notes-johns-hopkins-lacrosse-gets-two-more-commitments-from-freshmen-20131227-story.html. Accessed December 29, 2019.
48. DI Council adopts rules to curb early recruiting | NCAA.org - The Official Site of the NCAA. Available at: http://www.ncaa.org/about/resources/media-center/news/di-council-adopts-rules-curb-early-recruiting. Accessed December 29, 2019.
49. A career built on fighting takes its toll on a former enforcer - The Globe and Mail. Available at: https://www.theglobeandmail.com/sports/robert-frid-enforcer-fighter-stuggles-with-concussions-hockey/article28929084/. Accessed December 29, 2019.

Long-Term Neurocognitive, Mental Health Consequences of Contact Sports

Barry S. Willer, PhD[a],*, Mohammad Nadir Haider, MD[b],
Charles Wilber, MD[b], Carrie Esopenko, PhD[c],
Michael Turner, MBBS[d], John Leddy, MD[b]

KEYWORDS

- Concussion • Chronic traumatic encephalopathy
- Traumatic encephalopathy syndrome

KEY POINTS

- Case series studies that describe the neuropathology of chronic traumatic encephalopathy have generated a hypothesis that some former athletes may develop neurodegeneration later in life.
- Studies of aging retired contact sport athletes, generally including age-matched control groups, suggest early onset dementia is rare.
- Imaging studies of former contact sport athletes have yielded mixed results but PET studies seem close to being able to identify CTE in living persons.

INTRODUCTION

There has been a dramatic increase in understanding the long-term neurocognitive and mental health consequences of playing contact sports. This article begins by discussing the possible link between repetitive head injuries and neuropathologic and neurocognitive disorders. Then we discuss mental health problems commonly found in this population and their radiologic findings. Lastly, we review other causes of neurocognitive and mental health disorders in this population that are independent of repetitive head injuries.

[a] Department of Psychiatry, Jacobs School of Medicine and Biomedical Sciences, Concussion Management Clinic and Research Center, State University of New York at Buffalo, 160 Farber Hall, 3435 Main Street, Buffalo, NY 14214, USA; [b] UBMD Department of Orthopaedics and Sports Medicine, Concussion Management Clinic and Research Center, State University of New York at Buffalo, 160 Farber Hall, 3435 Main Street, Buffalo, NY 14214, USA; [c] Department of Rehabilitation & Movement Sciences, School of Health Professions, Rutgers Biomedical and Health Sciences, Rutgers University, 65 Bergen Street, Newark, NJ 07107, USA; [d] International Concussion and Head Injury Foundation, Institute of Sport, Exercise and Health, University College London, 170 Tottenham Court Road, W1T 7HA, UK
* Corresponding author.
E-mail address: bswiller@buffalo.edu

Clin Sports Med 40 (2021) 173–186
https://doi.org/10.1016/j.csm.2020.08.012
0278-5919/21/Crown Copyright © 2020 Published by Elsevier Inc. All rights reserved.
sportsmed.theclinics.com

CHRONIC TRAUMATIC ENCEPHALOPATHY
History

The links between head injuries during sports and impairments in neurocognitive and mental health have been studied since 1928 when forensic pathologist Harrison Martland wrote about the typical tremors, slowed movement, confusion, and speech problems found in boxers with dementia pugilistic.[1] The term chronic traumatic encephalopathy (CTE) was first used in 1949 to describe the "punch-drunk" syndrome in boxers,[2] and was initially believed to only affect boxers who took considerable blows to the head and not athletes who played other contact sports. In 1973 Corsellis and colleagues[3] described 15 cases where there was pronounced neuropathologic changes including ventricular dilatation, cavum septum pellucidum enlargement, and neurofibrillary tangles. The National Institutes of Health held a consensus meeting in 2015 to define the neuropathologic criteria for CTE diagnosis,[4] and concluded, with acceptable agreement (61%), that pathognomonic lesions for CTE were abnormal perivascular accumulation of tau in neurons, astrocytes, and cell processes in an irregular pattern at the depths of the sulci of the frontal, temporal, or parietal cortices.[5] Goldfinger and colleagues[6] re-examined the specimens of the brains studied by Corsellis and only found half of the 14 specimens qualified as CTE using the more recent National Institutes of Health–approved criteria. CTE is considered a neurodegenerative disorder but clearly there is not solid agreement on what pathologists should use as the gold standard for diagnosis.

Forensic pathologist Bennet Omalu in 2005 is credited for bringing attention to the disease in the nonboxer population when he published a case-report of a 50-year-old former National Football League (NFL) athlete with suspected CTE who presented with gross neurobehavioral impairments before dying by suicide.[7] There has been an exponential increase in research describing the long-term effects of repetitive head injuries since the first case-reports were published. In 2009, McKee and colleagues,[8] from the Boston University brain bank, described CTE in three more cases of former athletes, two of whom were boxers. In 2013, McKee and colleagues[9] described postmortem analysis of 85 former NFL and National Hockey League (NHL) athletes, most with a history of repetitive mild traumatic brain injury ranging in age from 17 to 98, and found 65 (76.5%) had CTE. The more recent research publication by Mez and colleagues[10] on the association of CTE and football, also from the Boston University group, reported that of 111 NFL players, 110 (99.1%) showed evidence of CTE on postmortem examination using the new 2015 criteria. In the total sample of 202 high school, college, and professional football players, various degrees of CTE were diagnosed in 177 of these players (87.6%). In a follow-up study Mez and colleagues[11] reported on 266 former American football players, where 233 (87.6%) met diagnostic criteria for CTE. They found a correlation between years played and severity of CTE. All of the athletes represented in the study had their brains donated to the brain bank managed by Boston University. All of the pathologic studies were conducted by the same pathologist, thus no evaluation of interrater reliability. There was no comparison group. The authors provided a discussion of ascertainment bias; simply stated, families of individuals with cognitive deficits were far more likely to donate the brain of their deceased family member for study. The collaborative effort led by Boston University to create a brain bank has been instrumental to the expansion of research on CTE. Their research suggests CTE is prevalent among athletes that play contact sports, especially at the professional level. However, the sample studied may not be representative of the entire population of former contact sport athletes.

Pathophysiology

The pathophysiology of CTE is complex, and we must begin with the classical finding of CTE.[12] The pathognomonic findings of CTE include abnormal perivascular accumulation of tau in an irregular pattern at the depths of the sulci of the frontal, temporal, or parietal cortices.[5] But where does this tau come from? Tau is a microtubule-associated protein present in the neuron.[13] It promotes the assembly and maintenance of microtubules, which are responsible for intracellular transport, axonal morphology, and cell physiology. Tau is a fundamental component in the brain, because it is responsible for maintaining neuronal integrity and axoplasmic transport.[9,13] Recent animal research has shown that traumatic brain injuries can cause shearing of microtubules,[14,15] releasing tau into the extracellular space that subsequently undergoes hyperphosphorylation and deposits in the cortex.[5] The hyperphosphorylated tau is unable to perform its normal function[16] and the brain does not have a system of removing excess tau.[17] Tau begins to accumulate and can even form widespread plaques in severe cases.[5] This can cause direct and indirect effects on the surrounding tissues, which can lead to further neurodegeneration.[17,18] Higher concentrations of tau correlate with greater neurocognitive dysfunction in severe cases of CTE[10]; however, the presence of tau on histochemical assessment is not specific to a history of repetitive head trauma or playing sports.[19,20] Rather, it is more suggestive of neurodegeneration than healthy aging.

TRAUMATIC ENCEPHALOPATHY SYNDROME
Definition

As a result of the research on former NFL athletes and the retrospective diagnoses of impaired cognitive and psychosocial function in athletes with autopsy-confirmed CTE, there has been a movement toward developing a clinical diagnostic criterion for individuals who experienced chronic exposure to repetitive head impacts presenting with cognitive and psychological complaints. That is, CTE is the neuropathologic determination of disease confirmed at autopsy, whereas traumatic encephalopathy syndrome (TES) represents the clinical symptoms, including behavioral, cognitive, and psychological complaints, in individuals who have experienced repetitive head trauma.[21,22] More work is needed to define the clinical diagnostic criteria for TES because recent work indicated that approximately 50% of a sample of men with clinical depression met the research criteria for TES.[19]

Is there a direct relationship between the diagnosis of CTE and behavioral decline and/or cognitive deficits? Gavett and colleagues[23] conducted interviews with friends and family members of people who had documented CTE. They described a consistent pattern of impairment in cognition, executive function, mood, behavior (impulsivity), and signs of motor neuron disease. Stern and colleagues[24] conducted a similar retrospective analysis of 36 deceased athletes (average age of death 56.8 years) with confirmed CTE (mostly former NFL athletes and a few former NHL athletes). Three of these athletes were asymptomatic, 11 had cognitive dysfunction, 13 had behavior alterations that gradually became mood changes, and 10 were diagnosed with dementia. Using next-of-kin interviews, Alosco and colleagues[25] studied 25 professional football players (mean age at death, 65 years) with autopsy-confirmed stage III or IV CTE. They found that 25 of 25 had cognitive symptoms and their age of cognitive decline was inversely related to their cognitive reserve.

In vivo studies in living, retired contact sport athletes have found conflicting results regarding the prevalence of TES. Hart and colleagues[26] compared 34 former NFL athletes (average age, 62) with 28 age and education matched control subjects. Control subjects were drawn from a larger sample of subjects from another study and were excluded if they had any cognitive impairments. Among the 34 retired NFL athletes they found eight to qualify as mild cognitive impairment and two had dementia. Of the two with dementia, one had vascular dementia associated with diabetes and stroke, whereas the other was of unknown cause. Casson and colleagues[27] examined 45 retired NFL players (average age, 45; average career of almost 7 years) and found no evidence of cognitive decline. Esopenko and colleagues[28] studied 33 former professional ice hockey players (average age, 54) and compared them with 18 age-matched control subjects. They found few differences on a full range of cognitive measures and no differences on critical cognitive factors, such as memory. They found that the athletes performed much better on all of the measures of cognition than the athletes expected they would perform. McMillan and colleagues[29] examined a sample of 52 former international rugby athletes (average age, 53) and 29 age-matched control subjects. They also found minimal differences; the only exception, athletes did poorly on one test of verbal learning. Importantly, the mean scores for both groups on almost every measure of cognition were in the average range for age and there were no differences in mental health or daily functioning between the retired athletes and the control group. Tarazi and colleagues[30] compared 45 retired Canadian Football League players (average age, 53) with 25 age-matched control subjects. They found no evidence of motor decline and found no differences on objective measures of memory, attention, or processing speed. However, they reported that the athletes perceived themselves as having cognitive problems. Despite the lack of any objective evidence of decline, the authors chose to emphasize the self-reported cognitive problems as evidence of modern CTE, as opposed to classic CTE, which would have also included motor decline. Willer and colleagues[31] published three papers from the same sample population in 2018. The authors compared 21 retired NFL and NHL players (average age, 54) with 21 age-matched, noncontact sport athletes. They did not find significant differences in executive functioning or mood disorders,[32] or the incidence of mild cognitive impairment.[33] The authors commented that the control subjects were recruited from an athletic population who were competitive in their youth and continued to remain active and competitive through their 50s, 60s, and 70s.[34] The Willer and colleagues[32] studies also reported that retired contact sport athletes self-described many more problems with cognition and executive function than was apparent on objective testing. They also found the former NHL/NFL athletes were anxious with most of that anxiety because of the belief that they might develop CTE and have a rapid decline in function.

The studies of cognitive and behavioral impairment in former contact sport athletes are summarized in **Table 1**. The number of subjects represented in these studies is 235, average age 54, yet only two were identified as having dementia, and only one of these as possible TES. There was no evidence across studies of cognitive impairment outside normal aging and mixed results with respect to behavioral functioning, with one study finding superior executive functioning and one finding inferior executive functioning. It is possible that, despite the best efforts to encourage participation, studies of retired athletes are only able to recruit the healthiest, thereby underrepresenting those with dementia. It is also possible that the prevalence of early onset dementia or TES is simply not as high as once believed.

Large epidemiologic studies have also failed to find an association between contact sport exposure and neurocognitive impairments. In one such long-term study,[35] they compared 834 men 65 years of age who had participated in American high school football with a sample of 1858 men from the same high schools who did not play

Table 1
Summary of studies that evaluated cognition and behavioral characteristics of former contact sport athletes

Author, Year	Athlete Sample	Mean Age	Control Sample	Cognitive Impairment	Behavioural Impairment
Hart et al,[26] 2013	NFL, N = 34	62	N = 28	8 MCI 2 Dementia	8 depressed
Casson et al,[27] 2014	NFL, N = 45	46	0	0 Dementia	9 depressed
Tarazi et al,[30] 2018	CFL, N = 45	53	N = 25	0 Dementia	Superior EF in athletes
Esopenko et al,[28] 2017	NHL, N = 38	54	N = 20	0 Dementia	Reduced EF in athletes
McMillan et al,[29] 2017	Rugby, N = 52	54	N = 29	0 Dementia	No differences
Willer et al,[32] 2018	NHL/NFL, N = 21	56	N = 21	8 MCI, 0 dementia	5 depressed, 7 anxious

Abbreviations: CFL, Canadian Football League; EF, executive function; MCI, mild cognitive impairment.

football and there were no differences in rates of cognitive impairment or depression. In a similar study, Janssen and colleagues[36] compared 296 high school football athletes (aged 60–80) with 190 athletes from the same high school and era who played noncontact sports. There were no differences in the rates of various neurologic diseases that would lead to dementia.[35] Recent work from the CARE Consortium, including data from 3422 current male American collegiate football players and 914 noncontact sport athletes, found that exposure to head contact before age 12 was not associated with neurocognitive deficits while in college.[37] The pattern of self-reported issues with cognition versus objective measures of cognitive decline turns out to be a common finding. A recent meta-analysis of studies published to-date suggests that a history of sports-related concussion impacts cognitive domains, such as psychomotor function, executive function, and memory.[38] However, the authors conclude that the cause and effect relationship between sports-related concussion and long-term health outcomes is limited by the lack of high-quality and adequately powered prospective studies in the field. This confirms that although there is now a stronger understanding of the potential mechanisms involved in the processes underlying concussion, the epidemiologic evidence, and the strength of this evidence, to support the long-term effects on cognition remains unclear. Understanding whether concussion in sport is significantly associated with worsening of cognitive function in later life is of paramount importance. Uncovering this possible association would have immediate repercussion on current play policy and regulations, and possibly on the listing of cognitive decline as an occupational disease for former players.

OTHER NEUROCOGNITIVE AND MENTAL HEALTH CONSEQUENCES

Epidemiologic studies have reported some evidence of neurodegenerative disease in contact sport athletes aside from CTE. In a cohort study of nearly 3500 NFL alumni, overall mortality rates were lower than the general US population; however, rates of Alzheimer disease and amyotrophic lateral sclerosis were three and four times higher, respectively, than the general population.[39] Similar results were found in a recent study examining cause of death in a large sample of former professional Scottish soccer players (N = 1180) compared with age-matched community-dwelling adults (N = 3807). The former professional soccer players showed a lower prevalence of all-cause mortality and ischemic heart disease, but showed a higher prevalence of death attributed to neurodegenerative disease (1.7% vs 0.5%).[40] These studies compared general and neurologic health outcomes in professional contact sport athletes with the general population. One recent study examined causes of death in former Major League Baseball players, who have little exposure to repetitive head trauma, to former NFL players.[41] The authors found that former NFL players had elevated all-cause mortality rates, and in particular, higher rates of death that included cardiovascular and neurodegenerative disease compared with former Major League Baseball players. Yet, it should be noted that other studies have failed to find an association between participating in American football at the high school level and neurodegenerative diseases, including Alzheimer disease, amyotrophic lateral sclerosis, or Parkinson disease.[36,42]

Mood disorders seem to be present in many members of the retired athlete population. In one of the earliest studies of psychosocial function in former NFL players, Guskiewicz and colleagues[43] found that a history of concussion was associated with lifetime diagnosis of depression, and moreover, that the prevalence of depression diagnoses increased in those with recurrent concussions. Furthermore, the risk of developing depression in former NFL players who have experienced concussions increases over time, ranging from 3% having a clinical diagnosis of depression in the no concussion group to 26.8% being diagnosed in the 10+ concussion group.[44] Similar results have been shown between self-reported depression, impulsivity, and aggression with concussion history in former collegiate Division I athletes.[45] In this sample, former athletes with three or more concussions were 2.4 times more likely to have moderate to severe depression and those with two or more concussions had higher mean impulsivity and aggression scores, compared with former athletes with no concussion history. Didehbani and colleagues[46] found increased symptoms of depression in retired NFL players when compared with healthy age- and education-matched participants, but also that the number of lifetime concussions was significantly related to depression total scores. Results from the United States based National Longitudinal Study of Adolescent to Adult Health, which followed athletes starting at 16 years of age for approximately 13 years, found playing American high school football did not impact cognitive abilities, depressive symptoms, or suicidal ideation.[47] However, there was a trend toward increased suicidal ideation in athletes with a history of contact sports, whereas the noncontact sport group showed a trend toward an increase in depressive symptoms. Most of the studies that suggest there is a significantly higher rate of depression in former contact sport athletes are postmortem studies.[9,48,49] Well-designed, longitudinal studies, however, have not found an increased rate, and some have even found a lower rate of suicide among retired contact sport athletes.[50]

RADIOLOGIC INVESTIGATIONS OF LONG-TERM CONSEQUENCES

Several imaging studies have been conducted to identify the possible long-term consequences of playing contact sports. Most of these studies have been performed with retired American football players and may not be generalizable to all contact sports. Koerte and colleagues[51] used MRI to compare structural differences in the brains of 72 retired professional football players and 12 noncontact athlete control subjects. They found that retired football players had a greater incidence of having an enlarged cavum septum pellucidum associated with brain atrophy. The finding was also found by Gardner and colleagues[52] in 17 retired professional football players and 17 matched control subjects. MRI studies have found other structural differences, with retired football players having greater cortical thinning[53] and significantly smaller bilateral hippocampal volume.[54] This cortical thinning is also seen in retired professional soccer players who have had a long history of heading.[55]

Some studies have not found a correlation between a lifetime history of concussion and structural differences. Terry and Miller[56] found no differences in cognitive function or brain volumes in those who had experienced two or more concussions compared with those with no concussion history, although better overall cognitive function was correlated with adjusted gray matter volumes. Importantly, their sample was matched for age, education, estimated premorbid IQ, and current concussion symptomatology. Additionally, in contrast to research suggesting that exposure to American football before the age of 12 was associated with greater cognitive impairment, Solomon and colleagues[57] found that years pre–high school football was not related to cognitive impairment or neurologic neuroradiologic abnormalities. Zivadinov and colleagues[58] performed multimodal radiologic assessment in 21 retired contact sport athletes (mean age, 56) and compared them with 21 age-matched noncontact sport athletes. The authors found no significant structural differences between the two groups. The noncontact sport group had a higher incidence of microbleeds that was not clinically significant.

Stern and colleagues[59] used flortaucipir PET to compare 26 former NFL athletes (mean age, 57) with 31 control subjects (mean age, 60). The athletes were carefully selected as high risk for CTE, based on years played and position played. The athletes also had objective signs of cognitive and neuropsychiatric impairment. The control subjects had no signs of impairment and no history of concussion. The athletes had higher p-tau levels measured by PET than control subjects. Importantly, the p-tau levels were highest in the regions of the brain that are potentially affected by CTE. The authors note that the results represent group differences and we are not at the point where elevated CTE-associated tau can be detected on an individual basis.

OTHER HEALTH CONDITIONS LEADING TO NEUROCOGNITIVE DECLINE

A lot of attention has been given to the neurocognitive and mental health consequences of head injuries in retired contact sport athletes, but little consideration has been given to other causes of neurocognitive decline, such as lifestyle issues or a history of musculoskeletal pain, that is not directly related to a history of head injuries. Athletes just starting out in their professional careers may lack proper dietary and lifestyle education for post-professional sport life and may develop improper habits during retirement. Haider and colleagues[34] compared the estimated energy expenditure and nutritional intake of 21 retired contact sport athletes with 21 age-matched athletic control subjects. They found retired contact sport athletes were significantly overweight and less physically active, important risk factors of cognitive decline. Lack of physical activity has been associated with brain atrophy,[60] neuroinflammation,[61] and vulnerability to trauma and disease,[62] whereas regular exercise has been linked to several neurocognitive benefits.[63] Willeumier and colleagues[64] studied 38 overweight and 38 healthy-weight retired NFL players (average age, 57 years) and showed that players with higher body mass index had significantly more cognitive decline, which suggests it is an independent risk factor in retired contact sport athletes. This higher body mass index was also associated with decreased activation of the prefrontal cortex.

Lastly, professional contact sport athletes train vigorously and often sustain orthopedic injuries, resulting in several sources of chronic pain and/or disability throughout their lives.[65] The sensory and emotional experience of pain, and its deleterious impact on mental health and cognitive functioning, could contribute to early neurocognitive decline. Increased pain intensity has been linked to impaired attention, reduced psychomotor speed, executive dysfunction,[66] and impaired working memory,[67] all of which are risk factors for early neurocognitive decline. Chronic pain may also lead to maladaptive coping mechanisms or substance abuse, further affecting neurocognitive functioning. High levels of pain in athletes have been linked to prior or recurrent injuries and/or multiple surgeries.[68,69] A systematic review[70] identified chronic pain to be significantly associated with abnormalities in neurobehavioral functioning (ie, deficits in memory, processing speed, and attention). It has also been shown that higher levels of chronic pain are strongly correlated with psychiatric manifestations, such as anxiety and depression.[71]

SUMMARY

Bennet Omalu published his first study[7] of an American football player showing CTE in 2005. Since then there has been significant interest in CTE and the risks of playing contact sport at the professional level and the amateur level. This interest has been generated by the politics of sport as much as the scientific pursuit of knowledge. The reactions of the professional sports world to the possibility of long-term damage from concussions was initially one of denial, thus polarizing the general public and to some extent the scientific community into CTE believers and those who were perceived to have affiliations with sports or sport teams (whether they have such an affiliation or not). A recent article in the Washington Post (Will Hobson, January 22, 2020) describes how Dr Omalu went from pathologist (as portrayed by Will Smith in the movie Concussion) to CTE activist.

The most supportive evidence of CTE has been generated by the studies conducted by Boston University, an organization that some have seen as having a bias. The brain bank at Boston University was cofounded by the Concussion Legacy Foundation, which has a primary purpose of creating safer sports through education and to end CTE through prevention and research.[72] CTE, therefore becomes a foregone conclusion for the Brain Bank cofounded by this organization. Most of the understanding, and resulting public discourse on CTE has come from their research, which has largely been a case series design with no control subjects.[73] This is considered to be the lowest level of evidence, that is, research that has a complete absence of any control groups and has no published evaluation of the reliability or validity of the diagnosis.[74] In general, this research is seen as hypothesis-generating rather hypothesis-testing.

The scientific studies of aging athletes in vivo, intended to evaluate TES, have fared only slightly better. They at least had comparison groups, although there are some important questions regarding the ideal control population to compare with professional athletes who played contact sports. These studies face similar difficulties to the pathology case series with identifying the extent to which the populations studied are representative of the population of contact sport athletes as a whole. The hypothesis of each of these studies is that some of the contact sport athletes will demonstrate characteristics of early onset dementia. When we combine the results of all of these studies we see little evidence of dementia; however, because each study relied on volunteer participation it is possible that athletes who were worried about their mental status or had been diagnosed with dementia did not wish to participate or did not have the means. When studies do not find a difference between the contact sport athletes and the comparison groups that does not necessarily mean that the two groups are the same. Rather, it could easily mean that the studies did not examine the variables that would be different between the groups. Still, the end result is that the in vivo studies of aging contact sport athletes produced results that are diametrically opposed to the case series results of the Boston University group.

The studies of former athletes using advanced imaging probably yield the best chance of providing meaningful answers to the questions about the long-term effects of concussion in those that played contact sports. The results thus far have been mixed, although the recent study by Stern and colleagues[59] using PET technology offers perhaps the best study to date to track TES in retired athletes who are still alive. There are unanswered questions with this study, such as whether the control group is a true comparison group, but a positive finding of hyperphosphorylated tau on PET scans being similar to the hypothesized locations based on the CTE case studies is encouraging. The representativeness of the former NFL athletes in this study is also in question but this type of research is certainly what is needed in the future.

The highly controversial nature of the topic of CTE has led to an unfortunate polarization of the public as a whole and many researchers and clinicians. It is safe to say that some former contact sport athletes will face some level of neurodegeneration because of their sport-related concussions. It is also likely, given the available research on living athletes, that the rates of neurodegeneration are low. Concerns about children and sports-related concussion and the likelihood of experiencing neurodegeneration are legitimate but there is insufficient evidence to countermand the known benefits of sport participation. Future research must somehow avoid the polarizing trap that allowed much of the current research to be misrepresented or misinterpreted. Otherwise future studies will suffer and the important questions that remain about the long-term effects of concussion on athletes will not be answered. In the meantime, the specter of CTE has at least played a significant role in establishing much better sport safety protocols and validated consensus of concussion management for amateur and professional athletes; albeit there is still room for improvement for recreational athletes. The proper and timely management of concussion is essential if one is to influence the long-term effects of concussion and that is the focus of most of the articles in this special compilation. With or without the fear of CTE, validated and independent research, in conjunction with the proper management of concussion, must be the foremost priority if future generations of children who want to be involved in sport are to be protected.

CLINIC CARE POINTS

- Concussion may have long term consequences or may not.
- The benefits of organized sports may be greater than the potential long term effects.
- The removal of bias in research will lead to more useful conclusions regarding the long term consequences of contact sports.

DISCLOSURE

The authors have nothing to disclose.

REFERENCES

1. Changa AR, Vietrogoski RA, Carmel PW. Dr Harrison Martland and the history of punch drunk syndrome. Brain 2017;141(1):318–21.
2. Critchley M. Punch-drunk syndromes: the chronic traumatic encephalopathy of boxers. In: Hommage a Clovis Vincent. Paris: Maloine; 1949. p. 131.
3. Corsellis J, Bruton C, Freeman-Browne D. The aftermath of boxing. Psychol Med 1973;3(3):270–303.
4. McKee AC, Cairns NJ, Dickson DW, et al. The first NINDS/NIBIB consensus meeting to define neuropathological criteria for the diagnosis of chronic traumatic encephalopathy. Acta Neuropathol 2016;131(1):75–86.
5. Kiernan PT, Montenigro PH, Solomon TM, et al, editors. Chronic traumatic encephalopathy: a neurodegenerative consequence of repetitive traumatic brain injury. Seminars in neurology. New York: Thieme Medical Publishers; 2015.
6. Goldfinger MH, Ling H, Tilley BS, et al. The aftermath of boxing revisited: identifying chronic traumatic encephalopathy pathology in the original Corsellis boxer series. Acta Neuropathol 2018;136(6):973–4.
7. Omalu BI, DeKosky ST, Minster RL, et al. Chronic traumatic encephalopathy in a National Football League player. Neurosurgery 2005;57(1):128–34.
8. McKee AC, Cantu RC, Nowinski CJ, et al. Chronic traumatic encephalopathy in athletes: progressive tauopathy after repetitive head injury. J Neuropathol Exp Neurol 2009;68(7):709–35.
9. McKee AC, Stein TD, Nowinski CJ, et al. The spectrum of disease in chronic traumatic encephalopathy. Brain 2013;136(1):43–64.

10. Mez J, Daneshvar DH, Kiernan PT, et al. Clinicopathological evaluation of chronic traumatic encephalopathy in players of American football. Jama 2017;318(4): 360–70.

11. Mez J, Daneshvar DH, Abdolmohammadi B, et al. Duration of American football play and chronic traumatic encephalopathy. Ann Neurol 2020;87(1):116–31.

12. Sundman M, Doraiswamy PM, Morey R. Neuroimaging assessment of early and late neurobiological sequelae of traumatic brain injury: implications for CTE. Front Neurosci 2015;9:334.

13. Lee VM, Goedert M, Trojanowski JQ. Neurodegenerative tauopathies. Annu Rev Neurosci 2001;24(1):1121–59.

14. Johnson VE, Stewart W, Arena JD, et al. Traumatic brain injury as a trigger of neurodegeneration. Neurodegenerative diseases. Springer; 2017. p. 383–400.

15. Zanier ER, Bertani I, Sammali E, et al. Induction of a transmissible tau pathology by traumatic brain injury. Brain 2018;141(9):2685–99.

16. Lindwall G, Cole RD. Phosphorylation affects the ability of tau protein to promote microtubule assembly. J Biol Chem 1984;259(8):5301–5.

17. Drubin DG, Kirschner MW. Tau protein function in living cells. J Cell Biol 1986; 103(6):2739–46.

18. Pîrşcoveanu DFV, Pirici I, Tudorică V, et al. Tau protein in neurodegenerative diseases: a review. Rom J Morphol Embryol 2017;58:1141–50.

19. Iverson GL, Terry DP, Luz M, et al. Anger and depression in middle-aged men: implications for a clinical diagnosis of chronic traumatic encephalopathy. J Neuropsychiatry Clin Neurosci 2019;31(4):328–36.

20. Bieniek KF, Blessing MM, Heckman MG, et al. Association between contact sports participation and chronic traumatic encephalopathy: a retrospective cohort study. Brain Pathol 2020;30(1):63–74.

21. Reams N, Hayward RA, Kutcher JS, et al. Effect of concussion on performance of National Football League Players. Int J Sports Physiol Perform 2017;12(8): 1100–4.

22. Montenigro PH, Baugh CM, Daneshvar DH, et al. Clinical subtypes of chronic traumatic encephalopathy: literature review and proposed research diagnostic criteria for traumatic encephalopathy syndrome. Alzheimers Res Ther 2014; 6(5):68.

23. Gavett BE, Stern RA, McKee AC. Chronic traumatic encephalopathy: a potential late effect of sport-related concussive and subconcussive head trauma. Clin Sports Med 2011;30(1):179–88.

24. Stern RA, Daneshvar DH, Baugh CM, et al. Clinical presentation of chronic traumatic encephalopathy. Neurology 2013;81(13):1122–9.

25. Alosco M, Kasimis A, Stamm J, et al. Age of first exposure to American football and long-term neuropsychiatric and cognitive outcomes. Transl Psychiatry 2017;7(9):e1236.

26. Hart J, Kraut MA, Womack KB, et al. Neuroimaging of cognitive dysfunction and depression in aging retired National Football League players: a cross-sectional study. JAMA Neurol 2013;70(3):326–35.

27. Casson IR, Viano DC, Haacke EM, et al. Is there chronic brain damage in retired NFL players? Neuroradiology, neuropsychology, and neurology examinations of 45 retired players. Sports Health 2014;6(5):384–95.

28. Esopenko C, Chow TW, Tartaglia MC, et al. Cognitive and psychosocial function in retired professional hockey players. J Neurol Neurosurg Psychiatry 2017;88(6): 512–9.

29. McMillan T, McSkimming P, Wainman-Lefley J, et al. Long-term health outcomes after exposure to repeated concussion in elite level: rugby union players. J Neurol Neurosurg Psychiatry 2017;88(6):505–11.

30. Tarazi A, Hussain MW, Alatwi MK, et al. The relationship between brain atrophy and cognitive-behavioural symptoms in retired Canadian football players with multiple concussions. Neuroimage Clin 2018;19:551–8.

31. Willer BS, Zivadinov R, Haider MN, et al. A preliminary study of early-onset dementia of former professional football and hockey players. J Head Trauma Rehabil 2018;33(5):E1–8.

32. Willer BS, Tiso MR, Haider MN, et al. Evaluation of executive function and mental health in retired contact sport athletes. J Head Trauma Rehabil 2018;33(5):E9–15.

33. Baker JG, Leddy JJ, Hinds AL, et al. An exploratory study of mild cognitive impairment of retired professional contact sport athletes. J Head Trauma Rehabil 2018;33(5):E16–23.

34. Haider MN, ODonnell K, Bezherano I, et al. Retired professional contact sport athletes are more sedentary and consume fewer brain healthy nutrients than non-contact sport controls. JSM Sports Med Res 2019. [Epub ahead of print].

35. Deshpande SK, Hasegawa RB, Rabinowitz AR, et al. Association of playing high school football with cognition and mental health later in life. JAMA Neurol 2017; 74(8):909–18.

36. Janssen PH, Mandrekar J, Mielke MM, et al, editors. High school football and late-life risk of neurodegenerative syndromes, 1956-1970. Mayo Clinic Proceedings. Rochester (MN): Elsevier; 2017.

37. Caccese JB, DeWolf RM, Kaminski TW, et al. Estimated age of first exposure to American football and neurocognitive performance amongst NCAA male student-athletes: a cohort study. Sports Med 2019;49(3):477–87.

38. Cunningham J, Broglio SP, O'Grady M, et al. History of sport-related concussion and long-term clinical cognitive health outcomes in retired athletes: a systematic review. J Athl Train 2020;55(2):132–58.

39. Lehman EJ, Hein MJ, Baron SL, et al. Neurodegenerative causes of death among retired National Football League players. Neurology 2012;79(19):1970–4.

40. Mackay DF, Russell ER, Stewart K, et al. Neurodegenerative disease mortality among former professional soccer players. N Engl J Med 2019;381:1801–8.

41. Nguyen VT, Zafonte RD, Chen JT, et al. Mortality among professional American-style football players and professional American baseball players. JAMA Netw open 2019;2(5):e194223.

42. Savica R, Parisi JE, Wold LE, et al, editors. High school football and risk of neurodegeneration: a community-based study. Mayo Clinic Proceedings. Rochester (MN): Elsevier; 2012.

43. Guskiewicz KM, Marshall SW, Bailes J, et al. Recurrent concussion and risk of depression in retired professional football players. Med Sci Sports Exerc 2007; 39(6):903.

44. Kerr ZY, Marshall SW, Harding HP Jr, et al. Nine-year risk of depression diagnosis increases with increasing self-reported concussions in retired professional football players. Am J Sports Med 2012;40(10):2206–12.

45. Kerr ZY, Evenson KR, Rosamond WD, et al. Association between concussion and mental health in former collegiate athletes. Inj Epidemiol 2014;1(1):28.

46. Didehbani N, Munro Cullum C, Mansinghani S, et al. Depressive symptoms and concussions in aging retired NFL players. Arch Clin Neuropsychol 2013;28(5): 418–24.

47. Bohr AD, Boardman JD, McQueen MB. Association of adolescent sport participation with cognition and depressive symptoms in early adulthood. Orthop J Sports Med 2019;7(9). 2325967119868658.

48. Scheuerman SB. The NFL concussion litigation: a critical assessment of class certification. FIU L Rev 2012;8:81.

49. Omalu BI, Bailes J, Hammers JL, et al. Chronic traumatic encephalopathy, suicides and parasuicides in professional American athletes: the role of the forensic pathologist. Am J Forensic Med Pathol 2010;31(2):130–2.

50. Iverson GL. Retired National Football League players are not at greater risk for suicide. Arch Clin Neuropsychol 2019;35(3):332–41.

51. Koerte I, Hufschmidt J, Muehlmann M. Cavum septi pellucidi in retired American pro-football players. J Neurotrauma 2016;33:346–53.

52. Gardner RC, Hess CP, Brus-Ramer M, et al. Cavum septum pellucidum in retired American pro-football players. J Neurotrauma 2016;33(1):157–61.

53. Goswami R, Dufort P, Tartaglia M, et al. Frontotemporal correlates of impulsivity and machine learning in retired professional athletes with a history of multiple concussions. Brain Struct Funct 2016;221(4):1911–25.

54. Strain JF, Womack KB, Didehbani N, et al. Imaging correlates of memory and concussion history in retired National Football League athletes. JAMA Neurol 2015;72(7):773–80.

55. Koerte IK, Mayinger M, Muehlmann M, et al. Cortical thinning in former professional soccer players. Brain Imaging Behav 2016;10(3):792–8.

56. Terry DP, Miller LS. Repeated mild traumatic brain injuries is not associated with volumetric differences in former high school football players. Brain Imaging Behav 2018;12(3):631–9.

57. Solomon GS, Kuhn AW, Zuckerman SL, et al. Participation in pre–high school football and neurological, neuroradiological, and neuropsychological findings in later life: a study of 45 retired National Football League players. Am J Sports Med 2016;44(5):1106–15.

58. Zivadinov R, Polak P, Schweser F, et al. Multimodal imaging of retired professional contact sport athletes does not provide evidence of structural and functional brain damage. J Head Trauma Rehabil 2018;33(5):E24–32.

59. Stern RA, Adler CH, Chen K, et al. Tau positron-emission tomography in former National Football League players. N Engl J Med 2019;380(18):1716–25.

60. Tseng BY, Uh J, Rossetti HC, et al. Masters athletes exhibit larger regional brain volume and better cognitive performance than sedentary older adults. J Magn Reson Imaging 2013;38(5):1169–76.

61. Pruimboom L, Raison CL, Muskiet FA. Physical activity protects the human brain against metabolic stress induced by a postprandial and chronic inflammation. Behav Neurol 2015;2015:569869.

62. Mattson MP. Energy intake and exercise as determinants of brain health and vulnerability to injury and disease. Cell Metab 2012;16(6):706–22.

63. Ahlskog JE, Geda YE, Graff-Radford NR, et al, editors. Physical exercise as a preventive or disease-modifying treatment of dementia and brain aging. Mayo Clinic Proceedings. Rochester (MN): Elsevier; 2011.

64. Willeumier K, Taylor D, Amen D. Elevated body mass in National Football League players linked to cognitive impairment and decreased prefrontal cortex and temporal pole activity. Transl Psychiatry 2012;2(1):e68.

65. Murray TA, Cook TD, Werner SL, et al. The effects of extended play on professional baseball pitchers. Am J Sports Med 2001;29(2):137–42.

66. Tamburin S, Maier A, Schiff S, et al. Cognition and emotional decision-making in chronic low back pain: an ERPs study during Iowa gambling task. Front Psychol 2014;5:1350.
67. Berryman C, Stanton TR, Bowering KJ, et al. Evidence for working memory deficits in chronic pain: a systematic review and meta-analysis. Pain 2013;154(8): 1181–96.
68. Schwenk TL, Gorenflo DW, Dopp RR, et al. Depression and pain in retired professional football players. Med Sci Sports Exerc 2007;39(4):599–605.
69. Cottler LB, Abdallah AB, Cummings SM, et al. Injury, pain, and prescription opioid use among former National Football League (NFL) players. Drug Alcohol Depend 2011;116(1–3):188–94.
70. Higgins DM, Martin AM, Baker DG, et al. The relationship between chronic pain and neurocognitive function: a systematic review. Clin J pain 2018;34(3):262–75.
71. Williams L, Jones W, Shen J, et al. Prevalence and impact of depression and pain in neurology outpatients. J Neurol Neurosurg Psychiatry 2003;74(11):1587–9.
72. Concussion Legacy Foundation. Available at: https://concussionfoundation.org/. Accessed September 14, 2020.
73. Riley DO, Robbins CA, Cantu RC, et al. Chronic traumatic encephalopathy: contributions from the Boston University Center for the Study of Traumatic Encephalopathy. Brain Inj 2015;29(2):154–63.
74. Burns PB, Rohrich RJ, Chung KC. The levels of evidence and their role in evidence-based medicine. Plast Reconstr Surg 2011;128(1):305.

Considerations for Athlete Retirement After Sport-Related Concussion

Julie C. Wilson, MD[a,b,c,]*, Tatiana Patsimas, MD[c],
Kathleen Cohen, DO[d,e], Margot Putukian, MD[d,e]

KEYWORDS

- Head injury • Athletic • Disqualification • Sports

KEY POINTS

- Athlete retirement after sport-related concussion (SRC) should be an individualized and informed decision for each athlete.
- An athlete's previous concussion history, as well as current concussion recovery trajectory, and results of neuroimaging and neuropsychological testing are considered in return-to-play decisions.
- Additional factors to consider include the importance of continued participation in sport for the athlete, the athlete's support system, and other external factors.
- The decision to retire after SRC is an example of shared decision making: the health care team shares information with the athlete, the athlete considers options, and together they make a decision.

INTRODUCTION

Sport-related concussion (SRC) is a common injury, especially in contact and collision sports.[1–3] Although the long-term consequences of SRC are still debated in the scientific community,[4–7] clinicians treating patients with concussion will inevitably encounter situations where athlete retirement should be considered. This article provides historical context for past retirement recommendations and examines various factors that may influence a retirement decision in the current landscape of SRC.

[a] Concussion Program, Orthopedics Institute, Children's Hospital Colorado, 13123 East 16th Avenue, B060, Aurora, CO 80045, USA; [b] Department of Orthopedics, University of Colorado School of Medicine, Aurora, CO, USA; [c] Department of Pediatrics, University of Colorado School of Medicine, 13123 East 16th Avenue, B060, Aurora, CO 80045, USA; [d] University Health Services, Princeton University, McCosh Health Center, 1st Floor, Washington Road, Princeton, NJ 08544, USA; [e] Rutgers-Robert Wood Johnson Medical School, New Brunswick, NJ, USA
* Corresponding author. Concussion Program, Orthopedics Institute, Children's Hospital Colorado, 13123 East 16th Avenue, B060, Aurora, CO 80045.
E-mail address: Julie.Wilson@childrenscolorado.org
Twitter: @juliewilsonmd (J.C.W.)

Clin Sports Med 40 (2021) 187–197
https://doi.org/10.1016/j.csm.2020.08.008
0278-5919/21/© 2020 Elsevier Inc. All rights reserved.

The question of whether to retire an athlete after SRC has traditionally been based on expert opinion and anecdotal evidence rather than on prospective studies. Adding to this complexity are evolutions in the definition of concussion and return-to-play (RTP) strategies, which have been modified in recent years as concussion research and knowledge have expanded. Much of the emphasis for retirement from sport in early recommendations was based on the number of concussions an athlete had sustained, either in a single season or over a lifetime, whereas more current recommendations highlight the importance of an individualized decision evaluating the nuances of each athlete's case and a shared decision-making model.

Historical Considerations

Many athletes, coaches, and health care providers are likely familiar with the 3-strike rule, a guideline adopted by many athletic organizations that recommends removing an athlete from contact sports for at least the remainder of a season after 3 concussions. Historically, this 3-strike rule was founded on an article published in 1952 by Augustus Thorndike.[8] Based on his experience caring for athletes at Harvard University, Thorndike[8] recommended that athletes retire from contact sports after 3 concussions of moderate severity. An important consideration is that definitions for concussion contemporary with Thorndike's[8] publication involved a loss of consciousness (LOC) or amnesia.[9] Although the definition for concussion has evolved in the decades following this publication,[10] the 3-strike rule has remained a commonly accepted indication for retirement among the general public and even some health care providers, despite its origin as expert opinion.

In the 1980s and 1990s, efforts were made to classify concussions based on severity and thereby assist clinicians in determining RTP timing and athlete retirement after SRC. At least half a dozen grading scales emerged during this period, most of which used the presence of confusion, amnesia, and LOC as factors to determine concussion severity.[11] Although some of these classification systems made recommendations for immediate management of concussions based on grade, most did not address athlete retirement. In 1998, Dr Robert Cantu[12] published guidelines (**Table 1**) for short-term and long-term retirement from contact sports using a concussion grading system he originally created in 1986.

In 2001, the inaugural International Conference on Concussion in Sport was held in Vienna to create consensus recommendations on the definition, diagnosis, and management of SRC.[13] This Concussion in Sport Group (CISG) defined concussion as a "complex pathophysiological process affecting the brain, induced by traumatic biomechanical forces."[13] Although the CISG acknowledged that there were strengths and weaknesses to contemporary concussion grading systems, they ultimately did not endorse a grading or classification system for concussions and instead recommended that health care providers treat each case of SRC individually and use clinical judgment to determine prognosis. Also in 2001, Paul McCrory[14] authored an editorial wherein he emphasized the lack of scientific evidence for the 3-strike guidelines and arbitrary exclusion periods. Echoing the sentiments of the CISG, he called for a more individualized approach to athlete disqualification and retirement based on thorough clinical and neuropsychological evaluation. As such, grading scales, the 3-strike rule, and other categorical retirement tools gave way to a more individualized approach.

Numerous factors may influence a sport retirement decision after SRC, including athlete age, relevant medical history, sport, position, and level of play, as well as severity and duration of concussion symptoms and results of neuroimaging and neuropsychological testing, if performed.[15] This article explores considerations pertaining

Table 1
Cantu[12] grading system for concussion

Grade	Grade 1 (Mild)	Grade 2 (Moderate)	Grade 3 (Severe)
Definition	No LOC and PTA <30 min	LOC <5 min or PTA ≥30 min but <24 h	LOC ≥5 min or PTA ≥24 h
Retirement recommendation	Terminate season after third concussion; may return to sport the following season if asymptomatic	Consider terminating the season after second concussion. Terminate season after third concussion; may return to sport the following season if asymptomatic	Terminate the season after second concussion; may return to sport the following season if asymptomatic. Consider lifetime retirement from contact sports after third concussion

Abbreviation: PTA, posttraumatic amnesia.
  Data from Cantu RC. Return to play guidelines after a head injury. Clin Sports Med. 1998;17(1):45-60.

to athletes' own medical and concussion histories, as well as external factors that influence sport participation. A summary of proposed contraindications to continued sports participation after SRC published in the last decade is given in **Table 2**.[15–20] Importantly, these are still based on expert opinion, and retirement after SRC remains an area for future research, which is likely to evolve with the understanding of SRC and related outcomes.

Concussion History

Despite the trend away from using only an athlete's total number of SRCs as the criterion for retirement, concussion history is typically still considered as 1 factor in the decision. For example, various experts suggest disqualification after multiple concussions in the same athletic season, although the exact number is debated.[15,17,20] Sedney and colleagues[17] recommended that 3 concussions, or 2 concussions with symptom duration longer than 1 week, sustained in a single season should result in disqualification for the remainder of the season. A more conservative approach has generally been advised in younger athletes, with experts advising retirement for the remainder of a sports season after 2 concussions sustained in a single season.[15,20] Presumably, this recommendation is intended to reduce head injury risk for the remainder of the season and allow the athlete to RTP in a future season, likely many months in the future. However, this recommendation does not take into account multi-sport athletes or athletes who participate in sports year-round, as is often encountered in a youth, high school, or collegiate sports setting. In these cases, health care providers may consider timing between injuries (ie, weeks or months) as a factor in return-to-sport decisions, rather than the specific sport season when the injuries occurred.

  Guskiewicz and colleagues[21] provided clinical evidence of a vulnerable period after return to sport in their 2003 study, because more than 90% of within-season repeat concussions in college football athletes occurred within 10 days of the initial injury, at an average interval of 5.6 days (average RTP at 3 days postinjury). Interestingly, a similar study published in 2020 suggests that a symptom-free waiting period (SFWP) before full return to sport, such as the RTP strategy published in the most

Table 2
Summary of proposed contraindications to sport participation following sport-related concussion

Factors Influencing Retirement	Cantu & Register-Mihalik,[16] 2011	Sedney et al,[17] 2011	Concannon et al,[20] 2014	Ellis et al,[15] 2016 (Pediatric SRC)	Laker et al,[19] 2016	Davis-Hayes et al,[18] 2018
Persistent symptoms (>3 mo)/prolonged recovery	Contraindication to returning to sports	Season or career ending	Relative contraindication	Season ending; consider RTP for following season if recovered	—	Relative contraindication
Diminished academic or athletic performance	—	Season or career ending	—	—	—	Relative contraindication
Decreased threshold or interval between injuries	Contraindication to returning to sports	Career ending	Relative contraindication	—	Absolute contraindication	Relative contraindication
Persistent focal neurologic deficits	Contraindication to returning to sports	—	Absolute contraindication	Strongly consider retirement depending on type and severity of deficit	Absolute contraindication	Relative contraindication
Persistent deficit on neuropsychological testing	—	—	Absolute contraindication	Individualized approach in consultation with neuropsychology	Absolute contraindication	Relative contraindication
Traumatic brain injury findings on neuroimaging (ICH, SAH, cerebral edema or contusion)	Contraindication to returning to sports	Career ending	Absolute contraindication	Absolute contraindication	Absolute contraindication	Absolute contraindication
Structural brain abnormalities found incidentally on neuroimaging (eg, arachnoid cyst, symptomatic Chiari malformation, hydrocephalus)	Contraindication to returning to sports	Career ending	Absolute contraindication	Individualized approach in consultation with neurosurgeon	Absolute contraindication	Absolute contraindication

recent CISG consensus statement,[3] can significantly reduce the overall number of repeat concussions in the same season and extend average time between within-season concussions to 56.4 days (average RTP time at 12 days postinjury, with mean SFWP of 6 days).[22] Note that concussion management has also become more conservative over the same time frame, in that athletes are not returned to play on the same day that they have sustained a concussion.[3] Further research is needed to understand optimal timing for RTP after SRC, especially for athletes with multiple injuries in the same season; however, the evidence discussed earlier supports the use of a graduated RTP strategy after recovery from SRC.

Concern has been raised for cumulative effects of multiple concussions, where athletes show an increased risk of subsequent concussion, worse symptom severity, and longer duration of recovery with increasing number of concussions.[23] Limited data in pediatric concussion suggest longer recovery when concussions occur less than 12 months apart, but more favorable recovery profiles when concussions were separated by more than a year.[24] In contrast, other studies have found faster recovery for subsequent concussions compared with initial injury,[25] or no difference in recovery for patients with and without history of previous concussion.[26] A few researchers have evaluated the effect of previous concussion history on preseason testing in an attempt to understand residual effects of concussion. Various studies in both high school and college athletes have found that history of 1 or more prior concussions did not influence preseason symptoms, neurocognitive performance, or postural stability, relative to athletes without history of concussion.[27–29] Notably, minimal evidence exists for athletes with more than 3 concussions, so further research is needed in this area to ascertain the impact of multiple concussions on athlete function and recovery.

Persistent Postconcussion Symptoms

The concept that athletes should not be returned to sport training or competition while still symptomatic from a concussion is broadly accepted in management of SRC.[2,3] For most athletes, recovery is rapid, within a few days to weeks, followed by return to sport after full recovery and completion of a graduated RTP strategy. Challenges arise when determining participation status in the setting of prolonged recovery. Historically, prolonged concussion symptoms have been proposed as criteria for sport retirement,[15,18,20] even once the athlete has fully recovered. Important to consider is that the criteria for prolonged symptoms have changed over the years, and have been inconsistently defined.[30] Although postconcussion syndrome has often been defined as symptoms greater than 3 months in duration following concussion,[31] currently experts favor terminology of persistent postconcussion symptoms (PPCS), which refer to symptoms persisting beyond the typical recovery period (10–14 days in adults, and up to 4 weeks in children).[32]

PPCS have a variety of causes, related to both injury and noninjury factors.[2,20] Pre-existing conditions, such as migraines, sleep disorders, depression, or anxiety, have been associated with higher symptom burden and longer recovery[3,32] and can complicate the determination of when an athlete has recovered from concussion. As such, involvement of a multidisciplinary team is often beneficial to help understand the contributing factors to PPCS and develop a management strategy. Given the complexity of PPCS, some experts propose that prolonged recovery from a single concussion by itself should not be grounds for retirement, as long as the athlete is fully recovered at the time of return to sport.[19] In contrast, a pattern of prolonged recovery occurring with each injury in the setting of multiple concussions or concern for decreased injury threshold may result in a retirement recommendation.[16–20,33]

Therefore, as the understanding of concussion progresses, it is apparent that concussion retirement guidelines must also evolve.

More recently, aerobic exercise has been identified as an effective intervention to reduce symptom severity and duration in the treatment of PPCS.[34,35] However, this can create a challenge for clinicians, because athletes and coaches may interpret initiation of a sub–symptom threshold aerobic exercise training program as the start of a graduated RTP strategy. As such, careful education and consistent follow-up are needed to ensure athletes engage in appropriate exercise type, duration, and intensity during recovery, and do not prematurely return to sport before medical clearance.

Neuroimaging

Neuroimaging is not required for diagnosis of SRC, and is not routinely indicated in the acute evaluation of SRC, given the lack of characteristic brain imaging findings with this injury.[3] However, a computed tomography scan may be used when there is concern for skull fracture or more severe brain injury in the acute setting after a head injury.[36] MRI may be considered in the setting of focal neurologic deficits, protracted recovery, or other atypical presentation of SRC.[15] Of note, many neuroimaging findings that are considered to be indications for retirement are related to more severe brain injury than a concussion, or are structural abnormalities that are unrelated to the injury but may have been found incidentally on neuroimaging studies performed after the injury (see **Table 2**). Athletes with abnormalities on neuroimaging, whether traumatic or not, may benefit from consultation with a neurosurgeon to help weigh the risks of return to sport specific to their individual case.[15]

Neuropsychological Evaluation

Neuropsychological testing may be undertaken for athletes with a history of multiple concussions or prolonged recovery, to help understand the impact on cognitive and psychological functioning. Incomplete recovery after concussion with respect to academic, cognitive, social, or psychological function may be objectively understood through neuropsychological testing and may help identify noninjury factors, such as preexisting conditions (eg, learning disability, attention deficit disorder, mood disorder), or external factors (eg, litigation, psychosocial stressors) that influence recovery.[19,32] Persistent impairment on neuropsychological testing following concussion is considered by many to be grounds for sport retirement.[15,19,20,33]

External Influences

Retirement from sport because of concussion is a complex decision, often influenced by the same people who supported the athletes during their playing careers. In addition to the athlete, family members, peers, coaching staff, and health care providers, including team physicians and athletic trainers, as well as concussion specialists, may contribute to the discussion leading to medical retirement.[18] Family and peer groups may both exert influence on youth and adult athletes alike in a retirement decision. The decisions of teammates or other prominent athletes within a given sport may influence an athlete's retirement decision. Several well-known athletes who sustained multiple concussions have withdrawn from play to prevent further injury; others have electively curtailed successful careers to preserve their health despite not sustaining major injuries. The impact of these highly publicized decisions is not well understood.

Coaching staff can also influence an athlete facing a potentially career-limiting injury. Because part of a coach's success depends on the health and maximal performance of the athletes, a coach may unduly influence athletes to push through injury and tolerate continued or compounding risk if an athlete's overall performance is not impaired by a current injury. A coach's preference regarding retirement may also influence health care providers when making decisions about return to sport.[37]

Amateur athletes pursuing professional athletic careers may make participation decisions based on their potential, both as a future athlete and a person with a life after sport. At times, a collegiate athlete may disagree with a disqualification decision and seek to transfer to a different institution willing to allow continued participation. Presently, a clear way for medical staff to communicate reasons for medical disqualification to other institutions does not always exist, especially in the setting of laws surrounding medical privacy.

Voluntary or athlete-initiated retirement may result in better outcomes for the athlete's psychosocial well-being.[38] The athlete's personal sport-related and nonathletic goals and risk tolerance directly affect this decision.[18] In general, the risk of future harm to an injured athlete is not precisely quantifiable and health care providers can help guide discussion surrounding this topic based on available evidence. The risk tolerance of health care providers varies and can influence their recommendations regarding an athlete's continued participation.[37]

Despite risks inherent in sport participation, the benefits of physical activity are numerous.[39] In addition, sport is often a core component of an athlete's identity, and medical retirement may be accompanied by poor adjustment or mood changes.[18] However, there exists a growing awareness of the public health concerns surrounding concussion and other leading causes of medical retirement.[40] Protection from further injury and minimizing risk of long-term complications remain common goals between self-retiring athletes and those athletes for whom health care providers mandated disqualification from play.[18] There may be a role for programs that help athletes adapt to life outside of sports, emphasize new pursuits, and provide resources for coping, and opportunities for connection and social support.[41] These efforts, along with follow-up care of medically retired athletes, are particularly important to protect and promote the health and well-being of the athletes.

Professional Athletes

The decision to retire from sport after SRC may be slightly different for professional athletes given the employment and career implications. Athletes may not want to disclose their histories if they think it will decrease their ability to be drafted and/or remain on the roster. Professional athletes whose financial stability depends on continued play may have an incentive to participate for as long as possible despite health risks. For example, under-reporting of concussions of National Football League players has been prevalent in the past.[42] Health care providers taking care of professional athletes should provide athletes with the information that they have regarding their injuries, and support the athlete's decision making related to risks and benefits of continued participation, using a shared decision-making model.[43]

Pediatric Athletes

Given the young age at which many athletes begin sports participation, as well as recent trends of increasing year-round sport participation and sport specialization in youth sports,[44] it is common for providers to encounter young athletes who have sustained multiple concussions. Consensus guidelines advise a more conservative approach for RTP in children and adolescents[3]; however, minimal evidence is available to guide decisions in this population. Similar to their adult counterparts, pediatric athletes should be managed on an individualized basis, taking into account the various factors mentioned earlier.[15] Other factors that may be relevant to consider in pediatric athletes include expected physical and cognitive growth and development,

---

Box 1
Questions to guide sport retirement decision making after sport-related concussion

Is there a reduced threshold for injury?	Concussions occurring closer together in time?[18,33]
	Concussion occurring with less force than would be expected to cause the injury?[16,18–20,33]
	Injuries becoming more severe/recovery taking longer with each subsequent injury?[16,18–20,33]
Has the athlete fully recovered?	Persistent symptoms/incomplete recovery?[16,18,20,33]
	Persistent neurologic deficit?[15,17–20]
	Persistent decline in neuropsychological function (academic/cognitive, social/emotional)?[15,17–20,33]
Are there abnormal findings on neuroimaging?	Evidence of previous traumatic injury?[15–20]
	Structural abnormalities that increase the risk of adverse events from a future head injury?[15–20]
What are the proposed risks and benefits of continued sports participation?	Anticipated future head injury risk in athlete's chosen sport?[18,19]
	Impact of future injuries to athlete's academic, work, social, or family function?[18,19]
	Athlete identity or aspirations?[18–20]
	Financial implications?[17,18,20]
	Influence of family, peers, and coaches?[17,37]

Data from Refs.[15–20,33,37]

---

competitive level, sport specialization, year-round participation, anticipated length of future risk exposure (ie, remaining competitive career), and the potential risk of head injury in other settings, including physical education class, recreational activities (riding a bicycle, jumping on a trampoline), as well as nontraditional sports such as skiing and snowboarding, skateboarding, and motocross. In some cases, young athletes may consider changing to a less competitive league, decreasing the amount of time spent in sport participation, or switching to a lower-risk position in their sport, as a means of modifying future head injury risk.[19]

Current recommendations indicate that there is no evidence to support a total number of concussions (lifetime or otherwise) that necessitates sport retirement in pediatric athletes.[15,45] However, health care providers should acknowledge the lack of evidence and assist the athletes and their parents in weighing the potential risks and benefits of continued sports participation in a shared decision-making model, with experts advocating that the future health of the patient be the major focus of the decision.[15,45] An important consideration for all athletes, but especially for youth athletes, is the potential negative consequences of sport retirement on regular physical activity. Given the increasing trend of sedentary behavior and obesity, and their associated health risks,[39] participating in regular physical activity in childhood and adolescence should be encouraged. Health care providers should help young athletes identify other athletic or physical activity pursuits in the event of contact/collision sport retirement. In addition, because previous concussion has been associated with emergence of mental health concerns,[46,47] for reasons that are not fully understood, the psychological health of young athletes should be monitored, especially in the setting of sport retirement.[19]

SUMMARY

There is insufficient evidence-based research that guides when to retire an athlete after SRC. The idea that a certain number of SRCs should determine retirement has not been validated. The authors recommend that the health care provider reviews with the athlete a series of questions that can help guide the retirement discussion (**Box 1**). These questions include (1) whether there is a reduced threshold for injury,[16–20,33] (2) whether there are persistent injury effects,[15–20,33] (3) whether there are abnormal findings on neuroimaging[15–20] (which may be unrelated to concussion), and (4) the potential risks and benefits of continued participation.[17–19,37] In reviewing these questions, the health care provider can provide information to the athlete, the athlete can consider the options, and, together, a shared decision can be made about retirement from sport.

DISCLOSURE

Dr J.C. Wilson, Dr T. Patsimas, and Dr K. Cohen have nothing to disclose. Dr M. Putukian reports that she is the Chief Medical Officer, Major League Soccer; Committee Member, National Football League, Head, Neck & Spine Committee; Principal Investigator, Princeton University site, NCAA & DoD Grand Alliance CARE study; Principal Investigator, Princeton University, Ivy League–Big Ten Concussion study.

REFERENCES

1. Bryan MA, Rowhani-Rahbar A, Comstock RD, et al. Sports- and Recreation-Related Concussions in US Youth. Pediatrics 2016;138(1). https://doi.org/10.1542/peds.2015-4635.
2. Harmon KG, Clugston JR, Dec K, et al. American Medical Society for Sports Medicine position statement on concussion in sport. Br J Sports Med 2019;53(4):213–25.
3. McCrory P, Meeuwisse W, Dvorak J, et al. Consensus statement on concussion in sport-the 5(th) international conference on concussion in sport held in Berlin, October 2016. Br J Sports Med 2017;51(11):838–47.
4. Stewart W, Allinson K, Al-Sarraj S, et al. Primum non nocere: a call for balance when reporting on CTE. Lancet Neurol 2019;18(3):231–3.
5. Manley G, Gardner AJ, Schneider KJ, et al. A systematic review of potential long-term effects of sport-related concussion. Br J Sports Med 2017;51(12):969–77.
6. Moore RD, Kay JJ, Ellemberg D. The long-term outcomes of sport-related concussion in pediatric populations. Int J Psychophysiol 2018;132(Pt A):14–24.
7. Yumul JN, McKinlay A. Do Multiple Concussions Lead to Cumulative Cognitive Deficits? A Literature Review. PM R 2016;8(11):1097–103.
8. Thorndike A. Serious recurrent injuries of athletes; contraindications to further competitive participation. N Engl J Med 1952;247(15):554–6.
9. Cantu RC. History of Concussion Including Contributions of 1940s Boston City Hospital Researchers. Semin Pediatr Neurol 2019;30:2–8.
10. Gurdjian ES, Volis HC. Congress of Neurological Surgeons Committee on head injury nomenclature: glossary of head injury. Clin Neurosurg 1966;12:386–94.
11. Cantu RC. Posttraumatic Retrograde and Anterograde Amnesia: Pathophysiology and Implications in Grading and Safe Return to Play. J Athl Train 2001;36(3):244–8.
12. Cantu RC. Return to play guidelines after a head injury. Clin Sports Med 1998;17(1):45–60.
13. Aubry M, Cantu R, Dvorak J, et al. Summary and agreement statement of the First International Conference on Concussion in Sport, Vienna 2001. Recommendations for the improvement of safety and health of athletes who may suffer concussive injuries. Br J Sports Med 2002;36(1):6–10.

14. McCrory P. When to retire after concussion? Br J Sports Med 2001;35(6):380–2.
15. Ellis MJ, McDonald PJ, Cordingley D, et al. Retirement-from-sport considerations following pediatric sports-related concussion: case illustrations and institutional approach. Neurosurg Focus 2016;40(4):E8.
16. Cantu RC, Register-Mihalik JK. Considerations for return-to-play and retirement decisions after concussion. PM R 2011;3(10 Suppl 2):S440–4.
17. Sedney CL, Orphanos J, Bailes JE. When to consider retiring an athlete after sports-related concussion. Clin Sports Med 2011;30(1):189–200, xi.
18. Davis-Hayes C, Baker DR, Bottiglieri TS, et al. Medical retirement from sport after concussions: A practical guide for a difficult discussion. Neurol Clin Pract 2018; 8(1):40–7.
19. Laker SR, Meron A, Greher MR, et al. Retirement and Activity Restrictions Following Concussion. Phys Med Rehabil Clin N Am 2016;27(2):487–501.
20. Concannon LG, Kaufman MS, Herring SA. The million dollar question: When should an athlete retire after concussion? Curr Sports Med Rep 2014;13(6): 365–9.
21. Guskiewicz KM, McCrea M, Marshall SW, et al. Cumulative effects associated with recurrent concussion in collegiate football players: the NCAA Concussion Study. JAMA 2003;290(19):2549–55.
22. McCrea M, Broglio S, McAllister T, et al. Return to play and risk of repeat concussion in collegiate football players: comparative analysis from the NCAA Concussion Study (1999-2001) and CARE Consortium (2014-2017). Br J Sports Med 2020;54(2):102–9.
23. Moser RS, Iverson GL, Echemendia RJ, et al. Neuropsychological evaluation in the diagnosis and management of sports-related concussion. Arch Clin Neuropsychol 2007;22(8):909–16.
24. Eisenberg MA, Andrea J, Meehan W, et al. Time interval between concussions and symptom duration. Pediatrics 2013;132(1):8–17.
25. Taubman B, McHugh J, Rosen F, et al. Repeat Concussion and Recovery Time in a Primary Care Pediatric Office. J Child Neurol 2016;31(14):1607–10.
26. Ellis M, Krisko C, Selci E, et al. Effect of concussion history on symptom burden and recovery following pediatric sports-related concussion. J Neurosurg Pediatr 2018;21(4):401–8.
27. Rosenblum D, Walton SR, Erdman NK, et al. If Not Now, When? An Absence of Neurocognitive and Postural Stability Deficits in Collegiate Athletes with One or More Concussions. J Neurotrauma 2020. https://doi.org/10.1089/neu.2019.6813.
28. Iverson GL, Brooks BL, Lovell MR, et al. No cumulative effects for one or two previous concussions. Br J Sports Med 2006;40(1):72–5.
29. Alsalaheen B, Stockdale K, Pechumer D, et al. Cumulative Effects of Concussion History on Baseline Computerized Neurocognitive Test Scores: Systematic Review and Meta-analysis. Sports Health 2017;9(4):324–32.
30. Tator CH, Davis HS, Dufort PA, et al. Postconcussion syndrome: demographics and predictors in 221 patients. J Neurosurg 2016;125(5):1206–16.
31. American Psychiatric Association. Diagnostic and statistical manual of mental disorders. 4th edition. Washington, DC: American Psychiatric Association; 1994.
32. Makdissi M, Schneider KJ, Feddermann-Demont N, et al. Approach to investigation and treatment of persistent symptoms following sport-related concussion: a systematic review. Br J Sports Med 2017;51(12):958–68.
33. Kirkwood MW, Randolph C, McCrea M, et al. Sport-Related Concussion. In: Kirkwood MW, Yeates KO, editors. Mild traumatic brain injury in children and

adolescents: from basic science to clinical management. New York: The Guilford Press; 2012. p. 341–60.

34. Leddy JJ, Cox JL, Baker JG, et al. Exercise treatment for postconcussion syndrome: a pilot study of changes in functional magnetic resonance imaging activation, physiology, and symptoms. J Head Trauma Rehabil 2013;28(4):241–9.

35. Leddy JJ, Kozlowski K, Donnelly JP, et al. A preliminary study of subsymptom threshold exercise training for refractory post-concussion syndrome. Clin J Sport Med 2010;20(1):21–7.

36. Kuppermann N, Holmes JF, Dayan PS, et al. Identification of children at very low risk of clinically-important brain injuries after head trauma: a prospective cohort study. Lancet 2009;374(9696):1160–70.

37. Kroshus E, Baugh CM, Meehan WP 3rd, et al. Personal subjectivity in clinician discussion about retirement from sport post-concussion. Soc Sci Med 2018; 218:37–44.

38. Stambulova N, Alfermann D, Statler T, et al. ISSP position stand: career development and transitions of athletes. Int J Sport Exerc Psychol 2009;7:395–412.

39. US Department of Health and Human Services. Physical activity guidelines for Americans. Washington, DC: US Department of Health and Human Services; 2018. Available at https://health.gov/sites/default/files/2019-09/Physical_Activity_Guidelines_2nd_edition.pdf.

40. Mannix R, Meehan WP 3rd, Pascual-Leone A. Sports-related concussions - media, science and policy. Nat Rev Neurol 2016;12(8):486–90.

41. Sidelined UA. Available at: https://www.sidelinedusa.org/. Accessed February 22, 2020.

42. Kerr ZY, Register-Mihalik JK, Kay MC, et al. Concussion Nondisclosure During Professional Career Among a Cohort of Former National Football League Athletes. Am J Sports Med 2018;46(1):22–9.

43. Baggish AL, Ackerman MJ, Putukian M, et al. Shared Decision Making for Athletes with Cardiovascular Disease: Practical Considerations. Curr Sports Med Rep 2019;18(3):76–81.

44. LaPrade RF, Agel J, Baker J, et al. AOSSM Early Sport Specialization Consensus Statement. Orthop J Sports Med 2016;4(4). 2325967116644241.

45. Rivara FP, Tennyson R, Mills B, et al. Consensus Statement on Sports-Related Concussions in Youth Sports Using a Modified Delphi Approach. JAMA Pediatr 2019. https://doi.org/10.1001/jamapediatrics.2019.4006.

46. Ellis MJ, Ritchie LJ, Koltek M, et al. Psychiatric outcomes after pediatric sports-related concussion. J Neurosurg Pediatr 2015;16(6):709–18.

47. Rice SM, Parker AG, Rosenbaum S, et al. Sport-Related Concussion and Mental Health Outcomes in Elite Athletes: A Systematic Review. Sports Med 2018;48(2): 447–65.

Future Directions in Sports-Related Concussion Management

Hamish Kerr, MD, MSc, CAQSM[a],*, Bjørn Bakken, MD[b],
Gregory House, MD[c]

KEYWORDS

- Biomarkers • Imaging • Video review • Accelerometers • Rule changes
- Injury epidemiology

KEY POINTS

- Despite continued efforts, there is no biomarker or imaging modality that can be used clinically to diagnose a sports-related concussion.
- Genetic testing is not a clinically useful tool for evaluation of sports-related concussion risk.
- Video review of mechanism of injury during elite sports performance has advantages for the team physician evaluating sports-related concussion on the sideline.
- Measurement of head acceleration shows promise, but clinical usefulness has yet to be established.
- Injury epidemiology should remain the backbone of changes in regulation and law enforcement, so that effects of interventions can be studied, and decisions can be based on data rather than expert opinion.

INTRODUCTION

Sports-related concussion (SRC) is an evolving field, and keeping abreast of the most recent literature and investigative findings remains a continual challenge. Some of the world's sports governing bodies have embraced this challenge by helping to fund an international consensus every 4 years, entailing experts reviewing the previous 4 years of research and meeting in person before disseminating the results. The most recent meeting took place in Berlin in 2016, and the next event is scheduled for 2021 in Paris.

[a] Sports Medicine, Department of Medicine, Albany Medical College, 1019 New Loudon Road, Cohoes, NY 12047, USA; [b] Department of Medicine, Albany Medical Center, 1019 New Loudon Road, Cohoes, NY 12047, USA; [c] Department of Family and Community Medicine, Albany Medical Center, 391 Myrtle Avenue, Albany, NY 12208, USA
* Corresponding author.
E-mail address: kerrh@amc.edu

Clin Sports Med 40 (2021) 199–211
https://doi.org/10.1016/j.csm.2020.08.009
0278-5919/21/© 2020 Elsevier Inc. All rights reserved.

Future directions of SRC can perhaps be best gauged from the discussion at each of these consensus meetings. Some topics have been discussed at almost every meeting and remain an area for optimism, despite not quite being ready for "prime time." Investigations exploring the use of imaging and biomarkers for SRC would fall into such categories and will be covered in this article. Alternative strategies ready for immediate implementation, such as the use of video review, change in regulation to allow proper field side evaluation, and law changes based on injury epidemiology and biomechanics are good examples.

IMAGING IN SPORTS-RELATED CONCUSSION

One of the major challenges of SRC management in current clinical practice is the lack of significant structural changes associated with concussion that can be identified with standard neuroimaging modalities. A defining feature of SRC highlighted at the 2016 Berlin Consensus underscores this point, namely that concussion "may result in neuropathological changes, but the acute clinical signs and symptoms largely reflect a functional disturbance rather than a structural injury and, as such, no abnormality is seen on standard structural neuroimaging studies."[1] To this end, there has been a general push to eschew obtaining unwarranted computed tomography images of the brain in closed head injuries in the emergency department per the Pediatric Emergency Care Applied Research Network.[2] There are, however, several more advanced imaging modalities currently available that have a greater sensitivity for subtle structural and functional brain changes associated with sport related concussion. These modalities have become the source of a great deal of recent clinical research. The possibility of using neuroimaging for the diagnosis and management of concussion has therefore gained increasing interest among clinicians in recent years, although debate remains regarding the validity of these modalities and the feasibility of using these tools in everyday practice.

Arguably, the 2 imaging modalities of greatest interest currently are functional MRI (fMRI) and diffusion-weighted MRI (also known as diffusion tensor imaging [DTI]). The fMRI has the ability to measure brain activity by detecting differences in cerebral blood flow, because it is known that blood flow increases to parts of the brain that are in use. This phenomenon is of particular interest in what is known as the default mode network, which is a network of interacting brain regions that demonstrates increased activity in healthy controls during rest and deactivation during attention demanding tasks. Several studies have demonstrated reduced network connectivity among key regions of the default mode network in concussed patients immediately following concussion.[3–7] Resting-state fMRI (rs-fMRI) is a further subset of fMRI that does not rely on task-based designs when obtaining imaging and has shown alterations in local connectivity acutely following SRC. Resolution of these imaging abnormalities seems to correlate with clinical recovery from SRC.[5,8,9] In addition, there seems to be a negative association between default mode network connectivity and the number of concussions an individual sustains.[3,10] One could argue that this factor makes rs-fMRI the more clinically applicable imaging modality, because it has the potential to predict patient recovery or development of persistent post-traumatic symptoms after an SRC.[11–13] Nevertheless, this modality remains challenging to apply to the clinical setting, because rs-fMRI studies generally reflect population-based functional changes as opposed to patient-specific alterations. The heterogenic nature of post-concussive symptoms also makes interpreting rs-fMRI a challenge, because there can be significant overlap between other psychological disorders including depression and post-traumatic stress disorder.[14]

DTI is another application of MRI that uses MRI sequences coupled with software that can estimate the directional diffusion patterns of water to generate contrast in MR images. This process provides an indirect pathway for measuring white matter axonal and myelin microstructure.[15] White matter changes have been observed in portions of the frontal, temporal, and parietal lobes of the brain in the initial postconcussion phase[16–20] with additional evidence to suggest that these white matter changes can persist beyond the medical clearance required for a return-to-play protocol, even up to 1 year after an injury.[21,22] The strength of DTI, however, may preferentially lie with its ability to detect chronic white matter changes associated with chronically concussed patients with persistent postconcussion symptoms.[23] There is a sizable body of evidence that demonstrates white matter changes in younger patients, those with multiple prior traumatic brain injuries, and those with protracted post-traumatic symptoms.[18,24–26] It is important to note, however, that there has also been recent evidence to suggest that postconcussion symptom reporting was not associated with white matter integrity in the subacute to chronic phase of recovery after a concussion.[27] This factor calls into question the validity of using DTI for diagnosis of concussion. A more practical challenge for the clinical application of DTI is the fact that this is a very high-cost modality.[28] Coupled with the fact that, like fMRI studies, the majority of DTI studies are reflective of population-based structural changes (given the high variability of DTI findings on an individual level),[29,30] DTI remains a research tool and does not seem to be a clinically relevant imaging modality for the diagnosis of concussion at the present time. According to the American Medical Society for Sports Medicine position statement, additional research will be required to determine the clinical usefulness of advanced neuroimaging in the setting of SRC.[31]

BIOMARKERS IN SPORTS-RELATED CONCUSSION

An exciting and evolving area of research in SRC is the role of fluid biomarkers in its diagnosis and prognosis. Multiple definitions of the term "biomarker" exist, including this one from the National Institutes of Health Biomarkers Definitions Working Group. A biomarker is "a characteristic that is, objectively measured and evaluated as an indicator of normal biological processes, pathogenic processes, or pharmacologic responses to a therapeutic intervention."[32] SRC is a disease state with a vast spectrum of presenting signs and symptoms and long-term outcomes that have previously been outlined in detail. The potential exists for devastating consequences as a result of premature return to play. There would be great usefulness, then in identifying biomarkers that can accurately and reliably diagnose and prognosticate SRC.

Proposed mechanisms exist in which neuronal axonal injury occurs releasing various proteins into the interstitial space within the central nervous system and subsequently the cerebrospinal fluid (CSF). A reasonable first place to attempt to obtain a sample, then, is the CSF via a lumbar puncture. However, because obtaining a lumbar puncture comes with a potential for injury and adverse events including, but not limited to infection, hematoma and prolonged CSF leak requiring further procedures, alternate sources of tissue are prudent. Because the normally highly selective blood–brain barrier seems to become more permeable during the SRC disease state, there are proteins released during axonal injury that cross into the peripheral circulation. A second proposed mechanism of central nervous system injury markers being present in the periphery is via the glymphatic system. This mechanism, reported by Plog and colleagues[33] and Brinker and colleagues[34] and summarized by Anto-Ocrah and colleagues,[35] describes proteins from axonal injury entering the brain's lymphatic system from the interstitial space, which then empties in to the peripheral circulation. An important consideration is that just as the peripheral lymphatic system may become occluded, so may the glymphatic system especially after an injury.[35]

A peripheral venous blood sample is a reasonable method of obtaining tissue for sampling for the purposes of SRC biomarker research. A consideration in the use of peripheral blood are the many potential confounding factors. The presence of normally circulating proteins, including albumin, immunoglobulins, and proteases can interfere with accurate detection, as can hepatic and renal clearance of biomarkers.[36] Furthermore, to truly realize the benefit of sideline evaluation, Anto-Ocrah and colleagues[35] propose that technology must be in place for a point-of-care analysis using capillary blood from a finger stick sample. This process would negate the necessity of having a phlebotomist on site for each practice, game, or other team activity. Until this is developed and perfected, however, a peripheral venous blood sample will remain the research standard.

According to a systematic review by McCrea and colleagues[37] published in 2017, there have been significant alterations found in 10 blood biomarkers with a correlation to SRC. These included α-amino-3-hydroxy-5-methyl-4-isoxazolepropionic acid receptor peptide, S100 calcium-binding protein B (s100B), total tau, marinobufagenin, plasma soluble cellular prion protein, glial fibrillary acidic protein, neuron-specific enolase, calpain-derived αII-spectrin N-terminal fragment, tau-C79, and metabolomics profiling.[37] Metabolomics, as defined by Klassen and colleagues,[38] is a method of identifying and comparing a set of specific metabolites found in biologic samples under both normal and altered states. In their review, they did identify moderate to high risk of bias, mostly owing to study design translating to poor generalizability.[37]

In another systematic review performed by O'Connell and colleagues,[39] 5 blood biomarkers were investigated from a total of 26 papers that were ultimately included in their review. In the words of the authors, the findings must be interpreted with caution because they identified limitations in the studies included.[39] Like other studies in this growing pool of literature, sample size among other factors, was partly responsible for this.

S100B has been identified as having the most promising data for use as a biomarker of SRC. S100B is a calcium-binding protein found mainly in astroglia and Schwann cells that help to regulate intracellular calcium concentration. It may also be found peripherally in adipocytes, melanocytes, bone, and injured muscle tissue.[35] Its concentration in both the CSF and serum increases after injury, but also after physical activity.[39,40] Tau protein and neuron-specific aldolase have been highly sought after targets of investigation. Tau protein is found both in the central nervous system and systemically, and neuron-specific aldolase can be found in smooth muscle and adipose tissue.[39] Again, this raises a challenge to prove that the elevated serum marker has a neuronal etiology.

Siman and colleagues[41] compared serum levels of calpain-derived αII-spectrin N-terminal fragment after concussion to preseason levels and found a significant increase after concussion. There did not seem to be an increase in levels after exertion alone without injury.[41] This finding lends itself to the possibility of αII-spectrin N-terminal fragment being used to confirm the diagnosis of SRC with greater specificity after a positive screening test with another biomarker such as S100B, which is perhaps not as specific to neuronal tissue, but more sensitive.[35]

There are multiple fluid biomarkers that are being used in the setting of trauma to the brain. In Europe, S100B has been used clinically. In the United States, the Food and Drug Administration has approved a 2-protein brain trauma indicator-glial fibrillary acidic protein and ubiquitin carboxy-terminal hydrolase L1. Both of these biomarkers have been shown to decrease frequency of computed tomography scan of the head in the emergency department.[31]

Much of the current literature is limited in its application to a broad population of athletes. Small sample sizes, sport-specific studies, or those limited to a particular level of competition or gender have predominated. The time to sampling is also a factor that makes generalizability challenging. Many of the current studies obtain samples no less than 1 hour after injury. To create an applicable diagnostic test, it would ideally be conducted immediately at the point of care. Although researchers are working diligently, fluid biomarkers do not yet have a practical role in the diagnosis or management of SRC.[31]

For athletes at all levels of competition, an accurate diagnosis and prognosis are important. With the growing foundation of knowledge regarding the lag between clinical and physiologic recovery from SRC, they become even more critical. Having objective data in the form of a fluid biomarker that can not only aid the clinical presentation in forming an accurate diagnosis, but to be able to trend that objective data along with the clinical course to inform physiologic recovery would be invaluable. It would help to ensure safe return to play for our youth and elite athletes and all levels in between.

GENETIC TESTING

Genetic testing is an important research tool but requires further validation to determine clinical usefulness in evaluation of SRC.[42] There is interest in genetics' influence on the prediction of the risk the of initial injury, prolonged recovery, and long-term neurologic health problems associated with traumatic brain injury, and repetitive head impact exposure in athletes. However, there is currently no scientific support for genetic testing in the evaluation and management of athletes with SRC, and additional research is needed to determine how genetic factors influence risk of injury and recovery after SRC.[37]

VIDEO REVIEW

It has been established that SRC can be difficult to diagnose owing to the often subtle presentation, lack of uniformity, and vague symptoms. This difficulty can be magnified in professional sports,[43] when medical staff are often expected to recognize athletes that may have sustained an injury and implement immediate management under the scrutiny of the watching public and the sport's governing body. Of course, it can be even more easily accomplished if you have multiple camera views, the option of watching the event repeatedly, and an opportunity to slow the movements. The Fifth International Concussion in Sport Group consensus incorporated the use of video review in recommendations for elite sport that may be being broadcast live, often allowing sideline physicians this opportunity.[42] World Rugby has included video review in the sports head injury assessment of potential concussion in elite-level matches for several years. A number of authors have suggested that video analysis can supplement the sideline evaluation of a rugby player and has the potential to decrease the incidence of missing head injuries.[44–46] Video review studies have also been conducted in other contact/collision sports such as rugby league,[47–50] ice hockey,[51] and Australian rules football.[52,53]

Gardner and colleagues[44] reviewed head impact events in more than 70 Australian rugby league matches. When there was no video review available, an unnoticed head impact events occurred once every 2 matches. With video review, this was reduced to an unnoticed head impact events every 4 matches, although the interobserver variability was weak (κ = 0.49; 95% confidence interval, 0.38–0.59). Gardner and associates[50] cautioned that further investigations are warranted to determine the reliability of identifying the objective signs of concussion when using video review.

Patricios and colleagues[43] identified 3 important components of video review:

1. Identification: video can help the clinician to identify suspicious events and evaluate the athlete's response immediately after the event.
2. Confirmation: video can support the confirmation of mandatory versus discretionary signs of SRC.
3. Management: video can support return to sport decisions if the off-field concussion screening is normal.

ACCELEROMETERS AND HEAD IMPACT SYSTEMS

It has long been recognized that the biomechanical characteristic of head trauma closest associated with brain injury is the acceleration of the brain tissue.[54–56] This kinetic variable has a close relationship with force of impact and the masses of the objects colliding (F = ma). Acceleration can be measured and is described as linear acceleration in a straight direction (meters/s/s) or angular/rotational acceleration (radians/s/s), which occurs around an axis of rotation.[57,58] Rotational acceleration has been more closely associated with traumatic brain injury.

Athletes participating in helmeted contact sports have been investigated using techniques to try and establish and quantify the acceleration inside the helmet during collisions. Harmon and colleagues[59] published a statement on helmeted and nonhelmeted impact monitors indicating that current impact sensor systems may not consistently record head impacts or forces transmitted to the brain. No device measuring angular acceleration can yet be used to diagnose concussion, and given the variability in threshold causing concussions, this modality may remain unlikely in the future.[60,61] Current impact measures are poor predictors of SRC,[62] and it may take better quantification of the number, location, density, and individual thresholds of head impacts to improve this process.

RULE CHANGES

Beaudouin and colleagues[63] claim a 29% lower incidence (incident rate ratio, 0.71; 95% confidence interval, 0.57–0.86; P = .002) in head injuries in male professional soccer since FIFA implemented a rule change in 2006 to consider that an intentional elbow–head contact result in a red card for the offending player (**Fig. 1**).

FIFA has not changed rules regarding heading in soccer; however, US Soccer implemented a regulation for youth soccer in 2016 banning heading the ball for players less than 10 years of age.[52] This rule is in place despite the fact that head injuries are very rarely reported in youth soccer.[64] O'Kane and coworkers[65] reported that 30% of concussions in female middle school soccer were related to heading. It would therefore perhaps have made more sense to institute regulation to instruct players to learn to head the ball properly, rather than banning them from doing so altogether until the age when they are actually at risk. In fact, stricter and more widespread application of the successful rule change in male professional soccer to include youth soccer and women's soccer in particular might have been a more sensible action (**Fig. 2**).

In contrast, ice hockey has based regulation change on studying the sports injury epidemiology and made decisions based on the evidence. Checking was banned for players less than 14 years of age based on epidemiologic studies conducted in Canada, which suggest that the incidence of SRC was reduced once checking was

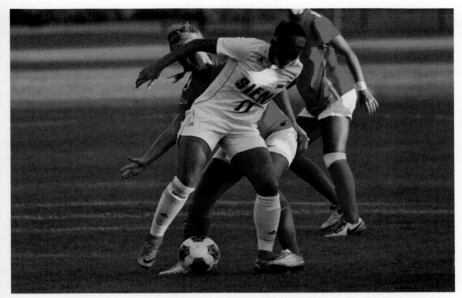

Fig. 1. Intentional use of the elbow in soccer to harm an opponent in collegiate women's soccer. (*Courtesy of* Stephen Ridler, Brunswick, New York, NY.)

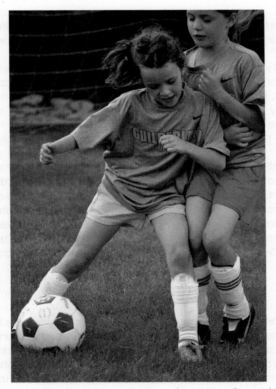

Fig. 2. Intentional use of the elbow in youth soccer. (*Courtesy of* Hamish Kerr, Albany, NY.)

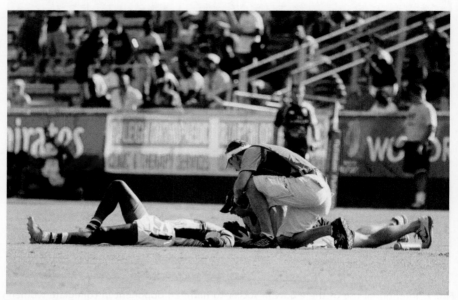

Fig. 3. On-field assessment of concussion in rugby. (*Courtesy of* USA Rugby, Lafayette, Colorado, CO.)

banned in younger age groups, and that the subsequent increase in injury once checking was introduced (≥14 years) was less than would otherwise have been anticipated.[53,66,67]

It is hoped that injury epidemiology will lay the foundation for future law changes and interventions. For example, the lacrosse world continues to contemplate girls' lacrosse helmets, but the evidence that helmets decrease SRC risk is lacking.[68] There are currently very few head impacts in girls high school lacrosse[69] and wearing helmets might actually increase the incidence of SRC if wearing a helmet results in more aggressive play from girls who currently wear a facemask only to protect from eye injuries.[70]

World Rugby altered regulations to develop a 10-min window for concussion evaluation, initially known as Pitch Side Concussion Assessment, then subsequently head injury assessment.[45] This regulation change allowed a player to be substituted while the concussion assessment was conducted and has been moderately successful in decreasing the incidence of players who sustain a concussion but was not recognized and being allowed to continue playing.[43,46,71] This practice is anticipated to be increased to a 15-minute evaluation window. Other sports might consider following suit (**Fig. 3**).

SUMMARY

At some time in the future, there may be an objective test to diagnose SRC on the sideline. This test does not currently exist, and clinical history and examination remain the only means to make the diagnosis. We can anticipate continued research eventually providing either a biomarker or an imaging modality that can be facilitated in the emergency department and may be able to provide concrete evidence that a concussive injury has been sustained. There is optimism that quantification of athletes' head acceleration may help with risk stratification, and there are continued efforts to scrutinize such data, so we know what the ultimate clinical manifestations are.

Until these efforts yield better diagnostic options, there are still many strategies that can help to prevent SRC. Including video review in the multimodal on field assessment can be helpful and permitting medical staff enough time to accomplish an evaluation seems to be sensible and warranted across all contact sports. Decreasing aggressive play, and rule enforcement to punish athletes whose actions have an intent to harm an opponent rather than just be assertive, have gained traction owing to injury epidemiology providing good evidence that such regulation is effective in decreasing the risk of SRC.

CLINICS CARE POINTS

- Do use a multimodal evaluation tool such as SCAT5 to diagnose SRC, but also consider video review as an adjunct if available.
- Accelerometer data have yet to become an established useful clinical tool.
- S-100B may be a useful biomarker for brain injury, and trials in Europe may suggest its use can help to minimize the use of computed tomography scans of the head in emergency department settings.

DISCLOSURE

The authors have nothing to disclose.

REFERENCES

1. Broglio SP, McCrea M, McAllister T, et al. A national study on the effects of concussion in collegiate athletes and US military service academy members: the NCAA-DoD Concussion Assessment, Research and Education (CARE) consortium structure and methods. Sports Med 2017;47(7):1437–51.
2. Puffenbarger MS, Ahmad FA, Argent M, et al. Reduction of Computed Tomography Use for Pediatric Closed Head Injury Evaluation at a Nonpediatric Community Emergency Department. Acad Emerg Med 2019;26(7):784–95.
3. Borich M, Babul AN, Yuan PH, et al. Alterations in resting-state brain networks in concussed adolescent athletes. J Neurotrauma 2015;32(4):265–71.
4. Zhou Y, Milham MP, Lui YW, et al. Default-mode network disruption in mild traumatic brain injury. Radiology 2012;265(3):882–92.
5. Zhu DC, Covassin T, Nogle S, et al. A potential biomarker in sports-related concussion: brain functional connectivity alteration of the default-mode network measured with longitudinal resting-state fMRI over thirty days. J Neurotrauma 2015;32(5):327–41.
6. Iraji A, Benson RR, Welch RD, et al. Resting state functional connectivity in mild traumatic brain injury at the acute stage: independent component and seed-based analyses. J Neurotrauma 2015;32(14):1031–45.
7. Johnson B, Zhang K, Gay M, et al. Alteration of brain default network in subacute phase of injury in concussed individuals: resting-state fMRI study. Neuroimage 2012;59(1):511–8.
8. Meier TB, Giraldo-Chica M, Espana LY, et al. Resting-state fMRI metrics in acute sport-related concussion and their association with clinical recovery: a study from the NCAA-DOD CARE Consortium. J Neurotrauma 2019;37(1):152–62.
9. Han K, Mac Donald CL, Johnson AM, et al. Disrupted modular organization of resting-state cortical functional connectivity in U.S. military personnel following

concussive 'mild' blast-related traumatic brain injury. Neuroimage 2014;84: 76–96.

10. Mayer AR, Mannell MV, Ling J, et al. Functional connectivity in mild traumatic brain injury. Hum Brain Mapp 2011;32(11):1825–35.

11. Militana AR, Donahue MJ, Sills AK, et al. Alterations in default-mode network connectivity may be influenced by cerebrovascular changes within 1 week of sports related concussion in college varsity athletes: a pilot study. Brain Imaging Behav 2016;10(2):559–68.

12. Chen JK, Johnston KM, Collie A, et al. A validation of the post concussion symptom scale in the assessment of complex concussion using cognitive testing and functional MRI. J Neurol Neurosurg Psychiatry 2007;78(11):1231–8.

13. Lovell MR, Pardini JE, Welling J, et al. Functional brain abnormalities are related to clinical recovery and time to return-to-play in athletes. Neurosurgery 2007; 61(2):352–9 [discussion: 359–60].

14. Parker RS. Recommendations for the revision of DSM-IV diagnostic categories for co-morbid posttraumatic stress disorder and traumatic brain injury. NeuroRehabilitation 2002;17(2):131–43.

15. Chenevert TL, Brunberg JA, Pipe JG. Anisotropic diffusion in human white matter: demonstration with MR techniques in vivo. Radiology 1990;177(2):401–5.

16. Lange RT, Panenka WJ, Shewchuk JR, et al. Diffusion tensor imaging findings and postconcussion symptom reporting six weeks following mild traumatic brain injury. Arch Clin Neuropsychol 2015;30(1):7–25.

17. Ling JM, Pena A, Yeo RA, et al. Biomarkers of increased diffusion anisotropy in semi-acute mild traumatic brain injury: a longitudinal perspective. Brain 2012; 135(Pt 4):1281–92.

18. Mayer AR, Ling JM, Yang Z, et al. Diffusion abnormalities in pediatric mild traumatic brain injury. J Neurosci 2012;32(50):17961–9.

19. Lipton ML, Kim N, Park YK, et al. Robust detection of traumatic axonal injury in individual mild traumatic brain injury patients: intersubject variation, change over time and bidirectional changes in anisotropy. Brain Imaging Behav 2012; 6(2):329–42.

20. Yallampalli R, Wilde EA, Bigler ED, et al. Acute white matter differences in the fornix following mild traumatic brain injury using diffusion tensor imaging. J Neuroimaging 2013;23(2):224–7.

21. Churchill NW, Caverzasi E, Graham SJ, et al. White matter during concussion recovery: comparing diffusion tensor imaging (DTI) and neurite orientation dispersion and density imaging (NODDI). Hum Brain Mapp 2019;40(6):1908–18.

22. Churchill N, Hutchison M, Richards D, et al. Brain structure and function associated with a history of sport concussion: a multi-modal magnetic resonance imaging study. J Neurotrauma 2017;34(4):765–71.

23. Miller DR, Hayes JP, Lafleche G, et al. White matter abnormalities are associated with chronic postconcussion symptoms in blast-related mild traumatic brain injury. Hum Brain Mapp 2016;37(1):220–9.

24. Churchill NW, Caverzasi E, Graham SJ, et al. White matter microstructure in athletes with a history of concussion: comparing diffusion tensor imaging (DTI) and neurite orientation dispersion and density imaging (NODDI). Hum Brain Mapp 2017;38(8):4201–11.

25. Messe A, Caplain S, Pelegrini-Issac M, et al. Structural integrity and postconcussion syndrome in mild traumatic brain injury patients. Brain Imaging Behav 2012; 6(2):283–92.

26. Wada T, Asano Y, Shinoda J. Decreased fractional anisotropy evaluated using tract-based spatial statistics and correlated with cognitive dysfunction in patients with mild traumatic brain injury in the chronic stage. AJNR Am J Neuroradiol 2012;33(11):2117–22.
27. Lange RT, Yeh PH, Brickell TA, et al. Postconcussion symptom reporting is not associated with diffusion tensor imaging findings in the subacute to chronic phase of recovery in military service members following mild traumatic brain injury. J Clin Exp Neuropsychol 2019;41(5):497–511.
28. Morgan CD, Zuckerman SL, King LE, et al. Post-concussion syndrome (PCS) in a youth population: defining the diagnostic value and cost-utility of brain imaging. Childs Nerv Syst 2015;31(12):2305–9.
29. Brandstack N, Kurki T, Tenovuo O. Quantitative diffusion-tensor tractography of long association tracts in patients with traumatic brain injury without associated findings at routine MR imaging. Radiology 2013;267(1):231–9.
30. Hulkower MB, Poliak DB, Rosenbaum SB, et al. A decade of DTI in traumatic brain injury: 10 years and 100 articles later. AJNR Am J Neuroradiol 2013; 34(11):2064–74.
31. Harmon KG, Clugston JR, Dec K, et al. American Medical Society for Sports Medicine position statement on concussion in sport. Br J Sports Med 2019;53(4): 213–25.
32. Biomarkers and surrogate endpoints: preferred definitions and conceptual framework. Clin Pharmacol Ther 2001;69(3):89–95.
33. Plog BA, Dashnaw ML, Hitomi E, et al. Biomarkers of traumatic injury are transported from brain to blood via the glymphatic system. J Neurosci 2015;35(2): 518–26.
34. Brinker T, Stopa E, Morrison J, et al. A new look at cerebrospinal fluid circulation. Fluids Barriers CNS 2014;11:10.
35. Anto-Ocrah M, Jones CMC, Diacovo D, et al. Blood-Based Biomarkers for the Identification of Sports-Related Concussion. Neurol Clin 2017;35(3):473–85.
36. Kawata K, Tierney R, Langford D. Blood and cerebrospinal fluid biomarkers. Handb Clin Neurol 2018;158:217–33.
37. McCrea M, Meier T, Huber D, et al. Role of advanced neuroimaging, fluid biomarkers and genetic testing in the assessment of sport-related concussion: a systematic review. Br J Sports Med 2017;51(12):919–29.
38. Klassen A, Faccio AT, Canuto GA, et al. Metabolomics: definitions and significance in systems biology. Adv Exp Med Biol 2017;965:3–17.
39. O'Connell B, Kelly AM, Mockler D, et al. Use of blood biomarkers in the assessment of sports-related concussion-a systematic review in the context of their biological significance. Clin J Sport Med 2018;28(6):561–71.
40. Townend W, Ingebrigtsen T. Head injury outcome prediction: a role for protein S-100B? Injury 2006;37(12):1098–108.
41. Siman R, Shahim P, Tegner Y, et al. Serum SNTF Increases in Concussed Professional Ice Hockey Players and Relates to the Severity of Postconcussion Symptoms. J Neurotrauma 2015;32(17):1294–300.
42. McCrory P, Meeuwisse W, Dvorak J, et al. Consensus statement on concussion in sport-the 5(th) international conference on concussion in sport held in Berlin, October 2016. Br J Sports Med 2017;51(11):838–47.
43. Patricios JS, Ardern CL, Hislop MD, et al. Implementation of the 2017 Berlin Concussion in Sport Group Consensus Statement in contact and collision sports: a joint position statement from 11 national and international sports organisations. Br J Sports Med 2018;52(10):635–41.

44. Gardner AJ, Kohler R, McDonald W, et al. The Use of Sideline Video Review to Facilitate Management Decisions Following Head Trauma in Super Rugby. Sports Med Open 2018;4:20.
45. Tucker R, Raftery M, Fuller GW, et al. A video analysis of head injuries satisfying the criteria for a head injury assessment in professional Rugby Union: a prospective cohort study. Br J Sports Med 2017;51(15):1147–51.
46. Fuller CW, Fuller GW, Kemp SP, et al. Evaluation of World Rugby's concussion management process: results from Rugby World Cup 2015. Br J Sports Med 2017;51(1):64–9.
47. Gardner AJ, Levi CR, Iverson GL. Observational review and analysis of concussion: a method for conducting a standardized video analysis of concussion in Rugby League. Sports Med Open 2017;3(1):26.
48. Gardner AJ, Howell DR, Levi CR, et al. Evidence of concussion signs in National Rugby League match play: a video review and validation study. Sports Med Open 2017;3(1):29.
49. Gardner AJ, Wojtowicz M, Terry DP, et al. Video and clinical screening of national rugby league players suspected of sustaining concussion. Brain Inj 2017; 31(13–14):1918–24.
50. Gardner AJ, Howell DR, Iverson GL. A video review of multiple concussion signs in National Rugby League match play. Sports Med Open 2018;4(1):5.
51. Putukian M, Echemendia RJ, Chiampas G, et al. Head injury in soccer: from science to the field; summary of the head injury summit held in April 2017 in New York City, New York. Br J Sports Med 2019;53(21):1332.
52. Chiampas G, Kirkendall D. Point-counterpoint: should heading be restricted in youth football? Yes, heading should be restricted in youth football. Sci Med Football 2018;2(1):80–2.
53. Emery C, Palacios-Derflingher L, Black AM, et al. Does disallowing body checking in non-elite 13- to 14-year-old ice hockey leagues reduce rates of injury and concussion? A cohort study in two Canadian provinces. Br J Sports Med 2020; 54(7):414–20.
54. Ommaya AK, Gennarelli TA. Cerebral concussion and traumatic unconsciousness. Correlation of experimental and clinical observations of blunt head injuries. Brain 1974;97(4):633–54.
55. Gennarelli TA. Mechanisms of brain injury. J Emerg Med 1993;11(Suppl 1):5–11.
56. Guskiewicz KM, Mihalik JP. Biomechanics of sport concussion: quest for the elusive injury threshold. Exerc Sport Sci Rev 2011;39(1):4–11.
57. Walilko TJ, Viano DC, Bir CA. Biomechanics of the head for Olympic boxer punches to the face. Br J Sports Med 2005;39(10):710–9.
58. Broglio SP, Sosnoff JJ, Shin S, et al. Head impacts during high school football: a biomechanical assessment. J Athl Train 2009;44(4):342–9.
59. Harmon KG, Clugston JR, Dec K, et al. American Medical Society for Sports Medicine Position Statement on Concussion in Sport. Clin J Sport Med 2019;29(2): 87–100.
60. Patricios J, Fuller GW, Ellenbogen R, et al. What are the critical elements of sideline screening that can be used to establish the diagnosis of concussion? A systematic review. Br J Sports Med 2017;51(11):888–94.
61. O'Connor KL, Rowson S, Duma SM, et al. Head-impact-measurement devices: a systematic review. J Athl Train 2017;52(3):206–27.
62. Broglio SP, Lapointe A, O'Connor KL, et al. Head impact density: a model to explain the elusive concussion threshold. J Neurotrauma 2017;34(19):2675–83.

63. Beaudouin F, Aus der Funten K, Tross T, et al. Head injuries in professional male football (soccer) over 13 years: 29% lower incidence rates after a rule change (red card). Br J Sports Med 2019;53(15):948–52.
64. Rossler R, Junge A, Chomiak J, et al. Soccer injuries in players aged 7 to 12 years: a descriptive epidemiological study over 2 seasons. Am J Sports Med 2016;44(2):309–17.
65. O'Kane JW, Spieker A, Levy MR, et al. Concussion among female middle-school soccer players. JAMA Pediatr 2014;168(3):258–64.
66. Emery CA, Kang J, Shrier I, et al. Risk of injury associated with body checking among youth ice hockey players. JAMA 2010;303(22):2265–72.
67. Black AM, Macpherson AK, Hagel BE, et al. Policy change eliminating body checking in non-elite ice hockey leads to a threefold reduction in injury and concussion risk in 11- and 12-year-old players. Br J Sports Med 2016;50(1):55–61.
68. Benson BW, Hamilton GM, Meeuwisse WH, et al. Is protective equipment useful in preventing concussion? A systematic review of the literature. Br J Sports Med 2009;43(Suppl 1):i56–67.
69. Caswell SV, Lincoln AE, Stone H, et al. Characterizing Verified Head Impacts in High School Girls' Lacrosse. Am J Sports Med 2017;45(14):3374–81.
70. Putukian M, Lincoln AE, Crisco JJ. Sports-specific issues in men's and women's lacrosse. Curr Sports Med Rep 2014;13(5):334–40.
71. Raftery M, Kemp S, Patricios J, et al. It is time to give concussion an operational definition: a 3-step process to diagnose (or rule out) concussion within 48 h of injury: World Rugby guideline. Br J Sports Med 2016;50(11):642–3.

Special Article

Perspectives on the Impact of the COVID-19 Pandemic on the Sports Medicine Surgeon: Implications for Current and Future Care

Kyle N. Kunze, MD, Peter D. Fabricant, MD, MPH,
Robert G. Marx, MD, MSc, Benedict U. Nwachukwu, MD, MBA*

KEYWORDS

- SARS-Cov-2 • COVID-19 • Sports medicine • Athletes • Orthopedics
- Practice management

KEY POINTS

- The COVID-19 (Coronavirus disease 2019) pandemic has presented considerable challenges for orthopedic sports medicine surgeons and their patients, requiring rapid adjustment.
- For sports medicine surgeons, major challenges have included navigating telemedicine, personal and institutional financial losses, and psychosocial impacts from providing care.
- For patients and athletes, major challenges have included delayed return to sport, incomplete or limited rehabilitation, and anxiety associated with traveling to health care settings.
- Clinicians must take the lessons learned thus far and continue to apply them now and for the future as a new normal evolves that consists of treating patients with injuries previously treated with traditionally normal methods.
- The authors speculate that practices will continue to adopt telemedicine as a standard of care, and distancing and transmission precautions will remain in place for the foreseeable future.

INTRODUCTION

The impact of the COVID-19 (Coronavirus disease 2019) pandemic has been immense and far reaching. At the time of this writing, almost 5 months after the effects of COVID-19 began to be recognized in the United States, the number of new cases remains uncontrolled in certain regions.[1] Coinciding with this pandemic have been numerous unforeseen effects, ranging from socioeconomic ramifications to significant

Department of Orthopaedic Surgery, Hospital for Special Surgery, New York, NY, USA
* Corresponding author. Hospital for Special Surgery, 535 East 70th Street, New York, NY 10021.
E-mail address: nwachukwub@hss.edu

Clin Sports Med 40 (2021) 213–220
https://doi.org/10.1016/j.csm.2020.08.014
0278-5919/21/© 2020 Elsevier Inc. All rights reserved.

sportsmed.theclinics.com

changes in the ways in which clinicians routinely evaluate and treat patients.[2–4] At this point, orthopedic surgeons, although returning to some degree of normalcy with regard to their practices, must be ready to permanently adapt the changes that this pandemic has imposed.

The subspecialty of sports medicine in particular has felt a significant impact. With essentially all sports, ranging from novice to professional levels, being canceled or postponed for the foreseeable future, it is difficult to conjecture what the future of sports participation will entail.[5] Patients with musculoskeletal injuries treated by sports medicine surgeons may have treatment delayed because of preventive measures introduced by health care institutions and prioritization of nonelective cases. From both patient and sports medicine surgeon perspectives, these barriers may also create significant financial crises. For example, restrictions on participation in sports and on performing elective surgeries may leave institutions with financial deficits or on the brink of bankruptcy.[4,6] Although many clinicians remain optimistic that these barriers will be gradually rescinded, it is only speculation as to whether and when health care practices will return to normal volumes and routines.

The COVID-19 pandemic has raised many questions that remain unanswered; however, the financial, psychosocial, and physical impacts are clear. This article highlights from both patient and physician perspectives the impact of the COVID-19 pandemic on sports medicine surgeons. These perspectives are reinforced using an evidence-based review of recent literature highlighting the various impacts of the pandemic. It is the primary aim of this article to enlighten both the academic community and general public as to how this pandemic has and continues to influence current sports medicine practice and thought, in addition to how it is poised to change future practice, perhaps permanently.

IMPACT ON SPORTS MEDICINE SURGEONS

The current health care landscape has transformed orthopedic sports medicine care. The global pandemic has required surgeons to cater to the musculoskeletal needs of their patients in a way that respects their overall health and mitigates the risk of COVID-19 transmission. Some of the ways that sports medicine surgeons and health care institutions have adapted to this landscape are highlighted here, along with a perspective on how this has affected care delivery.

Telemedicine: Treating Physical Problems Through Virtual Means

The use of telemedicine has been expanded to include a large portion of patient visits in order to respect the physical barriers instated by government and state officials such that the risk of COVID-19 transmission be minimized.[7,8] Specifically, the barriers associated with the provision of virtual musculoskeletal care have been removed in the wake of the COVID-19 global pandemic. Insurers now reimburse for telemedicine and legislature, which allows the provision of virtual care, even going as far as to allow the practice of telemedicine across state lines for some encounters in some jurisdictions. A health care industry analysis by Bestsenny and colleagues[9] suggested that in health care there had been a rapid adoption of telemedicine with high rates of both patient and provider satisfaction.

There are many benefits and challenges for sports medicine surgeons in engaging in virtual visits with patients. Major limitations to the use of telemedicine include technical difficulties resulting in lag or premature ending or disruption of a visit, concern for the quality of the encounter, and inability to perform a complete physical examination.[10] These limitations may negatively influence the diagnostic value of a new or return patient encounter. However, there are significant benefits to these visits, including decreased risk of COVID-19 transmission, saved travel time for patients, and potentially lower rates of no-shows.[11] A recent article by Tenforde and colleagues[12] sought to describe the results from a quality improvement initiative during a rapid adoptive phase of telemedicine for outpatient sports and musculoskeletal physicians where surveys were completed by 119 patients and 14 physiatrists. The investigators reported that telemedicine was primarily used for follow-up visits (70.6% of visits); patients rated their experience as excellent or very good between 91.6% and 95.0% of the time with regard to having concerns addressed, communication, treatment plan development, convenience, and satisfaction; the rate of no-show was only 2.7%; and the key barrier identified for the visits was technical issues.

Although telemedicine continues to expand and the efficiency and technical quality of visits will likely to continue to improve, the in-person physical examination is impossible to replicate, because this is a skill that is cultured and developed throughout training. Tanaka and colleagues[10] recently proposed a set of checklist items and systematic virtual examination techniques to help address these limitations. Their recommendations for a virtual checklist include (1) ensuring the camera is secured in a steady position; (2) numerous space and positioning guidelines for the knee, hip, shoulder, and elbow depending on the extremity that is the chief complaint; (3) lighting recommendations; (4) clothing recommendations depending on the extremity that is the chief complaint; and (5) ensuring that the location allows the patient to speak privately. For the systematic virtual examination, the investigators propose various maneuvers that patients can perform in conjunction with provider instruction in the comfort of their own homes, and provide approximate weights of household items that can be used during provocative strength tests. Because telemedicine is likely to remain common in the examination and evaluation of patients presenting for sports medicine evaluations, development of further examination maneuvers and new technology that will allow improved examinations will be imperative. Future directions may include standardized video instructions for patients, application of motion capture technology, and more reliance on diagnostic aids. Sports medicine surgeons will need to adapt their diagnostic algorithm in the virtual era in order to continue to provide the highest quality of care for their patients.

Financial Implications

High-volume orthopedic sports medicine centers have been forced to quickly absorb significant revenue losses that could not have been anticipated. Because these institutions were unprepared for such rapid financial losses, many are on the verge of bankruptcy and, for most, a large source of income (elective surgery) has been suddenly and dramatically curtailed.[4,13] As a result of financial pressures, many institutions have instituted pay decreases, furlough policies, and even orthopedic staff downsizing. In order to respond to these financial pressures and better align themselves with their institutional plight, hospital-employed surgeons may find themselves accepting pay decreases, and private-practice surgeons may seek out governmental loans to weather the financial storm. The elimination of elective surgery and by proxy income for sports medicine surgeons may have forced some to seek out alternative sources of income, including increased call and locum positions. As sports medicine surgeons return to a new normal, there is likely to be immense pressure to recoup the missed volume. However, the reality is that financial losses in the current fiscal year will have to be amortized in upcoming years and may have implications for surgeon decision making and workload.

The likely ripple effects of the current financial difficulties associated with COVID-19 are that financial disaster planning will become a part of institutional contingency planning. Specifically, institutions will pay increased attention to their cash flow, cash reserve, and maintaining a health account receivable. In addition, surgeons have become sensitized to the importance of having cash on hand to cover ongoing monthly expenditures in the absence of monthly income. Financial wisdom suggests 6 months of typical salary as appropriate liquidity.

Psychosocial Perspectives: Effects of Off-Service Deployment

With governmental and institutional focus on resuming patient care and returning to a new normal, the short-term and long-term effects of being immersed in a critical care environment may be overlooked. Many physicians were previously required to care for patients with COVID-19 or volunteered to do so, which has been shown to be a significant stressor and to impose a large psychological burden.[14,15] A recent worldwide study of the impact of COVID-19 on spine surgeons revealed that family health concerns and anxiety were common and significant stressors, and that loss of income, clinical practice, and extent of surgical management varied widely. It is plausible, and likely, that these trends exist for sports medicine surgeons as well. Because COVID-19 disproportionality affects individuals of an older age,[16–18] older sports medicine surgeons may be at risk of increased susceptibility and this too may have a psychological impact. Because sports medicine surgeons are required to be in hospital settings, this anxiety may be unavoidable and frequent. Such studies highlight the challenges experienced by orthopedic providers and the need for guidelines to be established for (1) psychosocial treatment of these providers, and (2) for anticipation of a second COVID-19 wave.

Research Productivity and Expectations

There has been a profound increase in research productivity during recent months, which coincides with diminishing clinical responsibilities. Furthermore, there is likely an academic "gold rush" to take advantage of the high rate of acceptance for articles pertaining to the COVID-19 pandemic. Gazendam and colleagues[19] recently described this phenomenon as the infodemic of journal publication. This group performed a systematic literature search and found that, over the 13-week period since the initial documentation of COVID-19, a total of 1741 articles pertaining to COVID-19 and severe acute respiratory syndrome–coronavirus-2 (SARS-CoV-2) were published in scientific journals, representing an exponential increase in academic productivity. This group also noted a short time from submission to publication, and a higher proportion of commentaries and opinion articles in journals with high impact factors.

Although a similar exploratory study has yet to be performed specifically for orthopedic research, similar trends are likely present. This trend would have benefits but also potentially negative consequences, if increased academic output is a function of sacrifices in quality. However, benefits of this trend include both personal and institutional gains in academic productivity and the potential to advance the field at a much more rapid pace. Institutions may seek to institute research infrastructures that give them the propensity to maintain the productivity observed during this era both now and in future years.

IMPACT ON PATIENTS AND ATHLETES

Although sports medicine surgeons have been greatly affected by the COVID-19 pandemic, challenges for their patients are also extensive and must be recognized.

Such challenges include enduring musculoskeletal pain and dysfunction in order to minimize travel and potential COVID-19 exposure, anxiety in association with traveling to and being in hospital settings, and return to sport. Some of these challenges, and the way in which sports medicine surgeons may contribute to addressing these challenges, are discussed here.

Anxiety, Pain, or Safety: Which Should Be Prioritized?

Patients have expressed significant concerns in coming into a hospital setting, whether this is for clinical evaluation or a surgical procedure. Although hospitals are prioritizing minimization of the risk of COVID-19 transmission, for patients not routinely part of hospital settings, this can be an overwhelming and anxiety-provoking experience.[20] In contrast, social isolation has been shown to be associated with increased anxiety and stress,[21] and the additional effects of musculoskeletal injuries in combination with this remains unknown. Because the balance of patient care, financial incentives, and COVID-19 risk is delicate, it will be imperative to appropriately counsel patients regarding this anxiety. The authors recommend taking advantage of clinical encounters in the telemedicine setting to prime patients to their experience in the hospital and to emphasize the precautions set in place to minimize the risk of COVID-19 transmission and the need to abide by these regulations. This approach may address anxiety through guiding expectations, addressing pain through conservative or surgical care in the inpatient setting, and ensuring the safety of all in these settings.

Returning to Sport, Eventually

Because amateur sporting events have been classified as low-priority events in the sequence of returning to a new normal, it is uncertain as to when, and the extent to which, sports will resume. Because athletes represent a large proportion of patients evaluated and treated by sports medicine surgeons, and because athletes remain sidelined, this has implications for both patients and providers.

There remain many questions for athletes. These questions include, (1) whether athletes who have contracted COVID-19 will experience long-term effects that influence their health and subsequently their game performance (and if so, what those long-term diseases and consequences are); (2) for those unaffected but that remain sidelined, how potential deconditioning or delayed treatment of a musculoskeletal injury will influence their propensity for return to sport and their performance; and (3) what the future of organized sports will look like. At the time of this writing, some professional sports, such as golf and mixed martial arts, have experienced some success in reinstating regular events because a surge of COVID-19 cases has not been observed (this may be a function of these sports being individual based). Hockey and basketball are sports with smaller teams, which may make this effort slightly less challenging than sports with large teams, especially because these sports were in the postseason. In order to facilitate a safe return to sport, some of these larger team sports organizations have explored the so-called bubble concept; however, professional baseball has experienced early setbacks, and other large spectator sports such as football may also if COVID-19 transmission cannot be adequately controlled. These complications indicate how difficult it will be for amateur sports, including high school and collegiate athletics, to resume regular schedules before the introduction of a widely available vaccine. It is hoped that future protocols can improve safety for these professional athletes and the staff that surround them.

It will be imperative for sports medicine surgeons to safely guide athletes to returning to sport, regardless of when that is or what it looks like. It will be essential for sports medicine surgeons and those involved in the care of athletes to counsel athletes to safely return to sport. In this way, clinicians may help their athletes to avoid injuries associated with returning to sport, such as ruptures of the Achilles tendon or anterior cruciate ligament. Close attention must be paid to fatigue and signs of imminent injury, such as pain with activity, and the athletes must be guided accordingly. Although clinicians are passionate about the return of sports and hope that athletes can soon return to doing what they love, their number 1 priority must be to facilitate a safe return.

The Impact of COVID-19 on Rehabilitation and Home Injury

Another unique cohort of patients being affected by the COVID-19 pandemic are those who underwent a surgical procedure in the period before the pandemic. These patients who required extensive rehabilitation and physical therapy were unable to receive it in most cases. Prohibiting this essential aspect of surgical recovery may predispose such patients to suboptimal outcomes compared with their counterparts who were able to successfully complete physical therapy and rehabilitation. It is also likely that such patients will endure a longer recovery than their counterparts accordingly. Sports medicine surgeons and physical therapists will need to be conscientious of this impact and help these patients experience the best clinical and functional outcomes possible.

As many individuals continue to seek ways of maintaining fitness and staying healthy during the pandemic, a trend in injuries related to home exercise programs may be observed. These patients may develop overuse tendinopathies of the biceps and rotator cuffs if they are not accustomed to performing these exercises regularly. As such, sports medicine surgeons are likely to continue to observe an increase in these types of injuries as long as gyms and fitness centers remain closed.

A TRANSIENT CHANGE OR NEW NORMAL?

There are many challenges that have been faced and new issues that will continue to be encountered as sports medicine surgeons care for patients and athletes in the midst of the evolving pandemic. Despite these challenges, they will endeavor to continue to provide the highest level of care to their patients and to get them back to what they love to do, whether that is walking along the river or hitting a buzzer beater. There will continue to be injuries regardless of the infectious burden imparted by COVID-19, and therefore clinicians have an obligation to their patients to find innovative and effective ways to treat them both mentally and physically. The rapidly evolving nature of the pandemic may make this process more challenging, because recommendations and epidemiologic data are dynamic; however, it is of the utmost importance to take the lessons learned thus far and continue to apply them now and for the future as a new normal evolves in the treatment of patients with injuries previously treated with traditionally normal methods. The changes that may be required cannot be predicted with any certainty, but the authors speculate that practices will continue to adopt telemedicine as a standard of care and that distancing and transmission precautions will remain in place for the foreseeable future.

DISCLOSURE

The authors have nothing to disclose.

REFERENCES

1. World Health Organization. Coronavirus disease 2019 (COVID-19). Situation Report April 29, 2020. Available at: https://nam03.safelinks.protection.outlook.

com/?url=https%3A%2F%2Fwww.who.int%2Fdocs%2Fdefault-source%
2Fcoronaviruse%2Fsituation-reports%2F20200429-sitrep-100-covid-19.pdf%
3Fsfvrsn%3Dbbfbf3d1_6&data=02%7C01%7Cr.mayakrishnan%40elsevier.com
%7C70ae398d1ef94726d77808d8566ccaac%
7C9274ee3f94254109a27f9fb15c10675d%7C0%7C0%
7C637354373097911192&sdata=baLhM3c%2FTL6Xpl4guVi5F3g%
2BLOp1JsInS3pIsnpgRiw%3D&reserved=0. Accessed July 30, 2020.

2. Khalatbari-Soltani S, Cumming RC, Delpierre C, et al. Importance of collecting data on socioeconomic determinants from the early stage of the COVID-19 outbreak onwards. J Epidemiol Community Health 2020;74(8):620–3.

3. Nicola M, Alsafi Z, Sohrabi C, et al. The socio-economic implications of the coronavirus pandemic (COVID-19): A review. Int J Surg 2020;78:185–93.

4. Vaccaro AR, Getz CL, Cohen BE, et al. Practice management during the COVID-19 pandemic. J Am Acad Orthop Surg 2020;28(11):464–70.

5. Schellhorn P, Klingel K, Burgstahler C. Return to sports after COVID-19 infection. Eur Heart J 2020. https://doi.org/10.1093/eurheartj/ehaa448.

6. Khullar D, Bond AM, Schpero WL. COVID-19 and the financial health of US hospitals. JAMA 2020. https://doi.org/10.1001/jama.2020.6269.

7. Hollander JE, Carr BG. Virtually perfect? telemedicine for covid-19. N Engl J Med 2020;382(18):1679–81.

8. Loeb AE, Rao SS, Ficke JR, et al. Departmental experience and lessons learned with accelerated introduction of telemedicine during the COVID-19 crisis. J Am Acad Orthop Surg 2020;28(11):e469–76.

9. Bestsenny O, Gilbert G, Harris A, et al. Telehealth: a quarter-trillion-dollar post-COVID-19 reality? McKinsey & Company; 2020. Available at: https://nam03. safelinks.protection.outlook.com/?url=https:%2F%2Fwww.mckinsey.com%2F~% 2Fmedia%2FMcKinsey%2FIndustries%2FHealthcare%2520Systems%2520and% 2520Services%2FOur%2520Insights%2FTelehealth%2520A%2520quarter% 2520trillion%2520dollar%2520post%2520COVID%252019%2520reality% 2FTelehealth-A-quarter-trilliondollar-post-COVID-19-reality.pdf&data=02%7C01% 7Cr.mayakrishnan%40elsevier.com%7C70ae398d1ef94726d77808d8566ccaac% 7C9274ee3f94254109a27f9fb15c10675d%7C0%7C0% 7C637354373097911192&sdata=a4sen1492tt% 2B92rS2dcSwW8oup7ElenAd83LaoY9dqM%3D&reserved=0. Accessed July 30, 2020.

10. Tanaka MJ, Oh LS, Martin SD, et al. Telemedicine in the era of COVID-19: the virtual orthopaedic examination. J Bone Joint Surg Am 2020;102(12):e57.

11. Atanda A, Pelton M, Fabricant PD, et al. Telemedicine utilisation in a paediatric sports medicine practice: decreased cost and wait times with increased satisfaction. J ISAKOS 2018;3(2):94.

12. Tenforde AS, Iaccarino MA, Borgstrom H, et al. Telemedicine During COVID-19 for outpatient sports and musculoskeletal medicine physicians. PM R 2020. https://doi.org/10.1002/pmrj.12422.

13. Gilat R, Cole BJ. COVID-19, Medicine, and Sports. Arthrosc Sports Med Rehabil 2020;2(3):e175–6.

14. Elbay RY, Kurtulmus A, Arpacioglu S, et al. Depression, anxiety, stress levels of physicians and associated factors in Covid-19 pandemics. Psychiatry Res 2020;290:113130.

15. Lai J, Ma S, Wang Y, et al. Factors associated with mental health outcomes among health care workers exposed to coronavirus disease 2019. JAMA Netw Open 2020;3(3):e203976.

16. Imam Z, Odish F, Gill I, et al. Older age and comorbidity are independent mortality predictors in a large cohort of 1305 COVID-19 patients in Michigan, United States. J Intern Med 2020. https://doi.org/10.1111/joim.13119.

17. Lloyd-Sherlock PG, Kalache A, McKee M, et al. WHO must prioritise the needs of older people in its response to the covid-19 pandemic. BMJ 2020;368:m1164.

18. Mueller AL, McNamara MS, Sinclair DA. Why does COVID-19 disproportionately affect older people? Aging (Albany NY) 2020;12(10):9959–81.

19. Gazendam A, Ekhtiari S, Wong E, et al. The "infodemic" of journal publication associated with the novel coronavirus disease. J Bone Joint Surg Am 2020; 102(13):e64.

20. Vindegaard N, Benros ME. COVID-19 pandemic and mental health consequences: Systematic review of the current evidence. Brain Behav Immun 2020. https://doi.org/10.1016/j.bbi.2020.05.048.

21. Xiao H, Zhang Y, Kong D, et al. Social capital and sleep quality in individuals who self-isolated for 14 days during the coronavirus disease 2019 (COVID-19) Outbreak in January 2020 in China. Med Sci Monit 2020;26:e923921.

Moving?

Make sure your subscription moves with you!

To notify us of your new address, find your **Clinics Account Number** (located on your mailing label above your name), and contact customer service at:

Email: journalscustomerservice-usa@elsevier.com

800-654-2452 (subscribers in the U.S. & Canada)
314-447-8871 (subscribers outside of the U.S. & Canada)

Fax number: 314-447-8029

**Elsevier Health Sciences Division
Subscription Customer Service
3251 Riverport Lane
Maryland Heights, MO 63043**

*To ensure uninterrupted delivery of your subscription, please notify us at least 4 weeks in advance of move.

Printed and bound by CPI Group (UK) Ltd, Croydon, CR0 4YY

08/05/2025

01864692-0003